CONTEMP<

CHRISTOPHER P. CANNON, MD
SERIES EDITOR

For other titles published in this series, go to
http://www.springer.com/7677

William Franklin Peacock ·
Christopher P. Cannon
Editors

Short Stay Management of Chest Pain

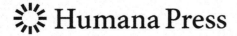 Humana Press

Editors

William Franklin Peacock
Department of Emergency Medicine
Cleveland Clinic Foundation
Mail Code E-19
9500 Euclid Ave
Cleveland, OH 44195
USA
peacocw@ccf.org

Christopher P. Cannon
Brigham & Women's Hospital
Cardiovascular Division
Harvard Medical School
350 Longwood Ave
Boston, MA
USA
cpcannon@partners.org

ISBN 978-1-4939-5720-0   ISBN 978-1-60327-948-2 (eBook)
DOI 10.1007/978-1-60327-948-2
Springer Dordrecht Heidelberg London New York

Printed on acid-free paper

Springer is part of Springer Science+Business Media (www.springer.com)

Preface

As the aging of America continues, ever increasing numbers of patients present to the hospital with signs and symptoms consistent with an acute coronary syndrome. This has challenged our health-care system, both in terms of sheer numbers and the complexity of their presentations. With increasing age, confounding comorbidities increase in a nearly logarithmic fashion. Noncardiac conditions can obscure the patient's ability to accurately report their symptoms, or mask a true cardiac presentation. This confluence of events results in the creation of a situation where the task of early emergency department risk stratification and diagnostic evaluation becomes increasingly difficult. In fact, the complaint of chest pain, once considered prima fasciae evidence of a potential acute coronary syndrome, has been replaced by the ischemic equivalent. Furthermore, in one recent large study, up to 30% of patients suffering a myocardial infarction had no chest pain whatsoever [1].

In 2008 it was estimated that 8% (11.2 million people) of all emergency department visits would be for chest pain. Considering the above data, more than 400,000 would be with myocardial infarction whose symptomatic manifestation does not even include chest pain. This is a problem for the ED. The currently available diagnostic tools are blunt and suspected ACS patients are at high risk of adverse outcomes. For emergency physicians, missed MI represents the single highest malpractice award. This creates a challenge as it is well established that coronary artery disease is the number one killer of Americans, that early diagnosis and intervention saves lives, and that if patients are discharged home while in the throes of an unsuspected myocardial infarction, their acute mortality is 30% higher than if accurately diagnosed.

Thus, this book was written to provide scientific and clinical insight on the management of patients who arrive at the hospital with a presentation consistent with a potential acute coronary syndrome. Who was this book written for? That would be the physicians and nurses working in the overcrowded emergency departments of the United States, where the majority of patients with suspected ACS present, the cardiologists and nurses who care for patients identified with possible ACS, and the hospital administrators charged with making it all work financially.

While at one extreme some clinical presentations are obviously low risk, some less clear presentations may result in sudden cardiac death. Separating these groups can be challenging. Yes, ST segment elevation myocardial infarction diagnosed by ECG rapidly identifies the highest risk population. However, a diagnostic ECG is found in not more than 4% of all chest pain presentations [2]. The remaining 96% fall into a gray zone where undefined risk of adverse outcomes drives a large number of individualized testing strategies.

The management of patients presenting to the hospital with a suspected acute coronary syndrome has undergone marked changes in the last decade. As little as 10 years ago, patients presenting to the hospital with suspected acute coronary syndromes were admitted to the coronary care unit for expensive and time-consuming evaluations. Despite this, as many as 5% of patients were discharged home to suffer an out-of-hospital acute myocardial infarction. Although some of this "misdiagnosis rate" was the result of technological limitations in testing and patient care process, the practice of emergency physicians evaluating suspected ACS patients and making admission and discharge decisions solely upon clinical grounds is clinically inaccurate. The bottom line is that the subjective impression is not good enough. Thus, the era of diagnostic inaccuracy resulted in medical errors, some with adverse outcomes, and emergency physicians had to collectively lower their admission threshold.

With the addition of rapid turnaround troponin assays in the mid-1990s, identification of high-risk patients became more objective. Although an improvement over the prior approach, it suffers a critical sensitivity deficit as an early isolated troponin measurement has no ability to discriminate all but the highest risk patients. While a positive troponin identifies the patient with an acute coronary syndrome, an undetectable troponin does not exclude an event. In fact, in an ED study of low-risk patients [3], despite a specificity of 99.2%, troponin's sensitivity was 9.5% for predicting acute adverse events. Therefore, with troponin we can confirm a diagnosis and identify the requirement for intervention (e.g., advanced antiplatelet therapy or the need for revascularization); however, we do not exclude an ongoing event. In the big picture, identifying that an acute event has already occurred (e.g., necrosis) is helpful; in the hierarchy of clinical value, it cannot stand as the sole diagnostic test.

To address the inability to exclude an acute coronary syndrome diagnosis, chest pain centers were developed. These units provide an environment where serial cardiac marker testing can be performed, and the potential for coronary perfusion deficits evaluated by provocative myocardial perfusion testing or radiographic imaging. Eligible candidates are the majority of patients with nondiagnostic ECG and troponin levels. The results have been impressive. Chest pain centers have markedly decreased adverse events. In one before-and-after study of their impact on 4,477 patients, Kugelmass et al. [4] reported that the implementation of CPC resulted in a 37% lower mortality, while simultaneously increasing the safe discharge rate by 36%.

Therefore, the current evaluation of a patient with a suspected acute coronary syndrome commonly consists of serial marker testing over several hours and possibly followed by an evocative test (e.g., stress testing) or coronary artery visualization (e.g., coronary artery-computed tomographic scanning). Medicolegal issues notwithstanding, this process rarely concludes with a discharged patient suffering a short-term adverse cardiac event, but only at significant cost in time, money, and ED resources.

As would be predicted by a simple noninvasive and accurate strategy, chest pain center use is skyrocketing and some centers report that 98% of all CPC test results are negative [5, 6] for acute coronary syndromes. Overall, ED physicians are 94.7% sensitive, 74% specific in identifying patients who were subsequently diagnosed with ACS within 30 days of ED visit [7]. It should be noted that while the exclusion of an acute coronary syndrome is valuable, and this book is focused on the cardiology aspects of chest pain, the chest pain center has evolved to now become a rapid diagnosis unit. It is commonly called the chest pain unit because this is how the undiagnosed patient presents, and it is only after a period of testing will those with high-risk acute coronary syndromes be identified. It is therefore inherent in the mission of these units that significant, but noncardiac, disease is identified (e.g., pulmonary embolism, aortic dissection, pneumonia). While not specifically covered by this book, it is important to recognize that the elimination of acute coronary syndromes from the list of probable diagnoses does not equate to the stability for discharge and further appropriate investigations are commonly necessary in the cohort of patients without an identified underlying cardiac cause of their symptoms.

The purpose of this book is to present the science and methodology that has allowed remarkable improvements in diagnostic accuracy and improved patient outcomes for the evaluation of patients presenting with suspected acute coronary syndromes. It will be of value to all acute care physicians, nurses, and hospital administrators charged with caring for this population.

Cleveland, OH   W. Frank Peacock, MD, FACEP
Boston, MA   Christopher P. Cannon, MD, FACC

References

1. Canto JG, Shlipak MG, Rogers WJ, et al. Prevalence, clinical characteristics, and mortality among patients with myocardial infarction presenting without chest pain. JAMA. 2000;283:3223–3229.
2. Pope JH, Aufderheide TP, Ruthazer R, Woolard RH, Feldman JA, Beshansky JR, Griffith JL, Selker HP. Missed diagnoses of acute cardiac ischemia in the emergency department. NEJM. 342(16); 2000, 1163–1170.
3. Peacock WF, Emerman CL, McErlean ES, et al. Prediction of short and long term outcomes by troponin-T in low risk patients evaluated for acute coronary syndromes. Ann Emerg Med. 2000;35:213–20.

4. Kugelmass AD, Anderson AL, Brown PP, et al. Does having a chest pain center impact the treatment and survival of acute myocardial infarction patients? Circulation. 2004;110:111–409.
5. Mitchell AM, Garvey JL, Chandra A, et al. Prospective multicenter study of quantitative pretest probability assessment to exclude acute coronary syndrome for patients evaluated in emergency department chest pain units. Ann Emerg Med. 2006;47:438–447.
6. Reilly BM, Evans AT, Schaider JJ, et al. Triage of patients with chest pain in the emergency department: A comparative study of physicians' decisions. Am J Med. 2002;112:95–103.
7. Christenson J, Innes G, McKnight D, et al. Safety and efficiency of emergency department assessment of chest discomfort. CMAJ. 2004;170:1803–7.

Contents

Contributors

Ezra A. Amsterdam MD Department of Internal Medicine (Cardiology), University of California, Davis, Medical Center, Sacramento, CA, USA, eaamsterdam@ucdavis.edu

Annitha Annathurai MMed (A&E) Emergency Medicine, Singapore General Hospital, Singapore, annitha19@hotmail.com

William J. Brady MD University of Virginia, Charlottesville, VA, USA, wb4z@hscmail.mcc.virginia.edu

Christopher P. Cannon MD, FACEP Harvard Medical School, Brigham & Women's Hospital, Boston, MA, USA; Cardiovascular Division, TIMI Study Group, Boston, MA, USA, cpcannon@partners.com

Anna Marie Chang MD Department of Emergency Medicine, Hospital of the University of Pennsylvania, Philadelphia, PA, USA, annamarie.chang@uphs.upenn.edu

Robert H. Christenson PhD, DABCC, FACB University of Maryland School of Medicine, Baltimore, MD, USA; Core Laboratories, Baltimore, MD, USA, rchristenson@umm.edu

Sean Collins MD, FACEP Department of Emergency Medicine, University of Cincinnati, Cincinnati, OH, USA, collinsp@ucmail.uc.edu, sean.collins@uc.edu

Shahriar Dadkhah MD, FACP, FACC Cardiology Research Department, Saint Francis Hospital, Evanston, IL, USA, dadkhahsc@aol.com

Deborah B. Diercks MD, MSc Department of Emergency Medicine, University of California, Davis Medical Center, Sacramento, CA, USA, dbdiercks@ucdavis.edu

Michael J. Gallagher MD Department of Cardiology, William Beaumont Hospital, Royal Oak, MI, USA, mgallagher@beaumont.edu

Chris A. Ghaemmaghami MD Department of Emergency Medicine, University of Virginia School of Medicine, Charlottesville, VA, USA, cg3n@virginia.edu

Louis Graff IV MD, FACP, FACEP Hospital of Central Connecticut, New Britain, CT, USA; University of Connecticut School of Medicine, Farmington, CT, USA, louisgraff4@aol.com

Elizabeth Harbison MD Department of Emergency Medicine, Vanderbilt University Medical Center, Nashville, TN, USA, harbison5@aol.com

Judd E. Hollander MD Department of Emergency Medicine, University of Pennsylvania, Philadelphia, PA, USA, Judd.hollander@uphs.upenn.edu

Jeffrey A. Holmes MD Department of Emergency Medicine, Maine Medical Center, Portland, ME, USA, drjeffholmes@gmail.com

Kay S. Holmes RN Society of Chest Pain Centers, Columbus, OH, USA, kholmes@scpcp.org

J Douglas Kirk MD, FACEP Department of Emergency Medicine, University of California, Davis, Medical Center Sacramento, CA, USA, jdkirk@ucdavis.edu

Michael C. Kontos MD Departments of Internal Medicine (Cardiology), Emergency Medicine, and Radiology, Virginia Commonwealth University, Richmond, VA, USA, mckontos@vcu.edu, mkontos@mcvh-vcu.edu

Ian McClure MD Department of Emergency Medicine, Vanderbilt University, Nashville, TN, USA, mcclureit@gmail.com

James McCord MD, FACC Heart and Vascular Institute, Henry Ford Hospital, Detroit, MI, USA, jmccord1@hfhs.org

Brian O'Neil MD, FACEP Department of Emergency Medicine, William Beaumont Hospital, Royal Oak, MI, USA, boneil@med.wayne.edu

Kelly Owen MD Department of Emergency Medicine, University of California, Davis Medical Center, Sacramento, CA, USA, kelly-owen@ucdmc.ucdavis.edu

William Franklin Peacock MD, FACEP Emergency Services Institute, Cleveland Clinic, Cleveland, OH, USA, peacocw@ccf.org

Gilbert L. Raff MD, FACC William Beaumont Hospital, Royal Oak, MI, USA, graff@beaumont.edu

Michael A. Ross MD, FACEP Department of Emergency Medicine, Emory University School of Medicine, Atlanta, GA, USA, michael.ross@emoryhealthcare.org

Sandra Sieck RN, MBA Sieck Health Care Consulting, Mobile, AL, USA, ssieck@sieckhealthcare.com

Korosh Sharain MA Cardiology Research Department, Saint Francis Hospital, Evanston, IL, USA, ksharain@gmail.com

Alan B. Storrow MD Department of Emergency Medicine, Vanderbilt University, Nashville, TN, USA, alan.storrow@vanderbilt.edu

Chapter 1
Epidemiology and Demography of Coronary Artery Disease

Shahriar Dadkhah and Korosh Sharain

Abstract The study of epidemiology is vital in identifying the connections which exist between lifestyle, environment, and disease, thus providing knowledge of the factors, distribution, and pathology of disease. As the leading cause of death in the United States since 1900, save 1918, coronary artery disease continues to overwhelm mortality and morbidity statistics. In the United States, 1 in 5 deaths are attributed to CAD, the leading cause of death of both males and females. In fact, CAD kills approximately five times more females than does breast cancer. The estimated direct and indirect cost of CAD in 2008 is $156 million. As a disease that manifests itself in the crib, it is not surprising that CAD is also the leading cause of death worldwide, becoming a pandemic. Coronary artery disease is a condition that is multifaceted, influenced by social status, genetics, lifestyle (culture), and environmental factors. The risk of development of CAD is said to increase with the transition of rural, agrarian, economically underdeveloped to urbanized, industrialized modern societies. Modernization leads to a more sedentary lifestyle, diets higher in calories, and psychosocial stresses. Risk factors such as hypertension, physical inactivity, tobacco use, and diet are modifiable risk factors, whereas genetics, age, race, and gender are nonmodifiable risk factors associated with CAD. Community education must continue to dominate efforts to reduce the major modifiable risk factors. As we continue to monitor the distribution of CAD in populations, epidemiology will provide us with better guidelines, which when applied appropriately can continue to decrease death rates caused by such a devastating disease worldwide.

S. Dadkhah (✉)
Cardiology Research Department, Saint Francis Hospital, Evanston, IL, USA
e-mail: dadkhahsc@aol.com

W.F. Peacock, C.P. Cannon (eds.), *Short Stay Management of Chest Pain*,
DOI 10.1007/978-1-60327-948-2_1,

Keywords Coronary artery disease · Heart disease · Cardiovascular disease · Epidemiology · Demography · Heart attack · Statistics · Stats · Risk factors · CAD · CHD

History of the Study of Epidemiology and Coronary Artery Disease

The study of epidemiology is vital in identifying the connections which exist between lifestyle, environment, and disease, thus providing knowledge of the factors, distribution, and pathology of the particular disease. A notable shift in the study of epidemiology occurred in the mid-twentieth century when epidemic studies began encompassing chronic noncommunicable diseases such as coronary artery disease (CAD) and lung cancer [1]. Infectious diseases were much easier to diagnose; therefore, epidemiological studies had more defined margins. On the other hand, noncommunicable diseases like CAD were much more difficult to diagnose and understand epidemiologically [1].

Coronary artery disease was a consequence of multiple factors with unpredictable onset and disease progression [1], resulting in atherosclerotic lesions, which could not be observed in the living patient [1]. In fact, a diagnosis of CAD in the beginning of the twentieth century could be made only after an autopsy. Therefore, it was difficult to assess prevalence and morbidity of CAD. Thus, the implementation of prospective cohort studies by the Framingham study sought to address this dilemma with CAD epidemiology.

In the late 1940s, post World War II studies were mostly case–control studies [1]. The Framingham study, which investigated heart disease epidemiology, was designed in 1947 as a longitudinal study intended to perform long-term follow-up of a population of individuals without known heart disease and assess the progression of CAD in these individuals [1]. Risk factor epidemiology emerged from the CAD methodology of epidemiology, which unlike prior noncommunicable disease epidemiology like lung cancer identified multiple risk factors for a single disease [1]. Coronary artery disease epidemiologists incorporated the multiple risk factor concept that insurance agencies had used previously [1].

After respective patient death, upon autopsy, a diagnosis would be made and thus retrospective review of the patient's history could provide clues as to the causes of that disease, namely CAD. This prospective and retrospective design allowed for the tracking of the progression and timeline of heart disease. (Box 1.1 provides a brief review of the pathophysiology of CAD.)

The study of epidemiology involves the cause and distribution of disease in a population. Understanding the epidemiology of CAD provides avenues for understanding disease progression, risk factors, treatment opportunities, education, and lifestyle impacts. Measuring such trends in populations allows for the assessment and re-evaluation of current guidelines.

Box 1.1 Pathophysiology of coronary artery disease

Pathophysiology of Coronary Artery Disease

Acute Coronary Syndrome (ACS) is a term used to describe the spectrum of conditions that include Unstable Angina, ST segment Elevation Myocardial Infarction, non ST segment Elevation Myocardial Infarction, and sudden cardiac death. The underlying atherosclerosis of CAD that precipitates ACS defines a disease sequelae that accounts for the leading cause of death in the world.

The pathophysiology of ACS is multifactorial, however, the key underlying component is the formation of a fatty streak. Injury or dysfunction of the endothelial lining of blood vessels caused by hypertension, smoking, and dyslipidemia, increases the permeability of the vessel. Lipids (LDL's) can enter the site of weakness and become oxidized. Oxidation of the LDL causes migration of smooth muscles cells and activates monocytes which phagocytose the lipid, ultimately resulting in the formation of a Foam cell or

fatty streak. The proliferation and differentiation of extracellular matrix proteins ultimately forms a fibrofatty atheroma consisting of a fibrous cap and necrotic center. The buildup of the atheroma leads to narrowing of the arteries and thus reduction in blood flow and oxygen delivery to the area. The atheroma can also rupture, blocking blood supply all together, causing a heart attack.

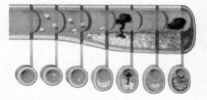

Libby P. *Circulation*. 2001;104:365-372

Currently the leading cause of death among both men and women [1], CAD was not clearly described until 1912 when James Herrick published his paper *Clinical features of sudden obstruction of the coronary arteries* [2]. But it was not until the 1950s that the weight of CAD in the medical community was realized. Random autopsies performed on American soldiers who died in the Korean War (1950–1953) showed surprising degrees of coronary atherosclerosis in soldiers who were in their teens and twenties [2]. It was hard to imagine a disease that presented itself clinically in the latter half of a person's life presenting itself biologically at such an early time.

There is little debate that atherosclerotic plaque and CAD begin in early stages of life. It is not surprising that a disease with such potential to do harm could become an epidemic. What is surprising is that the risk factors attributed to CAD have been well documented since the 1950s [1], yet CAD has remained the leading cause of death in the United States (US) every year since 1900, except 1918 because of the influenza pandemic (Fig. 1.1) [3].

Cardiovascular Disease Statistics

According to the 2008 American Heart Association Heart Disease and Stroke Statistics, an estimated 80.7 million American adults have at least one cardiovascular disease, which is approximately 1 in 3 Americans [3]! Only 38.2 million of these patients are over the age of 60 (Fig. 1.2) [3]. A common misconception is

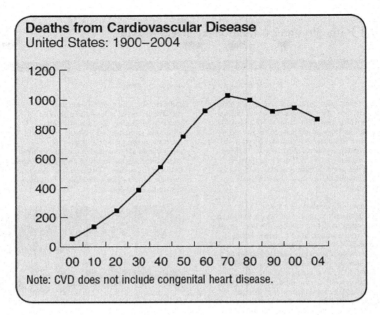

Fig. 1.1 Deaths from cardiovascular disease in the thousands [3]

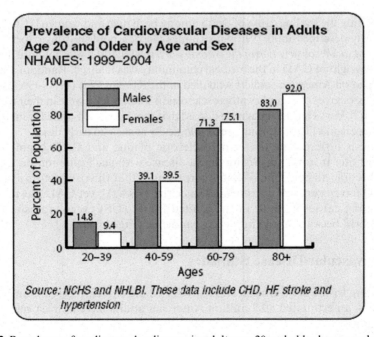

Fig. 1.2 Prevalence of cardiovascular diseases in adults age 20 and older by age and sex [3]

that cardiovascular diseases do not affect females as it does males. This could not be further from the truth. Cardiovascular diseases claimed the lives of 460,000 American females in 2004; by comparison, breast cancer took the lives of 40,954 American females (Fig. 1.3) [3].

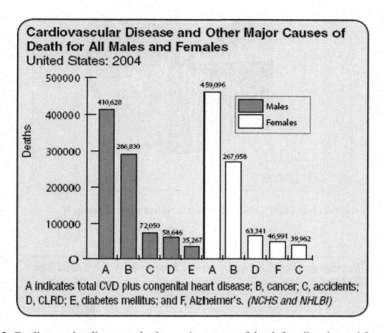

Fig. 1.3 Cardiovascular disease and other major causes of death for all males and females [3]

Coronary Artery Disease Statistics

Coronary artery disease accounts for over half of all the deaths caused by cardiovascular diseases (Fig. 1.4) [3]. In 2005, the estimated prevalence of CAD in adults age 20 and older was 16 million (8.7 million males and 7.3 million females) (Fig. 1.5) [3]. The magnitude of these numbers is inconceivable. By comparison, the population of New York, NY, in 2005 was 8.2 million [4]. It is also estimated that 770,000 Americans will have a new coronary attack and 430,000 will have a recurrent attack this year [3]. In fact, 1 in 5 deaths in the United States can be attributed to CAD, which is the largest killer of American males and females (Box 1.2) [3]. The economic impact of CAD is just as astonishing. The estimated direct and indirect cost of CAD in 2008 is projected to be $156 billion (Fig. 1.6) [3]!

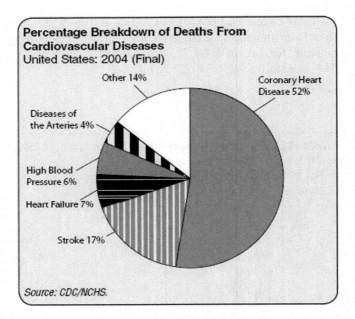

Fig. 1.4 Percentage breakdown of deaths from cardiovascular disease [3]

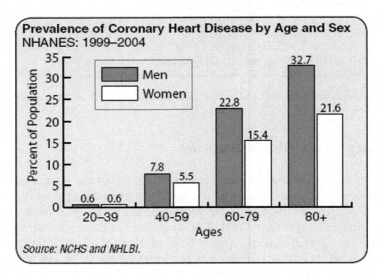

Fig. 1.5 Prevalence of coronary artery disease [3]

Box 1.2 Fast stats of coronary artery disease

Fast Stats CAD

- Every 26 seconds an American will suffer a Coronary event!

- Every minute, someone will die from a coronary event!

- 1 in 30 female deaths in the US is attributed to breast cancer, 1 in 6 is due to CAD!

- Average years of life lost due to a heart attack is 15 years!

- 1 in 5 individuals over age 40 who suffer a heart attack will die within one year, and 1 in 3 will die within 5 years!

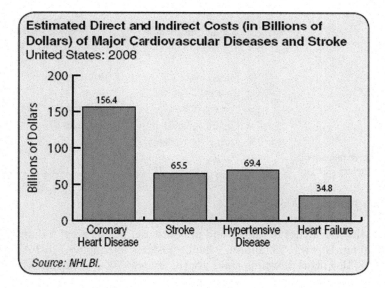

Fig. 1.6 Estimated direct and indirect costs of major cardiovascular diseases [3]

What's worse is that CAD has become a pandemic, being the world's leading cause of death [5]. It is estimated that 3.8 million men and 3.4 million women die each year from CAD worldwide [5].

Coronary artery disease is a condition that is multifaceted, influenced by social status, genetics, lifestyle (culture), and environmental factors. Coronary artery disease is less prevalent in countries such as Central and South America and Africa. In contrast, mortality from CAD is expected to increase in developing countries due to economic and societal changes that occur with advanced development [5]. The risk of development of CAD is said to increase with the transition of rural, agrarian, economically underdeveloped to urbanized, industrialized modern societies [5]. Modernization leads to a more sedentary lifestyle, diets higher in calories, and psychosocial stresses [6]. It was found that a population of Japanese people (Japan being a low-risk CAD location) who immigrated to the United States acquired an incidence of CAD that was similar to those native to the United States [5]. Changes in diet, lifestyle, and environment can be to blame. India, China, and the United States are among the countries with the highest deaths attributed to CAD [5].

Risk Factors of CAD

As mentioned before, the risk factors for CAD are well documented. Epidemiological studies have provided the medical community with determinants of CAD. It is interesting to report that approximately 90% of CAD patients have at least one major modifiable risk factor of the following: hypertension, physical inactivity, tobacco use, hyperlipidemia, overweight, and diabetes (Fig. 1.7) [3].

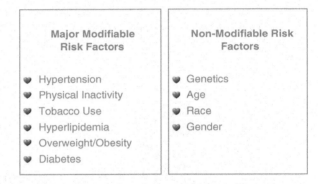

Fig. 1.7 Risk factors of coronary artery disease

Hypertension

In 2005, the prevalence of high blood pressure (defined as greater than or equal to 140/90 mmHg) was 73 million, which translates to roughly 1 in 3 Americans (Fig. 1.8) [3]. This is alarming since approximately 70% of people who have a first heart attack have blood pressures at or above that range. It has been calculated that the risk for cardiovascular disease doubles for every 10 point increase in diastolic and 20 point increase in systolic blood pressure [5].

Physical Inactivity

Physical inactivity is another major risk factor of CAD. Physical inactivity increases risk of CAD by 1.5 times [3]. In 2005, only 43.8% of males and 27.8% of female students in grades 9–12 met recommended levels of physical activity (Figs. 1.9 and 1.10) [3].

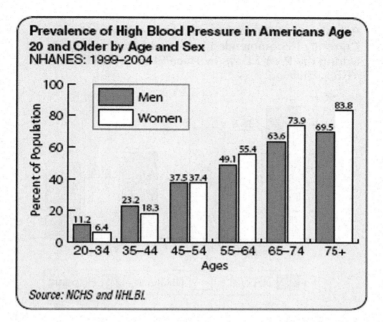

Fig. 1.8 Prevalence of high blood pressure in Americans age 20 and older by age and sex [3]

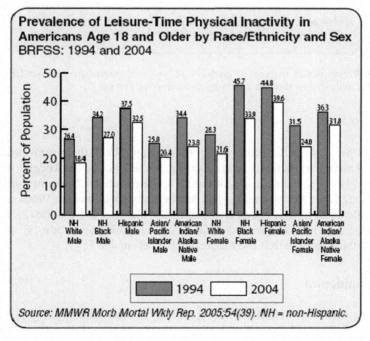

Fig. 1.9 Prevalence of leisure-time physical inactivity in Americans age 18 and older by race/ethnicity and sex [3]

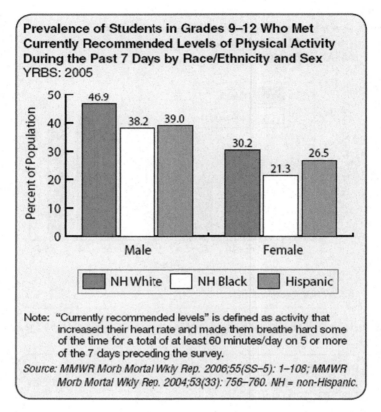

Fig. 1.10 Prevalence of students in grades 9–12 who met currently recommended levels of physical activity during the past 7 days by race/ethnicity and sex [3]

Tobacco Use

Smokers are 2–4 times more likely to develop CAD than nonsmokers [3]! With this high of a risk factor, it is upsetting that in 2005, of the students in grades 9–12, 31.7% of male and 25.1% of female students reported current tobacco use [3]. Although the rates of smoking has decreased by 50% since the 1960s, currently the prevalence of smoking of adults aged 18 and above is 46.6 million (25.9 million males and 20.7 million females) or 21% of the adult population [3]. Approximately 80% of people that use tobacco begin before age 18 [3].

Hyperlipidemia

The mean total blood cholesterol level among children aged 4–11 is 164.5 mg/dL and aged 12–19 is 161.7 mg/dL (Fig. 1.11) [3]. It is estimated that more than 106.7 million Americans have total blood cholesterol above 200 mg/dL, i.e., about 48% of the adult population [3].

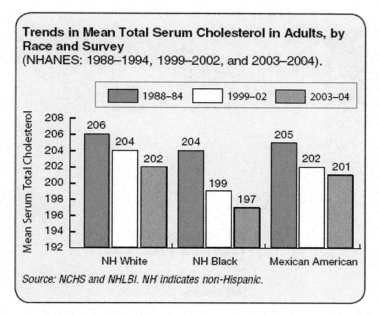

Fig. 1.11 Trends in mean total serum cholesterol in adults by race and survey [3]

Overweight and Obesity

Alarmingly, over 9 million children aged 9–16 were overweight and 142 million of US adults over the age of 20 were overweight, representing 66% of the adult population (Fig. 1.12) [3].

Diabetes

About 1.5 million new cases of diabetes were diagnosed in Americans age 20 and older in 2005. Worldwide, the trend of diabetes is increasing (Fig. 1.13) [3]. Approximately half of patients with diabetes are unaware that they have it [3].

There are also numerous nonmodifiable risk factors for CAD, including genetics, age, gender, and ethnicity. Risk categories for these nonmodifiable risk factors provide that much more motivation to reduce the risk factors of the things we can control such as diet, tobacco use, blood pressure, cholesterol intake, and physical activity.

Heart disease age-adjusted death rates have reduced by 25.8% since 1999, yet it is still the number 1 cause of morbidity and mortality in the United States, proving its immense impact [3]. The reduction in death rates can be attributed to research, improvements of medication and procedures, technology, and reduction in some risk factors such as smoking. But regardless of how well our

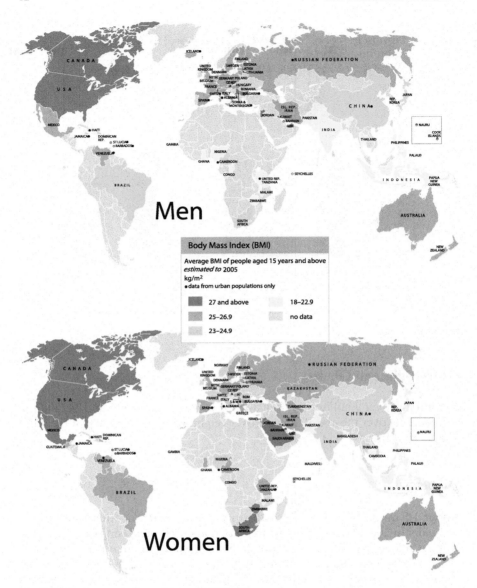

Fig. 1.12 Body mass index estimates in 2005 [5]

in-hospital diagnosing and treatment techniques are, approximately 60% of CAD deaths occur out of the hospital. Frighteningly, 50% of men and 64% of women who died suddenly of CAD in 2005 had no previous clinical symptoms of this disease, and just one-fifth of coronary attacks are preceded by long-standing angina [3]. These facts demonstrate the continual need for community

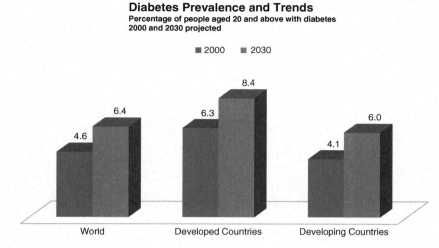

Fig. 1.13 Diabetes prevalence and trends [5]

education and awareness of the steps that can be taken to reduce the risk of such a destructive disease. Employing preventive care and community education has been and will continue to be a very important factor in the future trends of CAD in populations.

As we continue to monitor the distribution of CAD in populations, epidemiology will provide us with even better guidelines, which when applied appropriately can continue to decrease death rates caused by such a devastating disease worldwide.

References

1. Oppenheimer, Gerald M. Profiling Risk: The emergency of coronary heart disease epidemiology in the United States (1947–70). International Journal of Epidemiology. 2006; 35;720–730.
2. McConnel, Thomas, H. MD. The Nature of Disease, Pathology for the Health Professions. Lippincott Williams & Wilkins, Baltimore, MD, 2006. p. 302.
3. Heart Disease and Stroke Statistics. Our Guide to Current Statistics and the Supplement to our Heart and Stroke Facts. 2008 Update At-a-Glance. American Heart Association. americanheart.org/statistics.
4. http://www.census.gov/popest/archives/2000s/vintage_2005/05s_challenges.html
5. World Health Organization. Cardiovascular Disease Atlas. http://www.who.int/cardiovascular_diseases/resources/atlas/en/
6. Taylor, Herman A. Coronary heart disease epidemiology in the 21st century. Epidemiologic Reviews. 2000:22;7–13.

Chapter 2
Financial Impact of Acute Coronary Syndromes: The Need for New Care Delivery Models

Sandra Sieck

Abstract Evaluation and management of the acute chest pain patient in a cost-efficient manner that optimizes clinical outcomes remains a challenging and daunting task for the health-care system. The spectrum of chest pain patients presenting to the emergency department (ED) ranges from those with acute coronary syndrome (ACS) and potentially immediate life-threatening hemodynamic compromise to those without any underlying cardiac disease. The ideal health-care delivery structure is one that is poised to intercept any patient along this continuum at the point of entry and quickly and appropriately triage the patient to the most efficient, evidence-based treatment strategy: patients requiring high intensity of services are expeditiously identified and managed; those without significant disease are assessed to avoid unnecessary admissions; and those with hidden ischemia and potential impending cardiac events are evaluated to minimize inappropriate discharge. The chest pain unit (CPU) has evolved as an operational mechanism to optimally fulfill these clinical needs, improve quality, enhance clinical outcomes, and reduce overall costs.

Keywords Acute coronary syndromes · Reimbursement · Value-based purchasing · Cost · Front-loading care · Point of entry · Efficiency · Chest pain unit · Observation · Quality · Improvements · Outcomes · Y model · ABC model

Introduction

Evaluation and management of the acute chest pain patient in a cost-efficient manner that optimizes clinical outcomes remains a challenging and daunting task for the health-care system. The spectrum of chest pain patients presenting to the emergency department (ED) ranges from those with acute coronary

S. Sieck (✉)
Sieck HealthCare Consulting, 9431 Jeff Hamilton Road, Mobile, AL 36695, USA
e-mail: ssieck@sieckhealthcare.com

W.F. Peacock, C.P. Cannon (eds.), *Short Stay Management of Chest Pain*,
DOI 10.1007/978-1-60327-948-2_2,
© Humana Press, a part of Springer Science+Business Media, LLC 2009

syndrome (ACS) and potentially immediate life-threatening hemodynamic compromise to those without any underlying cardiac disease. The ideal health-care delivery structure is one that is poised to intercept any patient along this continuum at the point of entry and quickly and appropriately triage the patient to the most efficient, evidence-based treatment strategy: patients requiring high intensity of services are expeditiously identified and managed; those without significant disease are assessed to avoid unnecessary admissions; and those with hidden ischemia and potential impending cardiac events are evaluated to minimize inappropriate discharge. The chest pain unit (CPU) has evolved as an operational mechanism to optimally fulfill these clinical needs, improve quality, enhance clinical outcomes, and reduce overall costs.

The High Costs of Cardiovascular Disease

Health-care costs have been a major driving factor for change since the 1990s. Yet health-care costs continue to escalate at a rate that exceeds standard inflation [1]. Health care currently consumes 16.2% of the US GDP, estimated at $2.2 trillion in 2007. The Centers for Medicare and Medicaid Services (CMS) estimate that total spending on health care will grow at an average annual rate of 7.3%, to exceed $4 trillion by 2016, or almost $13,000 per US resident (Fig. 2.1). Over half of national expenditures arise from hospital care and physician services, 30.0 and 21.2%, respectively (Fig. 2.2). Not surprisingly, the hospital setting has been the target of multifaceted efforts for cost reduction strategies.

Despite marked advances in the diagnosis and treatment of cardiovascular disease, it remains the number one cause of mortality in the United States. Cardiovascular care accounts for approximately 14 % of the nation's health-care expenditures. Of the nearly 16 million people in the United States with coronary heart disease, 8 million will ultimately be diagnosed with acute coronary syndrome. Over the last two decades, annual inpatient admissions for coronary heart disease (CHD) as the primary diagnosis increased 5% to 1,828,000. The estimated total direct and indirect costs of care of CHD is expected to be $156.4 billion in 2008 [2]. Lost productivity from morbidity related to coronary disease accounts for $10.2 billion and lost productivity from mortality for $58.6 billion, or 6.5 and 38%, respectively, of total cardiovascular disease costs.

Cardiovascular disease impacts total hospital care and costs substantially. Emergency departments see over 5 million visits for chest pain suggestive of ischemia annually, resulting in $10 billion of hospital costs [3]. In 2007, ACS was responsible for 1.57 million hospital admissions. Total costs for coronary atherosclerosis care, including angioplasty and bypass surgery, are estimated to result in $51 billion of hospital charges in 2008. Any strategy that can positively impact quality of care for CHD in the hospital setting has potential for significant fiscal impact.

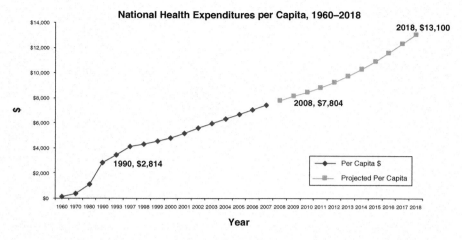

Fig. 2.1 Total expenditures of health care through 2016 (Kaiser Family Foundation, Trends in Health Care Costs and Spending, September 2007)

Notes Set 1:
1. The health spending projection were based on the 2007 version of the National Health Expenditures released in Jan 2009
2. 2000 base year. Calculated as the difference between nominal personal health care spending and real personal health care spending. Real personal health care spending is produced by deflating spending on each service type by the appropriate deflator (PPI, CPI, etc.) and adding real spending by service type.
3. July 1 Census resident based population estimates.
* Numbers and percents may not add to totals because of rounding.
*SOURCE: Centers for Medicare & Medicaid Services, Office of the Actuary.

Notes Set 2.
1. Census resident-based population less armed forced overseas and population of outlying areas. Source: U.S. Bureau of the Census.
2. U.S. Department of Commerce, Bureau of Economic Analysis.
* Numbers and percents may not add to totals because of rounding. Dollar amounts shown are in current dollars
*SOURCE: Centers for Medicare & Medicaid Services, Office of the Actuary, National Health Statistics Group; U.S. Department of Commerce, Bureau of Economic Analysis; and U.S. Bureau of the Census.

The Chest Pain Dilemma

Chest pain accounts for 5–6% of emergency department visits [4]. Eighty percent of chest pain patients actually present through the ED. Sixty to seventy percent of patients with chest pain are admitted, but only 10% have a diagnosis of acute myocardial infarction and 10% have unstable angina. Approximately three-fourths of chest pain patients presenting to the ED do not have ACS and would not require the intense and costly treatments afforded to ACS patients.

ACS patients are presenting to the ED earlier in the clot progression sequence, often making an accurate diagnosis in the early stages difficult. This

Fig. 2.2 Distribution of
national health expenditures
(Kaiser Family Foundation,
Trends in Health Care Costs
and Spending, September
2007)

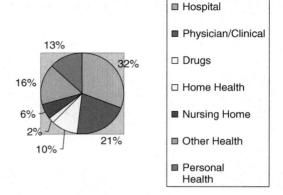

gives rise to a worrisome subgroup of 2–5% of chest pain patients who actually will have a myocardial infarction but who are discharged from the emergency department. This patient population has an unusually high subsequent incidence of poor outcomes [5].

At the inception of the coronary care unit, most chest pain patients with even a remote chance of potential for ACS were admitted to the CCU awaiting a "rule-in" or "rule-out" diagnosis of myocardial infarction. This practice was a time- and resource-inefficient method for finding those patients at highest risk. The goal of cardiac care today is to accurately and expeditiously identify the high-risk group for immediate interventions and cautiously, but efficiently, sort out the low-risk group who requires a substantially lower level of resource utilization. A well-designed chest pain unit (CPU) affords that opportunity.

Historical Perspective of CPU

Reimbursement forces in health care are moving many aspects of care delivery to the outpatient setting. Care in such settings is usually more efficient and less costly. The emergence of the chest pain center in the 1990s demonstrated a more efficient way of ruling out myocardial infarction for those patients in a low-risk population subset.

Traditionally, patients with chest pain have been evaluated in the emergency department and a decision is made to admit to the acute level of care hospital based on an assessment of the likelihood of a diagnosis of acute coronary syndrome. Because of the limitations of the sensitivity and/or the specificity of tests used in this evaluation—ECG, cardiac markers—the common practice has been to admit the majority of patients, even with a moderately low level of suspicion in order to avoid sending a patient home with an acute myocardial infarction. This practice has led to cost and resource inefficiencies since only 15–20% of patients admitted to the coronary care unit with chest pain are demonstrated to have sustained a myocardial infarction [6].

In an effort to reduce unnecessary admissions while reducing inappropriate discharges, the concept of the chest pain short-stay unit emerged and later developed into the chest pain unit or observation unit. CMS defined observation status as that commonly assigned to patients who present to the emergency department and who then require a significant period of treatment and/or monitoring before a decision is made concerning their next placement. This clinical decision unit is a 23-hour observation unit in which patients are assessed by a physician and a determination made of which patients need subsequent hospitalization. Such units focused on chest pain patients with low probability of acute coronary syndrome, expediting the evaluation to exclude ACS. This "rule-out MI" evaluation was a "telescoped" version of that provided in a traditional inpatient setting. The CPU is really a clinical decision unit (outpatient telemetry unit) that is designed to place the patient in the "correct" disposition. The unit should be viewed as a corrective action component through process improvement versus a stand-alone unit designed to merely generate revenue for the facility and physicians alike.

The original CPU served as a temporary holding area for the patient who was likely to be discharged without the evidence of ischemia. This triaging function allowed appropriate and expeditious care to the low-risk patient, while maintaining open bed availability in the inpatient units for patients requiring higher acuity care. The traditional CPU holding area resulted in cost savings predominantly by reducing the overall length of stay (LOS). Additionally, the ability to off-load chest pain patients from the ED helped to reduce ED overcrowding and gridlock [7], therefore enhancing ED throughput.

Chest pain units utilize a risk stratification approach in the immediate minutes of a patient's entry to make a decision on the subsequent clinical pathway. High-risk patients or those identified with ACS are admitted to the acute care facility or triaged directly to the catheterization laboratory for angiography and possible PCI. Low-risk patients remain in the CPU for further risk stratification with serial cardiac ischemia markers and exercise testing. The goal upon entry into the CPU is to render a decision on the pathway of the patient in an expeditious, but finite, amount of time. For instance, the decision to administer thrombolytics or divert ACS patients to a cath lab ideally should be done in less than 20–30 min. The decision to discharge the nonischemic chest pain patient can be made within 2–16 hours. The ultimate goal of the CPU is to transition many of the services now performed in the inpatient setting to the CPU for earlier treatment—the true "short-stay coronary care unit or (outpatient telemetry)."

Forces Affecting Cardiac Care Reimbursement

Multiple external and internal forces are affecting cardiac care delivery in the United States. Increasing third-party regulation and oversight impacts what care will be reimbursed.

Medicare is probably the most significant force in this reimbursement transformation, and many third-party payers follow Medicare's lead.

Medicare is increasingly pushing for evidence-based *and* cost-effective care. Demonstration projects have been created to gather objective data on the current system as a basis for future change efforts. Key pieces of current government focus include elimination of waste, reallocation of payment structures, quality accountability, fraud detection, and consumer accountability [8].

For the future, however, CMS is proposing to transform Medicare from a passive payer of claims to an active purchaser of care. In looking at care provided, CMS is centering its focus on clinical outcomes that are attained (or not) as a result of care provided. Simple provision of services will not suffice for optimal reimbursement in upcoming years. To that end, CMS is planning to base reimbursement on outcomes measures (e.g., morbidity, mortality, complication rates), risk-adjusted ICD-9 codes, and value-based purchasing programs.

The MS-DRG (Medicare Severity DRG) severity-adjusted payment system represents an attempt to alleviate a disparity in payments based on the old one-size-fits-all DRG payments for several conditions [9]. The previous set of 538 DRG codes has been expanded to 745 to take into consideration disease severity. The difference in reimbursement can be substantial, based on the presence or the lack of certain complications or comorbidities. For ACS, the initial reimbursement stratification point is based on coding a DRG for STEMI versus non-STEMI, and then further stratification is based on the types of interventions performed. It is critical for the acute care facility to accurately code ICD-9-CM and CPT codes to reflect the patient's severity in order to obtain appropriate reimbursements for the intensity of care provided.

Improving cost-efficiency and quality of care are no longer buzz words. Medicare has targeted inpatient care of acute myocardial infarction as one of the conditions for which quality of care indicators is being measured [10]. Five of the Medicare's ten quality process indicators focus on STEMI [11]. In 2007, CMS introduced a new quality effort that puts hospital payments at risk. The new program submitted by Congress would reduce payments to hospitals, with hospitals later "buying back" monies through high performance on quality measures. This new design is a value-based purchasing program whereby a defined percentage of a hospital's DRG payment will be based on the facilities meeting a set of performance measures. It is likely that this system will evolve over several years, with initial payments based on a hospital merely reporting the relevant data to CMS. Over time, increasing percentages of facility payments will be based on performance measures. Theoretically, ultimately the entire payment could be performance based.

Additionally, Medicare is targeting areas at high risk for payment errors. The Program to Evaluate Payment Patterns Electronic Report (PEPPER) is an initiative looking at hospital claims likely to have errors [12]. Target areas for this project include 1-day stays, hospital readmissions, and several DRGs known to have a high rate of errors. DRG 143, chest pain, was one of the top 20 DRGs nationwide for 1-day stay discharges in 2007. Just over 40% of these

Table 2.1 Volume of 1-day stays for DRG 143 (chest pain)

	2004	2005	2006	2007
One-day DRG 143	105,418	99,412	91,008	43,709
All DRG 143	245,146	234,089	217,418	103,691
One-day stay (%)	43.0	42.5	41.9	42.2

admissions involve 1-day discharges (Table 2.1). One-day stays are a focus of the initiative, as these short stays stand out as a potential area of improvement where medically necessary care might have better been provided on an out-patient basis or in an observation unit.

These reimbursement initiatives make it critical for acute care facilities to enhance data-capturing capabilities, improve coding accuracy, apply risk stratification to care pathways, and focus on clinical outcomes in order to remain financially sound.

Reimbursement for Chest Pain and ACS

CMS is the payer for a majority of acute cardiac patients who are largely of Medicare age. In its reimbursement policies, CMS is trying to shift unnecessary inpatient volume back to the point of entry for more efficient risk stratification, assessment, and intensive treatment. This influence, attained through reimbursement initiatives, has evolved rapidly over the last 5 years.

In 2002, CMS established a new coding and separate payment system for observation status for the diagnoses of chest pain, asthma, or heart failure if they met certain criteria for diagnostic testing, minimum and maximum time limits for observation, and documentation in the medical record. APC 0339 was designed to relieve some of the pressures of treating CHF, chest pain, and asthma patients aggressively on the front end of the care process versus admitting them to an acute care setting. Most diagnostic tests ordered during this observation stay were separately reimbursable, resulting in optimal reimbursements for the acute care facility. Another benefit of APC 0339 was that any revisits within 30 days or hospital admission after an OU stay were reimbursable when meeting medical necessity, unlike when the patient was admitted directly as an inpatient initially. This new coding system resulted in a financially favorable reimbursement for low-risk chest pain patients who could be discharged from the observation unit or CPU. Over the next 4 years, observation unit claims increased substantially (Table 2.2).

In 2008, CMS deleted the code, APC 0339, and created two composite APCs for extended assessment and management, of which observation care is a component. CMS views this as "totality of care" provided for an outpatient encounter (Table 2.3). The new codes are as follows:

Table 2.2 Observation unit claims

Year	Claims
2003	56,000
2004	77,000
2005	124,000
2006	271,000

- **APC 8002 Level I:** Extended Assessment and Management (observation following a direct admission or clinic visit) reimbursed at $351
- **APC 8003 Level II:** Extended Assessment and Management (observation following an emergency level four or five visits) reimbursed at $639.

Additionally, the use of an observation status is no longer limited to chest pain, heart failure, and asthma. Any medical condition that meets medical criteria can be placed in such status. Although the overall reimbursement for an ED plus observation status episode of care has been reduced slightly from 2007 to 2008, an expected increase in volume will offset this reduction. Now patients with a lengthy ED stay, 1-day stays, and a traditional inpatient observation could receive this beneficial change.

These recent changes have significant potential impact on acute care facilities. In order to remain financially viable in caring for chest pain and ACS patients, the hospital must develop new care delivery models, utilize evidence-based pathways, optimize point of service efficiency, and enhance data analytic capabilities. Front-loading care will allow facilities to have greater control over the variables that introduce out-of-range variations within daily operations.

Clinical and Fiscal Rational for a CPU

The success of the CPU depends on the provision of at least equivalent clinical outcomes compared to inpatient stays, but at reduced costs. Studies show that observation of carefully selected emergency chest pain patients results in improved clinical outcomes. One study showed that the use of an observation unit resulted in a tenfold decrease in the error rate for missed diagnosis of myocardial infarction [13]. The Chest Pain Evaluation Registry (CHEPER) study reported a significant reduction in missed MIs from 4.5 to 0.4%, a change that enhances quality, reduces the risk of potential high-cost medical/legal payouts, and decreases readmissions from erroneous diagnoses [14].

The current CPU is not merely a holding area for low-risk patients and a conduit to the cath lab for high-risk ischemic patients. The use of a CPU has been shown to demonstrate resource advantages over the typical hospital admission, even when the same tests are performed. For typical lowrisk chest pain patients admitted to the hospital, the average length of stay is 2–3 days, while for an observation unit or CPU, the average is 12–18 hours [15]. Each outpatient CPU bed frees 2.2–3.5 inpatient beds that can then be allocated to high-acuity patients [16].Additionally, from a DRG standpoint, all charges

Table 2.3 New observation unit payment summary 2008

Year	ED visit level	ED w/ OBS (criteria met)	Direct admit (criteria met)	ED & direct admit (criteria not met)	Diagnosis
2007	Level V $325	Level V $325 APC0339 $442 Pmt $768 + Ancillaries $$ (30% penetration)*	APC 0604 $442	APC 0604 $51 (70% penetration)*	Chest pain CHF Asthma
2008	Level IV or V $348	Level IV or V $0 APC 8003 $0 Comp pmt $639 + Ancillaries $$ (70% penetration)*	APC 8002 $351	APC 0604 $53 (30% penetration)*	Any medically necessary diagnosis (excl. status "T" and "V")**
Pmt impact	Inc $23	Dec $129	Dec $91	Inc $2	

*Note penetration of claims shift in 2008 to higher payment.
**Postprocedure or postsurgery codes.

originating in the ED are debited from the total payment for which the patient is admitted. The difference between coding DRG 14 (chest pain) now MS-DRG 313 versus DRG 140 (unstable angina) now MS-DRG 311 could potentially cause the hospital opportunity revenue losses from $4000 to $6000 per case.

The current shift in patients from the traditional inpatient treatment protocol to a more efficient plan of care initiated in a CPU has resulted in a significant economic impact on the acute care facility (see Table 2.4) [17].One multicenter study showed that the use of a CPU resulted in a lower incidence of missed MI (0.4 versus 4.5%, P<0.001) and a lower final rate of hospital admission (47 versus 57%, P<0.001). These clinical benefits were accompanied by an average saving of more than $120 per patient [18]. In a prospective, randomized trial of patients seen at a CPU, there were no cases of missed primary cardiac events or erroneous discharges and resource utilization was more efficient when ACS patients were seen in the CPU than when they were admitted to the coronary care unit [19].

Another potential benefit to the acute care facility is the reduction in ED burden resulting from a CPU. A study by Pines at the University of Pennsylvania evaluated the clinical impact of overcrowding in the ED on outcomes in ACS patients [20]. Of 6646 patients presenting with chest pain, 831 had an ACS diagnosis. Patients were more likely to have a complication or adverse outcome when the ED was crowded. Pines concluded that ED overcrowding is not solely an issue for the ED, but it is a measure of a more global system-wide dysfunction. The ED crowding puts pressures on all parts of the hospital—lab, X-ray, housekeeping, etc.—and has a domino effect on services for inpatients as well.

These preliminary data suggest that a well-designed CPU affords the hospital a mechanism to streamline care of the chest pain patient more efficiently, expeditiously, and scientifically appropriately with resulting improved quality of care indicators, overall reduced costs compared to the traditional approach, and with more favorable reimbursements.

Re-engineering the Chest Pain Delivery Model—New Solutions

As reported in the Institute of Medicine's Report Brief in June of 2006, tools developed from engineering and operations research have been successfully applied to a variety of businesses, from banking and airlines to manufacturing companies.

These same tools have been shown to improve the flow of patients through hospitals, increasing the number of patients that can be treated while minimizing delays in their treatment and improving the quality of their care. One such tool is queuing theory, which by smoothing the peaks and valleys of patient admissions has the potential to eliminate bottlenecks, reduce crowding, improve patient care, and reduce cost. Another promising tool is the clinical decision unit, or 23-hour observation unit, which helps ED staff determine whether certain ED patients require admission. Hospitals should use these

Table 2.4 Acute myocardial infarction financial outcomes

AMI financial outcomes:

Core measure: AMI	#Patients	Average LOS	Total cost	Average cost per case
Feb–June 2005 (pre-EPA)	319	5.41	$ 6,286,443.02	$ 19,707
Feb–June 2006 (post EPA)	269	5.25	$ 5,106,669.57	$ 18,984
Comparison		↓ 0.16 days		Savings per case $ 723 Total Savings $ 194,487

AMI clinical outcomes:

Core measure: AMI	# Patients	# Complications	Complications (%)	# Readmits	Readmits (%)
Feb–June 2005 (pre-EPA)	319	35	10.97	6	1.88
Feb–June 2006 (post EPA)	269	21	7.81	2	0.74
Comparison			↓ 3.16		↓ 1.14

tools as a way of improving hospital efficiency and, in particular, reducing ED crowding [21].

It is becoming increasingly clear that improving hospital efficiency and patient flow is a critical piece in improving the delivery model of acute level of care that can result in better quality and reduce costs of care. Implementing small changes to the current inefficient hospital structure will not afford the degree of impact that will enhance long-term viability of health-care systems in today's marketplace. Only the introduction of innovative new models will insure success. To that end, tools commonly used in the business and engineering world to improve operational efficiencies are now finding their way into the halls of medicine [22].

The Y model is an approach that allows facilities to closely examine different aspects of operations within their systems [23]. It encompasses the concept of health-care delivery along a continuum from the point of entry into the "system" through to discharge. The Y model is a vertical process, in which patients are "pulled through" rather than "pushed through." It attempts to align clinical and financial balance to find an optimal breakeven point. The Y model is best applied to the overall operations of the hospital systems. But initial projects can target one specific disease or condition, such as ACS. By applying variations of the Y model, which all focus on two endpoints, quality and cost, facilities can recognize ways to turn ACS from a negative contribution margin to one that breaks even or contributes favorably.

Understanding the application of the Y model to the health-care setting involves comparing health-care services to the industrial setting. Industrial facilities can detail the exact route from raw material to finished product with detailed accuracy. The end-product is priced to the market based on the operating costs within the process. If the manufacturing process varies greatly over time, costs of production rise and are passed on in a higher market price. In order to keep prices down, actions must be taken to get the variances under control. If not, the contribution margin is eroded and eventually could become negative. The objective is to keep the contribution margin at its maximum without compromising quality.

This model can be similarly applied to an ACS patient routing through the health-care delivery setting. Patients receive services within different "care units" within the acute hospital setting. These care units are analogous to the industrial setting's business units. By understanding how each care unit's operational strategies affect each subsequent care unit from point of entry to discharge, a seamless transfer of patient care in both outpatient and inpatient settings can optimize quality improvement and positive economic value. Without each care unit providing vital information to others in this holistic approach, moving patients efficiently through the system is challenged.

The current processes in the health-care delivery for most patients in a hospital setting are more characteristic of a "zigzag model " (Fig. 2.3). For example, an ACS patient usually enters through the ED and receives treatments and evaluations through multiple disconnected service sectors or "care units" (known as business units in the commercial sector). These care units are represented by nursing, EKG department, radiology department, pharmacy,

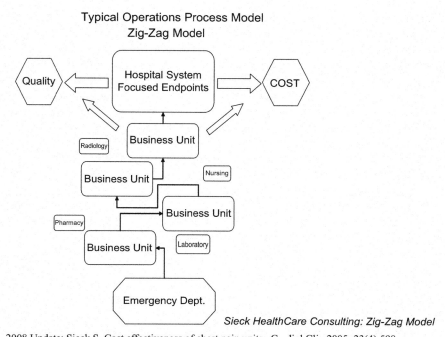

Fig. 2.3 Zigzag model of care (2008 Update: Sieck S. Cost effectiveness of chest pain units. Cardiol Clin 2005; 23(4):598)

laboratory, etc. Each of the care units is viewed and acts as a single independent business unit from the standpoint of the hospital. The outputs of these care units' activities are collated by the provider, usually once the patient has been admitted to the acute hospital bed. It is then—at the "back end" of the process— that care treatment plans are decided upon. The zigzag model is disconnected and fragmented, which can adversely impact quality, costs, efficiency, patient satisfaction, and clinical outcomes.

The Y model represents a different approach and provides a framework to facilities to optimize a disease management model covering costs of care by placing the proper resources at the "front end" of the point-of-care entry. This concept begins at the point of entry and ends at discharge and marries a clinical and financial strategy that meets quality indicators while producing desirable profit margins. Beginning in the ED, this concept emphasizes an efficient, rapid assessment and action centered on a seamless integration of ancillary services such as the laboratory, diagnostic imaging, and skilled nursing while understanding the economic impacts on decisions made as the patient is directed through the system.

Accurate data analysis is a critical piece toward successfully implementing the Y Model. Baseline analysis of ED admissions drills down on the exact volume of cases by ICD-9 codes instead of the inpatient DRG, providing a more accurate picture of the number of patients that are passing through the outpatient door within a system. With this analysis and the proper guidance, facilities can target individual diseases more effectively. Patients who require an inpatient admission are properly admitted and those who could be effectively treated in the outpatient setting are treated and properly released. The placement of more critical patients in the inpatient acute care setting impacts the case mix index (a currently used severity of illness adjustor) positively because the patients are simply sicker and require more resources.

Creating a new care delivery system for the ACS patient that is based on the Y model can positively impact the contribution margins when ACS patients are carefully identified, risk stratified, and given appropriate early treatment during the interaction (Fig. 2.4). This model emphasizes a multidisciplinary team approach to align the "care units" that affect an ACS patient's progress through the current system. Additionally, low-risk patients that are evaluated and discharged from the CPU reduce unnecessary resource utilization, thereby efficiently "saving" such resources that are required for high-risk-only patients.

The emphasis of the Y model is on front-end compliance that sets up the pathway the patient will follow (Fig. 2.5). A patient is not "arbitrarily" admitted to an inpatient bed, treated, and then discharged. A decision is made up front on the most ideal care venue for the risk-stratified patient to be admitted to and undergo tailored treatment. It also initiates the financial pathway with identified markers throughout the patient interaction that allows facilities to know

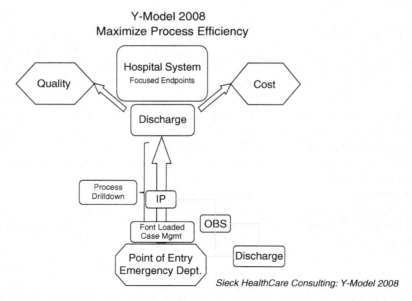

Fig. 2.4 Y model using risk stratification and ABC approach (2008 Update: Sieck S. Cost effectiveness of chest pain units. Cardiol Clin 2005;23(4):597)

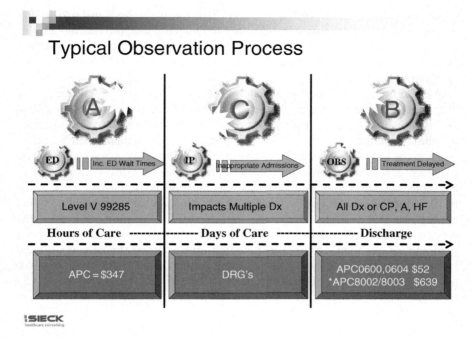

Typical Observation Process

Fig. 2.5 ACB process

the ramifications of making random decisions versus following a protocol designed to emphasize quality while optimizing economic results. The Y model places an emphasis on process improvement while targeting the endpoints of quality and contribution margin.

One medical center has successfully implemented part of the model for an Acute Coronary Syndrome (ACS) Process Improvement Project [24]. Prior to the initiative the hospital had a "zigzag" model of care. Patients entered through the ED and were admitted to the acute care bed, diagnostics completed, and treatment was then initiated. With initiation of the Y model, stratification was performed and appropriate therapy initiated in the ED with point-of-care testing in a patient-centric improvement effort. The new design resulted in improvements in turnaround time for therapy, reduced LOS, enhanced patient placement in the most appropriate bed venue (e.g., CCU, telemetry, or clinical decision unit), and improved patient satisfaction. Improvements demonstrated in the ACS redesign can be translated to the ADHF setting. Similar to the ACS patient, not every HF absolutely requires inpatient admission. And similarly, not all HF patients are candidates for the OU. Point-of-entry triaging to the most appropriate care unit where an individualized treatment plan is rendered allows a facility to better merge quality care with positive financial outcomes [25, 26].

Improvements demonstrated in the ACS redesign can be translated to any patient who would otherwise be admitted to the acute hospital setting. Similar to the ACS patient, not every patient absolutely requires a critical care, telemetry, or even medical-surgical bed. And similarly, not all ACS patients are candidates for the CPU.

An additional component of a redesign strategy involves the ABC model of outpatient observation unit care. The ABC model defines a new approach to observation unit or chest pain unit processes. The current care flow in most hospitals is actually an "ACB" process (Fig. 2.5). The patient spends several hours in the ED (A), after which is admitted to the hospital (C), and only then are treatment and observation initiated (B). Overall there is not only treatment delay but increased backlog in the ED. Essentially most of the "front-end" time in the ACB sequence is inefficiently wasted—both clinically and financially. When appropriate care and treatment are "front-loaded," the more efficient ABC process can take place (Fig. 2.6). In this case, the ED stay is shortened to a minimum of less than 2 hours—just enough time to assess the patient's clinical status and triage to the next point of care—either the CPU for those low-risk patients who are likely to be discharged or to the cath lab, telemetry or the CCU for higher risk patients.

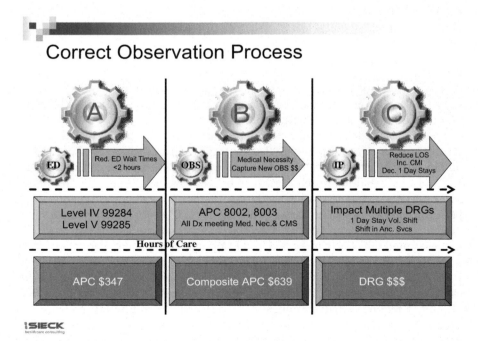

Fig. 2.6 Current location of the indeterminate patient

The observation status of the CPU can be equated with an outpatient telemetry unit in function. The patient with chest pain is not any less "cared for" in this unit than he/she would be on the telemetry unit. In fact, the level of care and observation is the same, but with enhanced efficiency resulting in a more timely disposition and resolution to final diagnosis and ultimate treatment. In the ABC model, the use of clinical pathways or treatment protocols is front-loaded with the assistance of case management. In this instance, the case manager plays an integrative role early in the evaluation and care of the chest pain patient rather than late in the course of hospitalization when most of the intensive resources have already been utilized and there is little opportunity for enhanced efficiencies beyond merely expediting discharge of the patient.

The use of the ABC and Y models also reduces ED crowding by expediently enhancing flow through the ED. Additionally, they reduce unnecessary admissions by truncating the total evaluation time for low-risk patients. Finally, LOS for inpatient admissions is reduced because there are no treatment initiation delays. Since almost half of chest pain patients can be safely evaluated and treated in the CPU, the financial implications of this model can be substantial (Fig. 2.7).

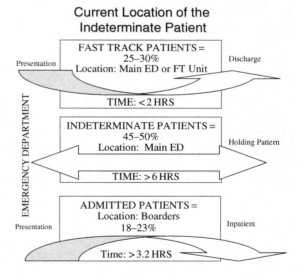

Fig. 2.7 ABC process

As noted in Fig. 2.8, Beta site testing and results demonstrated clinical and financial benefits of front-loaded care. In one facility applying components of the model to core measure conditions, quality ranking of the index facility compared to all other facilities within their system resulted in moving from being 25th out of 26 facilities to becoming number 1 [27]. ED volume increased from 47,000 to 60,000 patient visits annually, while the rate of patients leaving without being seen decreased from 10.1 to 3.2%, and full ED status fell from 10 days/month to 2 days/month. On the inpatient side, LOS decreased from

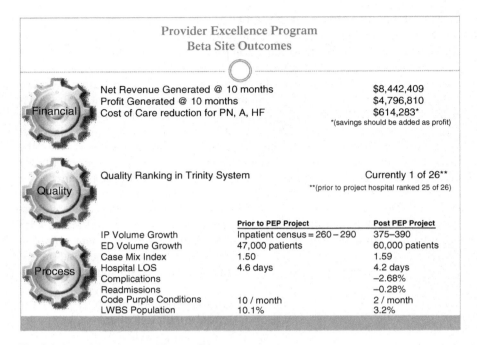

Fig. 2.8 Beta site outcomes: Fresno, CA

4.6 to 4.2 days, readmissions dropped by 0.28%, complications decreased by 2.68%, and their case mix index increased from 1.50 to 1.59%. It should also be noted that specifically AMI data improved overall, see Fig. 2.5.

While both the Y model (disease management) and ABC model (observation) appear inherently understandable and conceptually "easy" in overall structure and objective, the actual implementation of the specific design and the management of the change process required for alignment of incentives, stakeholder buy-in, and participation are the critical factors upon which the success of such a project hinges. Although the final objective of merging quality and resource efficiency is the goal of any organization, the specific implementation plan and strategy must be individualized to each hospital based on a complete analysis of the baseline processes, time and resource constraints, training needs, and willingness to change of the participants.

Measuring Changes Is Critical

Finally, the importance of data is crucial. The critical success factor in the implementation of any of the preceding programs is the knowledgeable use of accurate metrics [28]. Prior to the initiation of any redesign, a detailed assessment must be conducted of the current processes in place, patient flow patterns, and clinical practice patterns. From this assessment, a key set of measurable indicators related to the proposed process improvement is then measured at baseline. It is important to select the most appropriate measurements that will impact objectives rather than merely using standard metrics that may be routinely measured for other initiatives (e.g., HEDIS), which may not always be appropriate for the new initiatives. As the programs are implemented, metrics are utilized to gauge and manage the change process. If a change process cannot be adequately measured, it will not be effectively or successfully managed.

Conclusion

Although death rates for acute coronary syndromes declined between 1999 and 2006 due to the impact of pharmacologic and interventional treatments, the numbers of patients with chest pain and ACS are likely to increase over the next decade as the Baby Boomer generation "comes of age" [29]. Expensive advances in diagnostic and therapeutic alternatives add to the economic burden of chest pain and ACS. With ACS representing a large volume of ED patients, changes in the care delivery model afford the opportunity for economic and outcomes benefit. Thus, it has been a major area of focused activity over the last 5 years.

Increased patient volumes and overcrowding of EDs have already impacted care for emergent medical conditions [30]. From 1997 to 2004, the average wait times for AMI patients increased 11.2% per year compared to 4.1% for all ED patients. An 8-minute wait time from ED door-to-care in 1997 increased to 20 minutes by 2005. More alarming, one out of four AMI patients experienced a wait of almost 1 hour before receiving care after arrival in the ED. Add these ED problems to the difficulties that are encountered when trying to create a system of acute cardiac care regionalized centers for AMI patients, and you have a health-care system that, if not broken already, is certainly in trouble and destined to be unable to deliver the quality care that is scientifically available to cardiac patients [31].

The 2001 Institute of Medicine report on Crossing the Quality Chasm describes a health-care system that is in need of a major redesign, not small changes:

As medical science and technology have advanced at a rapid pace, however, the health care delivery system has floundered in its ability to provide consistently high-quality care to all Americans [32].

The health care system as currently structured does not, as a whole, make the best use of its resources.

The costs of waste, poor quality, and inefficiency are enormous. If the current delivery system is unable to utilize today's technologies effectively, it will be even less able to carry the weight of tomorrow's technologies and an aging population, raising the specter of even more variability in quality, more errors, less responsiveness, and greater costs associated with waste and poor quality.

To meet the demands of the current forces in the health care, such as, increased quality, continued resource efficiency, and cost reductions in the face of severity-adjusted and value-based reimbursements, the hospital must be ready to totally redesign the flow of care from the ED to an individualized optimal care pathway. The CPU is one step in this major overhaul redesign process.

References

1. Kaiser Family Foundation, Trends in Health Care Costs and Spending, September 2007, http://www.kff.org/insurance/upload/7692.pdf (accessed January 13, 2008)
2. Heart Disease and Stroke Statistics, 2008 Update at a Glance, American Heart Association, 2008 http://www.americanheart.org/downloadable/heart/1198257493273HS_Stats%202008.pdf (accessed January 14, 2008)
3. Ewy GA, Ornato JP. Emergency cardiac care: Introduction. J Amer Coll Cardiol 2000;35:825–880
4. Quin G. Chest pain evaluation units, Western Journal of Medicine 2000 December; 173(6):403–407
5. McCarthy BD, Beshansky JR, D'Agostino RB, Selker HP. Missed diagnoses of acute myocardial infarction in the emergency department: Results from a multicenter study. Annals of Emergence Medicine 1993;22:579–582
6. UC Davis Health System: First-class training from first-class emergency medicine physicians. http://www.ucdmc.ucdavis.edu/emergency/chestpaineval.html
7. Joint Commission Resources, Managing Patient Flow:Strategies and Solutions for Addressing Hospital Overcrowding, 2004, p. 11
8. www.cms.hhs.gov http://www.cms.hhs.gov/DemoProjectsEvalRpts/downloads/MMA-demolist.pdf
9. See Wynn et al., "Evaluation of Severity-adjusted DRG Systems: Interim Report," RAND: Santa Monica, CA., WR-434-CMS, 2007 (available at www.rand.org/pubs/working_papers/WR434/)
10. www.cms.hhs.gov; http://www.cms.hhs.gov/HospitalQualityInits/downloads/Hospital HQA2004_2007200512.pdf
11. Jacobs AK, Antman EM, Ellrodt G, et al. Recommendation to develop strategies to increase the number of ST-segment elevations myocardial infarction patients with timely access to primary percutaneous intervention—The American Heart Association's acute myocardial infarction (AMI) Advisory Working Group. Circulation 2006;113:2152–2163
12. Short-Term Acute Care Program for Evaluating Payment Patterns Electronic Report (ST PEPPER) User's Guide October 2007 http://www.hpmpresources.org/LinkClick.aspx?fileticket = H5IICGIqbvM%3d&tabid = 1059&mid = 1052
13. Graff LG, et al. Impact on the care of the emergency department chest pain patient from the Chest Pain Evaluation Registry (CHEPER) study. American Journal of Cardiology 80:563–568, 1997
14. Graff LG, Dallara J, Ross MA, Joseph AJ, et al. Impact on the care of the emergency department chest pain patient from the Chest Pain Evaluation Registry (CHEPER) study. American Journal of Cardiology 1997;80(5):563–568
15. Pope J et al. New England Journal of Medicine 2000:342;1163–1170
16. Ross M et al. The impact of an ED observation unit on inpatient bed capacity. Annals of Emergency Medicine 2001;8:576
17. Sieck S, ACS Best Practice. Journal of Critical Pathways in Cardiology 2002;1(4):225

18. Graff LG, Dallara J, Ross MS, Joseph AJ, et al. Impact on the care of the emergency department chest pain patient from the Chest Pain Evaluation Registry (CHEPER) study. American Journal of Cardiology 1997;80(5):563–568
19. Farouh ME, Smars PA, Reeder GS, et al. A clinical trial of a chest pain observation unit for patients with unstable angina. Chest Pain in the Emergency Room (CHEER) Investigators. New England Journal of Medicine 1998;339(26):1882–1888
20. Pines JM, Hollander JE. Association between cardiovascular complications and ED crowding. American College of Emergency Physicians 2007 Scientific Assembly; October 8–11, 2007; Seattle, WA.
21. The Future of Emergency Care in the United States Health System reports are available from the National Academies Press, 500 Fifth Street, N.W., Lockbox 285, Washington, DC 20055; (800) 624–6242 or (202) 334–3313 (in the Washington metropolitan area); Internet, http://www.nap.edu. The full text of this report is available at http://www.nap.edu
22. Institute of Medicine. The Future of Emergency Care: Hospital Based Emergency Care at the Breaking Point. June 2006
23. Sieck HealthCare Consulting – www.sieckhealthcare.com
24. Holland J, Holt T, Nord G, et al. Enhancing outcomes of acute coronary syndrome. Abstracts from the Eighth Annual Society of Chest Pain Centers Scientific Sessions. Critical Pathways in Cardiology: A Journal of Evidence-Based Medicine 2005;4(4):193–194.
25. Sieck, SG. The process and economics of heart failure. Short Stay Management of Heart Failure 2006, (5):39–53
26. Holland J, Holt T, Nord G, et al. Enhancing Outcomes of Acute Coronary Syndrome. Abstracts from the Eighth Annual Society of Chest Pain Centers Scientific Sessions. Critical Pathways in Cardiology: A Journal of Evidence-Based Medicine 2005; 4(4):193–194.
27. Sieck HealthCare Consulting – beta site: Saint Agnes Medical Center, Fresno, CA; 2006–2007
28. Kornecki Z. What Gets Measured Gets Managed. February 2008
29. Fox KAA, Steg PG, Eagle KA, et al. Decline in death and heart failure in Acute Coronary Syndromes, 1999–2006. JAMA 2007;297:1892–1900
30. Waits to See an Emergency Department Physician: US Trends and Predictors, 1997–2004. Health Affairs 2008 January 15
31. Kereiakes DJ. Specialized centers and systems for heart attack care. American Heart Hospital Journal 2008;6:14–20
32. Institute of Medicine, Crossing the Quality Chasm: A New Healthcare System for the 21st Century. 2001

Chapter 3
Why Have a Chest Pain Unit?

Annitha Annathurai and Michael A. Ross

Abstract Acute coronary syndromes are a leading cause of death in the United States with most patients presenting to the emergency department with chest pain. From the physician's perspective, chest pain is a "high-volume, high-risk, and high-liability" symptom. From the health-care system's perspective, chest pain evaluation is costly and difficult to complete in a timely manner using traditional approaches. To address these issues, chest pain centers have been developed as a means of providing quality care, ensuring patient safety, while maintaining cost-effectiveness. The concept of a chest pain "unit" has been expanded to a chest pain "center," which represents a hospital-wide designation rather than a unit. Chest pain centers are now accredited based on standardized criteria that cover the full spectrum of care for acute coronary syndrome patients – from EMS to the hospital and back to the community. Within that framework, the chest pain unit generally focuses on the management of "low-risk" chest pain patients. The goal is to avoid inadvertent discharge of occult ACS patients in a cost-effective manner. This involves patient selection or risk stratification, serial testing to identify myocardial necrosis, and then provocative testing with or without imaging to identify unstable angina. Studies have shown this approach to be associated with several benefits – lower rates of missed acute coronary syndromes, reduced unnecessary inpatient admissions, reduced cost and length of stay, improved patient and physician satisfaction, improved patient quality of life, improved hospital resource utilization and inpatient bed capacity , decreased ambulance diversions, and fewer patients leaving the ED without being seen. Several of these benefits may be tied to economic benefits for the hospital, as well as benefits for those paying for health-care services. This chapter examines the justification for a chest pain unit in a hospital and its benefits to the health-care system.

A. Annitha (✉)
Department of Emergency Medicine, Singapore General Hospital, Singapore
e-mail: annitha19@hotmail.com

W.F. Peacock and C.P. Cannon (eds.), *Short Stay Management of Chest Pain*,
DOI 10.1007/978-1-60327-948-2_3,
© Humana Press, a part of Springer Science+Business Media, LLC 2009

Keywords Chest pain center · Costs and cost analysis · Acute coronary syndrome · Emergency service hospital

Background on Why Chest Pain Units Are Needed

As a condition seen in the emergency department, chest pain is a "high-volume, high-risk, and high-liability" symptom. In 2006 the most common specific principal reasons given by adult patients (aged 15 years and older) for visiting the ED were, in descending frequency, abdominal pain, chest pain, back pain, headache, and shortness of breath [23]. Chest pain is the symptom that most patients with an acute coronary syndrome present with. Coronary artery disease is the "top killer" of Americans [13]. Based on 2004 statistics, it caused one of every five deaths in the United States in 2004 [13]. Every 26 seconds an American will suffer a coronary event, and every minute one will die from a coronary event [13]. About 38% of those who have experienced a coronary attack in a given year will die [13]. The estimated average number of years of life lost due to a heart attack is 15 years [13]. There are racial disparities in these numbers as well, with 2004 CHD death rates per 100,000 population of 223.9 for black males, 194.2 for white males, 148.7 for black females, and 114.7 for white females [13]. People who survive the acute stage of an MI have 1.5- to 15-fold greater risk of illness or death than the general population [13]. On a more encouraging note, progress has been made in decreasing death rates from CHD. Between 1950 and 1999 the CHD death rate decreased by 59%; however, between 1994 and 2004 the number of deaths declined only by 18%. It has been suggested that the declining percentages may be due to increased awareness, lifestyle changes, and early detection and therapeutic interventions [13].

From the hospitals' perspective, the estimated 2008 total cost, both direct and indirect, of CHD is $156.4 billion [13]. In 2005 an estimated 1.27 million people had undergone inpatient angioplasty procedures, 1.32 million had inpatient diagnostic cardiac catheterizations, 98,000 had inpatient implantable defibrillators, and 180,000 had inpatient pacemaker procedures in the United States [13]. There was a total of 1.41 million discharges with an acute coronary syndrome diagnosis, 838,000 with a myocardial infarction diagnosis, and 558,000 with an unstable angina diagnosis [13]. Amongst those patients who were admitted and discharged from hospitals, the leading principal hospital discharge diagnoses were nonischemic heart disease (7.6%) and chest pain (5.7%) [23]. Out of the 13.9 million people admitted to the ED and discharged from hospital, a total of 2.3 million were diagnosed with noncardiac chest pain (chest pain, heart disease excluding ischemic heart disease) [23]. Only 20% of the 2.3 million were discharged with the diagnoses of ischemic heart disease, suggesting that the other 80% were non-CHD related [23]. The cost for negative inpatient cardiac evaluations has been estimated to be $6 billion a year [5, 6].

From the physicians' perspective, failure to diagnose or treat acute myocardial infarction represents the largest percentage of malpractice claims paid against emergency physicians for any one condition [33]. Losses from malpractice litigation of this condition in the ED account for 20–39% of all malpractice dollars awarded [5, 6, 18]. This is in large part because roughly 1 in 20 patients experiencing an acute MI does not present in a typical manner. As a frame of reference, MI is diagnosed when a patient has two of three criteria – chest pain suggestive of AMI, a rise and fall in cardiac markers, and an ECG which is diagnostic for AMI. Unfortunately one-third of MI patients never present with chest pain. MI patients that present without chest pain are likely to be older, female, diabetic, and have a history of CHF. If an MI patient presents without chest pain, they are 2.2 times more likely to die while they are in the hospital. Furthermore, less than half of MI patients will present with diagnostic cardiac markers on arrival, and roughly half of AMI patients will not have a diagnostic ECG. In fact 8% of patients having an AMI present with a completely normal ECG [40]. As a result of this, studies have reported that roughly 2–8% of patients with an acute MI are inadvertently discharged home from the ED [18, 24]. Pope showed that relative to ACS patients that are admitted, inadvertently discharged patients with MI are 90% more likely to die. Inadvertently discharged patients with unstable angina are 70% more likely to die. In a separate study, Lee showed that the short-term mortality rate for MI patients mistakenly discharged from the ED is about 25%, which is almost twice of what would be expected if they were admitted [19]. Henceforth, the responsibility of reducing missed MI or ACS discharge rates while ensuring appropriate and necessary admissions to the hospitals falls largely on the shoulders of emergency physicians.

So Why Not Admit All "Suspect" Chest Pain Patients?

While the clinical and medicolegal risks of chest pain patients might drive one to simply admit all patients to the hospital as an inpatient, there is evidence that this is not the optimal solution. Studies have demonstrated that the approach of admitting chest pain patients is associated with inpatient length of stays of roughly 2–3 days, with lower rates of completed testing than care in a chest pain observation unit. The 2005 NHAMCS Survey 2005 ED Summary reported that roughly 80% of the 2.1 million patients admitted for chest pain evaluation were discharged with non-ACS diagnoses such as "heart disease nonischemic" and "chest pain." Only 20% were diagnosed with "ischemic heart disease" [23].

Unwarranted admissions also further compound the problem of "boarders" and hospitals at full capacity with no beds, resulting in hospital diversions, an increase in ED crowding, and related issues. In the past 10 years there has been a disturbing trend in ED visits compared with hospital capacities. From 1996 to 2006, the annual number of ED visits increased from 90.3 to 119.2 million (up by 32%). This represents an average increase of about 2.9 million visits (3.2%) per year. There were, on average, about 227 visits to US EDs every minute during 2006. As the number of visits to the ED increased, the number of hospital EDs has decreased from 4,019 to 3,833 (a 4.6% decrease), thus increasing the annual number of visits per ED from 1996 to 2006. This has led to an increase in ED "boarding" or holding admitted patients in the ED that do not have an available bed [15]. Boarding has been shown to be associated with delays in care, ambulance diversion, increased hospital lengths of stay, medical errors, increased patient mortality, financial losses to hospital and physician, and medical negligence claims [1]. In a discussion of high-impact solutions to this crisis, the American College of Emergency Physicians report on boarding recommended an expansion of what has been called "observation medicine" to improve utilization of limited hospital resources [1]. This may occur by avoiding unnecessary admissions, while avoiding inappropriate discharges.

What Is a Chest Pain Center? What Is a Chest Pain Unit?

Similar to the trauma center concept, chest pain centers have been developed over the last 25 years to address issues facing ACS patients. These centers standardized processes identified as being critical to the care of these patients. They include protocols related to the timely diagnosis and reperfusion of STEMI patients, chest pain diagnostic protocols to avoid inadvertent discharge of ACS patients, public outreach efforts to bring patients suffering with ACS to the hospital sooner, appropriate staffing and resources, and an effective interface with both emergency medical services and hospital administration.

A survey published by Zalenski in 1995, which focused on emergency department (ED)-based chest pain centers in the United States, found a chest pain centers prevalence of 22.5%, which yielded a projection of 520 centers in the United States in 1995. EDs with centers had higher overall patient volumes, greater use of high-technology testing, lower treatment times for thrombolytic therapy, and more advertising (all p <0.05) [41]. Hospitals with centers had greater market competition and more beds per annual admissions, cardiac catheterization, and open heart surgery capability (all p <0.05). Logistic regression identified open heart surgery, high admission volumes, and nonprofit status as independent predictors of hospitals having chest pain centers. Thus, chest pain centers had a moderate prevalence, offered more services and marketing efforts than standard EDs and tend to be hosted by large nonprofit hospitals [41].

In 1998, the Society of Chest Pain Centers (SCPC) was established, involving a collaboration of physicians, nurses, and health-care experts from cardiology, emergency medicine, nuclear medicine, and clinical pathology [44]. Through literature review and expert consensus, the society developed standardized criteria for chest pain center (CPC) accreditation. To achieve accreditation, an institution must submit documentation and participate in a site visit conducted by SCPC reviewers. To achieve accreditation, a hospital is required to both document and demonstrate compliance with eight key elements related to the care of patients with acute coronary syndromes [32] (Table 3.1). In June 2003, the first hospital

Table 3.1 Eight key elements. To earn accredited chest pain center status, a facility confirms performance of the processes in the following eight (8) key areas (www.scpcp.org)

1. Emergency department integration with the emergency medical system
2. Emergency assessment of patients with symptoms of possible ACS – timely diagnosis and treatment of ACS
3. Assessment of patients determined to have low to moderate risk for ACS
4. Functional facility design
5. Personnel, competencies, and training
6. Organizational structure
7. Process improvement orientation
8. Community outreach program

chest pain center was accredited. By August 2008, there were 400 accredited CPCs in the United States. A 2008 study compared compliance with CMS core measures for the treatment of patients with acute myocardial infarction [32]. Hospitals are required to report these core measures. To provide reliable comparison groups, a multivariate logistic regression model using a propensity-score adjustment factor was used. This study found that accredited chest pain centers were associated with better compliance with Centers for Medicare and Medicaid Services core measures and saw a greater proportion of patients with AMIs [32].

While a chest pain center represents a hospital-wide designation, covering a wide spectrum of services, a chest pain unit represents a dedicated geographic unit within a hospital – where a component of a chest pain centers' services is provided. The chest pain unit is generally where patients at low to intermediate risk of having an acute coronary syndrome are managed. Different models can be utilized for this approach. The unit may be located in the ED or adjacent to the ED, or it may be located remotely in an inpatient unit. It may be managed by emergency physicians alone, cardiologists or internists alone, or a combination of these specialties. Many choose the ED location since the ED is where most chest pain patients enter the hospital. The unit may be a pure chest pain unit or a unit where chest pain is one of the several conditions managed in a general "observation unit" or a "clinical decision unit." Chest pain units generally use a standardized approach that includes initial ED risk stratification or patient selection, admission to the CPU with CPU protocol orders that include serial testing (cardiac markers and ECGs) to identify STEMI and NSTEMI, followed by some type of provocative testing (stress test with or without imaging) to identify unstable angina [7, 8, 25–28, 36, 38]. These topics will be reviewed individually in subsequent chapters.

Why Have a Chest Pain Unit?

Based on the published literature and the experience of chest pain units, there are several beneficial reasons why a hospital should consider having a chest pain unit. They are listed in Table 3.2.

Table 3.2 Beneficial reasons for why a hospital should consider having a chest pain unit

- Reduction in mortality and morbidity risk for ACS patients
- Reduction in unnecessary inpatient admissions, costs, and length of stay for chest pain patients
- Improved patient satisfaction and quality of life with a chest pain unit
- Improved physician satisfaction
- Improved hospital resource utilization – increased capacity, decreased ambulance diversion, fewer patients that leave ED without being seen.
- Economic benefits – more cost-effective, decreased compliance risk, more equitable admissions, new service line, marketing advantage, decreased liability risk

Reduction in Mortality and Morbidity Risk for ACS Patients

Earlier studies of CPU protocols monitored the outcomes of these patients and reported that they had exceedingly low rates of mortality or morbidity [8, 19, 20, 22, 25, 38]. A 1997 landmark study by Graff examined the impact of having a chest pain observation unit on the care of chest pain patients [12]. Specifically such units would increase the proportion of chest pain patients with an extended evaluation for cardiac ischemia ("rule-out MI evaluation"), decrease the number of missed MIs, and decrease costs [12]. This was a multiple site registry study of eight established chest pain observation units compared with previous studies on chest pain evaluation without the use of observation (five studies, 12,405 patients). A total of 23,407 chest pain patients were included in the study group, representing 5.3% of ED visits. In the chest pain observation units, 153 of 2,229 patients (6.9%) were found to have acute MI. Most of the observation chest pain patients (76%) were discharged home without hospital admission. Compared to previous studies of chest pain patients, a higher proportion of patients underwent a "rule-out MI evaluation" (67 vs 57% $p < 0.001$) equal to 2,250 additional patients completely evaluated ($1,219,500 additional costs). A lower proportion of MIs were missed (0.4 vs 4.5%, $p < 0.001$). Compared to previous studies, final hospital admission rate was lower (47 vs 57%, $p < 0.001$), equal to 2,314 hospital admissions avoided in the study population ($4,093,466 saved costs). Calculated true costs overall were lower by $2,873,966 at the study hospitals, i.e., $124 per patient for all 23,407 evaluated at the study hospitals. The authors concluded that chest pain observation units increased the proportion of chest pain patients thoroughly evaluated, decreasing the rate of missed MI, while lowering the portion of patients eventually admitted to the hospital and lowering overall costs [12].

The lower rate of missed MI is largely due to the fact that admission to a CPU is easier to accomplish than admission to an inpatient bed. This effectively lowers a physicians' threshold to perform a complete evaluation on the "lower risk" patients. In doing so the atypical MI patients are not discharged home, but are detected while still in the ED. In fact, Graff showed that there is an inverse correlation between the rate of missed MI and the admit rate in an "at-risk" undifferentiated chest pain population [12] (Fig. 3.1). One might argue that by

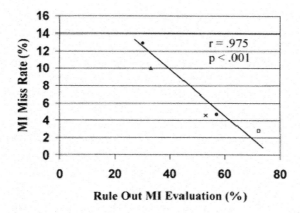

Fig. 3.1 An inverse relation exists between the percentage of patients with a "rule-out MI evaluation" (hospital admission) and the missed MI rate. The analysis includes all previous studies that quantified the disposition of all emergency department chest pain patients, the number of MI patients, and the percentage of missed MIs. Reprinted from American Journal of Cardiology, 1997 Vol 80(5), Graff et al., Impact on the care of the Emergency Department Chest pain patients from the Chest Pain Evaluation Registry (CHEPER) study, pages 563–568 [12]

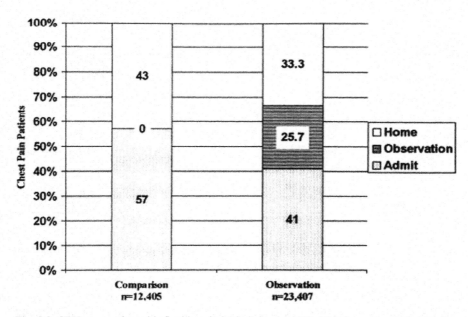

Fig. 3.2 CPU approach avoids final hospital admission by 10%. This figure shows the practice pattern for ED disposition of chest pain patients. Varies significantly between the study population using CPU and the comparison population. Reprinted from American Journal of Cardiology, 1997 Vol 80(5), Graff et al., Impact on the care of the Emergency Department Chest pain patients from the Chest Pain Evaluation Registry (CHEPER) study, pages 563–568 [12]

keeping 10% of chest pain patients that previously might have been discharged from the ED, to lower the missed MI rate, one is increasing the overall cost of care for these patients. However, the CPU approach also avoids final hospital inpatient admission by 10%. The cost savings of this group more than offsets the added costs of patients that might have been directly discharged from the ED (Fig. 3.2). Additionally, studies have shown that patients enrolled in a CPU diagnostic protocol are more likely to receive stress testing prior to discharge than if they were admitted to a general inpatient bed. This increases the likelihood that patients with unstable angina will be detected [10]. This is important since studies have indicated that most ACS patients identified in a CPU are detected by stress testing or imaging [22, 39].

Reduction in Unnecessary Inpatient Admissions, Costs, and Length of Stay for Chest Pain Patients

The impact of a CPU on inpatient admissions has been demonstrated in several studies beyond the Graff study described above. There have been several studies documenting the beneficial impact of a CPU on cost, admission avoidance, and length of stay. These are listed in Table 3.3. A few are notable and worth reviewing in more detail.

Table 3.3 Beneficial impact of CPU on cost

Author/year	Savings/ pt	Study design	Costing method
Kerns/1993 [17]	$1,873	Contemporaneous	Charges
Hoekstra/1994 [14]	$1,160	Contemporaneous	Charges
Hoekstra/1994 [14]	$2,030	Contemporaneous	Charges
Rodriguez/1994 [30]	$1,564	Contemporaneous	Charges (mean IP)
Stomel/1999 [37]	$1,497	Contemporaneous	Costing
Mikhail/1997 [22]	$1,470	Historical	Costing
Sayre/1994 [35]	$1,449	Contemporaneous	Engineered std.
Gomez/1996 [9]	$1,165	Historical	Charges
Gomez/1996 [9]	$624	Randomized	Charges
Gaspoz/1994 [4]	$698	Contemporaneous	Costs (detailed)
Roberts/1997 [29]	$567	Randomized	Costs (detailed)

In 1997, Mikhail reported his results of a prospective observational case series of 502 CPU patients [22]. Admitted and discharged patients were followed through chart review and telephone survey, respectively. Of the 502 patients transferred to the CPC, 477 (95%) completed follow-up at 14 days. Of the CPC admissions, 410 (86%) were discharged home. Those discharged after diagnostic evaluation yielded negative findings and had 100% survival and zero diagnosis of AMI at 5-month follow-up. Overall mortality and incidence of AMI on long-term follow-up for all patients transferred to the CPC were 0.4 and 0.2%, respectively. Sixty-seven patients (13%) were admitted from the CPC, of whom 44 (66%) had a final diagnosis of ischemic heart disease (IHD) or AMI. Twenty-four patients with IHD were identified only on further stress testing. This represented 55% of confirmed ACS patients. Of these patients, seven underwent percutaneous transluminal coronary angioplasty or coronary artery bypass grafting during hospitalization. All were discharged home without major morbidity. Overall, 424 patients (84%) underwent stress testing. The cost of mandatory stress testing to identify one patient with IHD after AMI was ruled out was $3,125. An average cost-per-case savings of 62% was achieved for each patient transferred to the CPU who otherwise would have been hospitalized. They concluded that mandatory stress testing was a safe, cost-effective, and valuable diagnostic and prognostic test in CPU patients [22].

In a 1996 prospective study by Gomez, 100 chest pain patients were randomized to either an inpatient admission or a CPU admission [9]. Myocardial infarction or unstable angina occurred in 6% of patients within 30 days; no diagnoses were missed. By intention to treat analysis (n = 50 in each group), the hospital stay was shorter and charges were lower with the rapid protocol than with routine care (p = 0.001). Among patients in whom ischemia was ruled out, those assigned to the rapid protocol had a shorter hospital stay (median 11.9 vs 22.8 h, p = 0.0001), less initial hospital charges ($893 vs $1,349, p = 0.0001), and lower 30-day hospital charges ($898 vs $1,522, p = 0.0001) than did patients given routine care. Prior to study initiation, historical control data were collected. Historical control subjects had a hospital stay that was even longer (median 34.5 h, p = 0.001 vs either group) and charges greater (median $2,063, p = 0.001 vs rapid protocol, p = 0.02 vs routine care group) [9].

In 1997, Roberts performed a prospective randomized study of 165 patients who presented to the ED with clinical findings suggestive of AMI or acute cardiac ischemia but at low risk using a validated predictive algorithm [29]. Their CPU protocol was called an "accelerated diagnostic protocol" or "ADP." The hospital admission rate for CPU vs control patients was 45.2 vs 100% (P<.001). The mean total cost per patient for CPU vs control patients was $1528 vs $2095 (P<.001). Of note the distribution of costs for CPU vs inpatient admission showed that CPU cost had two peaks – one in a low cost range for patients that were discharged and another in a higher cost range for admitted patients (see Fig. 3.3). The mean LOS measured in hours for CPU vs control patients was 33.1 hours vs 44.8 hours (P<.01). In their study, the CPU saved $567 in total hospital costs per patient treated. They found that the use of an ED-based CPU protocol could reduce hospitalization rates, LOS, and total cost for low-risk patients with chest pain needing evaluation for possible AMI or ACI [29].

In 1998, Farkouh performed a prospective, randomized trial of the safety, efficacy, and cost of admission to a CPU as compared with those of regular hospital admission for patients with unstable angina who were considered to be at intermediate risk for cardiovascular events in the short term [3]. A total of 424 eligible patients were randomly assigned to routine hospital admission (a monitored bed under the care of the cardiology service) or admission to the CPU managed by the emergency department staff. Patients whose test results

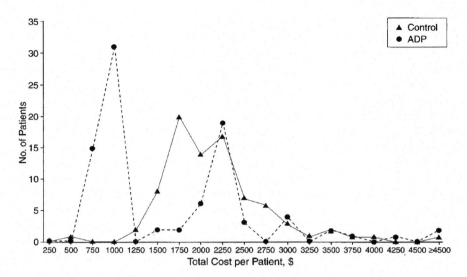

were negative were discharged, and the others were hospitalized. The 212 patients in the hospital admission group had 15 primary events (13 myocardial infarctions and 2 cases of congestive heart failure), and the 212 patients in the CPU group had 7 events (5 myocardial infarctions, 1 death from cardiovascular causes, and 1 case of congestive heart failure). There was no significant difference in the rate of cardiac events between the two groups. No primary events occurred among the 97 patients who were assigned to the CPU and discharged. Resource use during the first 6 months was greater among patients assigned to hospital admission than among those assigned to the CPU admission ($P<0.01$ by the rank-sum test). They concluded that a CPU located in the emergency department can be a safe, effective, and cost-saving alternative to inpatient admission [9].

In a 2004 study, Goodacre performed a cluster-randomized controlled trial [10]. In this study, 442 days were randomized to either chest pain observation unit care days or routine care days. Their objective was to measure the effectiveness and cost-effectiveness of providing care in a chest pain observation unit compared with routine care for patients with acute, undifferentiated chest pain. This was a British study of 972 patients with acute, undifferentiated chest pain (479 attending on days when care was delivered in the chest pain observation unit, 493 on days of routine care). Patients were followed for over 6 months. They found that the use of a chest pain observation unit reduced the proportion of chest pain patients admitted from 54 to 37% ($P <0.001$) and the proportion discharged with acute coronary syndrome from 14 to 6% (P = 0.264). Rates of cardiac event were unchanged. Care in the chest pain observation unit was associated with improved health utility during follow-up (0.0137 quality-adjusted life years gained, P = 0.022) and a saving of 78 British pounds per patient (P = 0.252). They concluded that care in a chest pain observation unit can improve outcomes , may reduce costs and that it seems to be more effective and more cost-effective than routine care [10].

Improved Patient and Physician Satisfaction

Patient satisfaction is an essential outcome measure in the diagnosis and treatment of any patient in the hospital or emergency department. In general patients that are otherwise healthy would rather go home after a period of evaluation than being admitted as an inpatient for several days. Inpatient admission is associated with a sense of loss of control of ones' life, a decline in functional status in the elderly, exposure to iatrogenic risks and nosocomial infections, temporary loss of work productivity, and can be associated with considerable anxiety among chest pain patients.

In a 1997 study, Rydman compared patient satisfaction with a CPU diagnostic protocol to standard inpatient hospitalization [34]. In his prospective study, 104 low-risk chest pain patients were randomized to a CPU or inpatient bed and assessed for satisfaction by means of an interview before hospital discharge. The CPU protocol patients scored higher in all four summary ratings of overall patient satisfaction. They concluded that patients were more satisfied with a rapid diagnosis in the CPU than with inpatient stays for acute chest pain. Furthermore, beyond clinical and cost issues, this benefit must be considered when deciding how chest pain patients are managed [34].

In a 2004 British study, Goodacre studied patient and primary care physician (PCP) satisfaction with CPU care and routine care [11]. In this prospective randomized study, 972 patients were given a self-completed patient satisfaction questionnaire 2 days after their hospital visit. In addition, 601 PCPs were sent a self-completed satisfaction questionnaire. They found that CPU care was consistently associated with higher scores across all patient satisfaction questions, from the perceived thoroughness of examination to care received to an overall assessment of the service received. CPU care achieved small improvements in only 2 of 10 PCP satisfaction questions concerning overall management of the patient and the amount of information about investigations performed. However, PCP satisfaction was not found to be inferior to traditional care. They also found that patient satisfaction did not predict PCP satisfaction. Emergency physicians may be more satisfied with care in a CPU simply because it becomes easier to complete the evaluation of low-risk chest pain patients, thus providing peace of mind. For some this means less liability fear, for others it provides reassurance that their patients are receiving appropriate care [11].

Improved Hospital Resource Utilization – Increased Capacity, Decreased Ambulance Diversion, Fewer Patients that Leave ED Without Being Seen

Both the Institute of Medicine Report on the future of emergency services and the ACEP Task Force Report on boarding recommend the use of an observation unit as part of the solution to hospital and ED overcrowding [1, 15]. It is not difficult to imagine that if patients avoid admission, then inpatient beds will be made available for patients that really need these beds. In a trickle-down effect, this will decongest the emergency department, which in turn will decrease the number of hours of ambulance diversion and patients that walk out before being seen by a physician due to prolonged waits in a congested ED. Regarding these claims there are a few studies to consider.

In 2001, Kelen looked at the impact of a hybrid ED observation unit called an "Acute Care Unit" (ACU) on ED overcrowding and the use of ambulance diversion [16]. They prospectively collected data on rates of patients who left without being seen (LWBS) and ambulance diversion before and after opening this unit. Over the study period there were 1,589 patients seen in the ACU during the first 10 weeks of operation, representing about 14.5% of the ED volume (10,871). About 33% could be classified as post-ED management (observation), 20% as admission processing, and the rest as primary evaluation. The number of patients who LWBS decreased from 10.1% of the ED census 2 weeks prior to opening of the ACU, and from 9.4% during the previous year, to 5.0% (range 4.2–6.2%) during the ensuing 10 weeks post opening. Ambulance diversion was a mean of 6.7 hours per 100 patients before the unit opened and 5.6 hours per 100 patients during the same time in the previous year and decreased to 2.8 hours per 100 patients after the unit opened. Both differences were statistically significant. A 6-month pre- and 2-month postexamination revealed that the mean monthly hours of ambulance diversion for the ED decreased by 40% ($p < 0.05$) in contrast to a mean increase of 44% (186 hours vs 266 hours) ($p < 0.05$) experienced by four proximate hospitals. It was their conclusion that an ED-managed ACU can have significant impact on ED overcrowding and ambulance diversion [16].

A 2001 study by Martinez looked at the impact of a 12-bed ED observation, which managed multiple conditions, not only chest pain, on inpatient admissions over 3 years, and compared this with the 3 years preceding its creation (Martinez). Among the 7,507 patients admitted to the observation unit over 3 years, 6,334 (85%) were discharged home within 23 hours [21]. Total inpatient medical admissions fell by a similar number (n = 5,366) during the 3 years of operation of the observation unit when compared with the 3 preceding years. Analysis of local area trends suggested that the use of the observation unit was the sole contributor to reduced hospital admissions, rather than regional census changes. It was their conclusion that an ED observation unit can reduce inpatient admissions [21].

An analysis by Ross attempted to look at the length of stay of patients admitted to an EDOU and compared this with the length of stay of patients with the same conditions that were admitted as an inpatient [31]. Conservative estimates were made using the lower 95th and 65th confidence interval length of stay, rather than the average, for the inpatient comparison group. These inpatient length of stays were applied to EDOU patients, and the number of bed days used for each group was then calculated and compared. Using these numbers, it was estimated that having one EDOU bed essentially "opened" either 2.35 or 3.16 IP beds – using each respective confidence interval estimate [31].

Economic Benefits – More Cost-Effective, Decreased Compliance Risk, More Equitable Admissions, New Service Line, Marketing Advantage, Decreased Liability Risk

There are several economic benefits to having a chest pain unit. A hospital may see a shift in admission volume and profile that is economically favorable. There are several ways in which this occurs. If one works from the assumption that without a CPU 2–8% of patients with ACS are being discharged from the ED, then this represents a significant number of lost admissions. Reimbursement for acute myocardial infarction and unstable angina has historically been favorable for hospitals. Knowing the baseline number of patients with ACS admissions to a hospital from the ED would allow one to estimate the number of gained admissions there might be if there were a decrease in the rate of missed ACS from 5 to 0.5% as was reported in the CHEPER study [12].

A related economic benefit that is often viewed as "intangible" is a decrease in medical malpractice costs by decreasing the rate of missed myocardial infarction and its associated complications. While this is a medicolegal benefit, it is more importantly a bridge to better care. No physician wants to miss this diagnosis, regardless of liability issues.

When considering the economic impact of a CPU bed, an analysis that involves a simple subtraction of costs from payments may significantly underestimate the financial value of a CPU admission. One needs to account for the impact of the CPU on opening inpatient beds, which a busy hospital may then backfill with better paying DRGs. In a 2008 analysis by Baugh using the economic principles of stock options, opportunity costs, and net present value, an analysis was described that captured the value generated by admitting a patient to an observation unit [2]. This approach captures more of the complexity of observation finance than the simple difference between payments and costs. When "backfill" admissions were taken into account, as well as lower incremental profit for DRGs that an ED observation unit might capture, the value of a single observation unit admission was about $2,908, which was 40% higher than expected. In general, however, the positive value generated by an observation unit bed must be considered in the context of other projects available to hospital administrators. Table 3.4 compares

A. Annitha and M.A. Ross

Table 3.4 Compares the trade-off value of observation admission versus backfilled admission. From: Baugh and Bohan. Inpatient revenue and cost summary [2]. Baugh CW, Bohan S. Estimating Observation Unit Profitability with Options Modeling, Academic Emergency Medicine 2008 Vol 15(5) pages 445–452, Copyright (2008) Blackwell Publishing.

Condition	Diagnosis-related group (DRG)	DRG payment ($)	Hospital cost ($)	Average LOS (Days)	Net profit (Loss)	Net profit (Loss) per hospital-day
Observation						
Chest pain/cardiac	140/143	2,410.64	3,553.30	2.25	(1,142.66)	(507.85)
GI/abdominal	183/189	2,673.67	3,961.01	3.00	(1,287.34)	(429.11)
Asthma/respiratory	80/88/97/100/102	3,161.17	4,457.90	3.64	(1,296.73)	(356.24)
General aliments/medical	278/421	3,192.28	4,370.15	4.00	(1,177.87)	(294.47)
Dehydration	297	2,202.96	3,285.57	3.00	(1,082.61)	(360.87)
Psychiatric/social services	425/430/432	4,726.77	4,909.13	6.77	(182.36)	(26.95)
Syncope/near syncope	142	2,772.34	5,070.73	2.50	(2,298.39)	(919.36)
Congestive heart failure	127	5,376.35	6,740.41	5.10	(1,364.06)	(267.46)
Head injuries	29/32	3,035.09	4,798.48	2.85	(1,763.39)	(618.73)
Kidney problems	321/326/332	2,551.28	3,728.88	3.10	(1,177.60)	(379.87)
Average		3,210.25*	4,487.55*	3.62*	(1,277.30)	(416.09)
Transfer						
Post-cardiopulmonary arrest	129/144	6,283.29	5,565.64	4.15	717.65	172.93
Overdose	449/450	3,168.60	3,136.22	2.85	32.38	11.36
Acute respiratory failure	87/99/101/475	9,102.39	7,494.39	6.10	1,608.00	263.61
Abdominal catastrophe	154/164/165/170/478	14,889.20	12,047.34	8.44	2,841.86	336.71
Seizures/epilepsy	24/25	4,118.66	3,960.58	3.90	228.08	58.48
GI bleeding	174	5,216.15	4,802.67	4.70	413.48	87.89
Aortic dissection	104/110/478	29,157.67	22,866.03	9.83	6,291.64	639.83
Smoke Inhalation	449/450	3,168.60	3,136.22	2.85	32.38	11.36
Fractures (not major trauma)	211/219/224/22	4,531.12	4,620.58	3.05	(89.46)	(29.33)
Sepsis	416	9,081.57	8,205.62	7.50	875.95	116.79
Average		8,878.72	7,583.53	5.34	1,295.20	166.97*

GI = gastrointestinal; LOS = length of stay.
*Used in the final calculation.

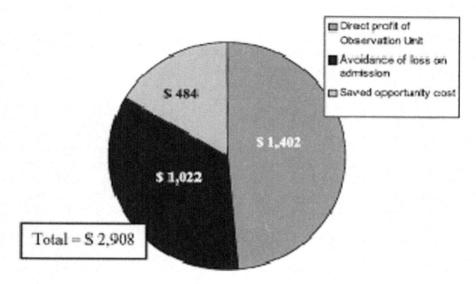

Fig. 3.4 Increment cost benefit of each component. Contribution to observation patient value. Direct profit of observation unit – payment on charges. Avoidance of loss on admission – avoidance of poor profit on short-stay admissions. Saved opportunity cost – gained inpatient admissions, which are more profitable. From Baugh and Bohan [2]. Baugh CW, Bohan S. Estimating Observation Unit Profitability with Options Modeling, Academic Emergency Medicine 2008 Vol 15(5) pages 445–452, Copyright (2008) Blackwell Publishing. All rights reserved

the trade-off value of observation admission vs backfilled admission, and Fig. 3.4 demonstrates the increment cost benefit of each component to be considered [2].

Another economic benefit of a CPU is cost minimization in a setting of fixed reimbursement as occurs with Medicare APCs, capitated contracts as occurs with managed care companies, or no reimbursement as occurs with uninsured patients. As has been described above, studies have demonstrated substantial cost reductions with the approach taken in a CPU. In all the above settings, a lower cost approach is more equitable for hospitals. However, the equitability of a CPU assumes that hospital services cost less in the CPU than care in a traditional inpatient bed. If it does not, then it is not an equitable alternative.

Over the past two decades, health care has steadily shifted from the inpatient setting to the outpatient setting. This has been driven by innovations in the practice of medicine as well as health-care policy and market forces. More recently the Center for Medicare and Medicaid Services has begun to focus on 1 day inpatient length of stays – initially through audits known as the "PEPPER reports" and subsequently through Recovery Audit Contractors known as the "RACs." In a demonstration project, the RACs recovered nearly one billion dollars from three states over a couple years. One of the leading sources of overpayment they collected was for 1-day inpatient admissions that should have been billed as observation. A CPU clearly allows hospitals to avoid this compliance risk and its associated penalties [42, 43].

A final economic benefit to hospitals that open a CPU is the opportunity to draw more patients by marketing this service line. Zalenski reported that chest pain center hospitals were more likely to market and that they were more likely to practice in competitive markets [41].

Summary

Health-care costs from ACS will continue to rise if we are merely focused in treating the end outcomes of this disease. Health is a continuum and efforts must be directed toward earlier detection and treatment. Many complications of heart disease can be prevented by creating health awareness and providing a means through which investigations are done promptly to identify those who present with symptoms earlier in the progression of the disease process. This allows early intervention to prevent the development of complications that may occur if the diagnosis was initially missed. Chest pain units are one way that can aid in the secondary prevention of disease progression.

References

1. ACEP Task Force Report on Boarding. April 2008. Emergency Department Crowding: High-Impact Solutions. www.acep.org
2. Baugh CW, Bohan S. Estimating observation unit profitability with options modeling. Acad Emerg Med. 2008;(15):445–452.
3. Farkouh ME, Smars PA, Reeder GS, et al. A clinical trial of a chest pain observation unit for patients with unstable angina. Chest Pain Evaluation in the Emergency Room (CHEER) Investigators. N Engl J Med. 1998;339:1882–1888.
4. Gaspoz JM, Lee TH, Weinstein MC, et al. Cost-effectiveness of a new short-stay unit to "rule out" acute myocardial ischemia in low risk patients. J Am Coll Cardiol. 1994;24:1249–1259.
5. Gibler WB, et al. A rapid diagnostic and treatment center for patients with chest pain in the Emergency Department. Ann Emerg Med. 1995;(25):1–8.
6. Gibler WB, et al. Chest pain centers: Diagnosis of acute coronary syndromes. Ann Emerg Med. 2000;(35):449–461.
7. Goldman L, Cook EF, Brand DA, et al. A computer protocol to predict myocardial infarction in emergency department patients with chest pain. NEJM. 1988;318:797–803.
8. Goldman L.Weinberg M, Weisberg M, et al. A computer-derived protocol to aid in the diagnosis of emergency room patients with acute chest pain. NEJM. 1982;307:588–596.
9. Gomez MA, Anderson JL, Karagounis LA, et al. An emergency department-based protocol for rapidly ruling out myocardial ischemia reduces hospital time and expense: Results of a randomized study (ROMIO). J Am Coll Cardiol. 1996;28:25–33.
10. Goodacre SW, Nicholl J, et al. Randomised controlled trial and economic evaluation of a chest pain observation unit compared with routine care. BMJ. 2004;328(7434):254.
11. Goodacre SW, Quinney D, et al. Patient and primary care physician satisfaction with chest pain unit and routine care. Acad Emerg Med. 2004;11(8):827–833.
12. Graff LG, Dallara J, Ross MA, et al. Impact on the care of the emergency department chest pain patient from the Chest Pain Evaluation Registry (CHEPER) Study. Am J Cardiol. 1997;(80):563–568.

13. Heart Disease and Stroke Statistics – 2008 Update American Heart Association www. americanheart.org/statistics
14. Hoekstra JW, Gibler WB, Levy RC, et al. Emergency department diagnosis of acute myocardial infarction and ischemia: a cost analysis. Acad Emerg Med. 1994;1:103–110.
15. IOM Report (www.iom.edu) : For report (http://www.nap.edu)
16. Kelen GD, Scheulen JJ, et al. Effect of an ED managed acute care unit on ED overcrowding and emergency medical services diversion. Acad Emerg Med. 2001; 8(11):1095–1100.
17. Kerns JR, Shaub TF, Fontanarosa PB. Emergency cardiac stress testing in the evaluation of emergency department patients with atypical chest pain. Ann Emerg Med. 1993;22:794–798.
18. Lee TH, et al. Clinical characteristics and natural history of patients with acute myocardial infarction sent home from the emergency room. Am J Cardiol. 1987;(60):219–224.
19. Lee TH, et al. Evaluation of the Patient with Acute Chest Pain. NEJM. 2000; 342(16):1187–1193.
20. Lee G, Cook EF, et al. Prediction of the need for intensive care in patients who come to the Emergency Departments with acute chest pain. NEJM. 1996;334:1498–1504.
21. Martinez E, Reilly BM, et al. The observation unit: a new interface between inpatient and outpatient care. Am J Med. 2001;110(4):274–277.
22. Mikhail MG, Smith FA, et al. Cost-effectiveness of mandatory stress testing in chest pain center patients. Ann Emerg Med. 1997;(29):88–98.
23. Nawar EW, Niska RW, Xu J. National Hospital Ambulatory Medical Care Survey: 2005 Emergency Department Summary Advance data from vital and health statistics; no. 386. Hyattsville, MD: National Center for Health Statistics. 2007.
24. Pope JH, et al. Missed diagnoses of acute cardiac ischemia in the emergency department. NEJM. 2000;342:1163–1170.
25. Pozen MW, D'Agostino RB, Mitchell JB, et al. The usefulness of a predictive instrument to reduce inappropriate admissions to the coronary care unit. Ann Intern Med. 1980;92:239–242.
26. PozenMW, D'Agostino RB, Selker HP, et al. A predictive instrument to improve coronary care unit admission practices in acute ischemic heart disease: a multi-center clinical trial. N Engl J Med. 1984;310:1273–1278.
27. Reilly B, et al. Impact of a clinical decision rule on hospital triage of patients with suspected acute cardiac ischemia in the emergency department. JAMA. 2002;288:342–350.
28. Reilly B, et al. Performance and potential impact of a chest pain prediction rule in a large public hospital. Am J Med. 1999;106:285–291.
29. Roberts RR, Zalenski RJ, Mensah EK, et al. Costs of an emergency department-based accelerated diagnostic protocol vs hospitalization in patients with chest pain: A randomized controlled trial. JAMA. 1997;278:1670–1676.
30. Rodriquez S, Cowfer JP, Lyston DJ, et al. Clinical efficacy and cost effectiveness of rapid emergency department rule out myocardial infarction and non invasive cardiac evaluation in patients with acute chest pain. J Am Coll Cardiol. 1994:23(suppl);284A.
31. Ross MA, Wilson AG, McPherson M. The impact of an ED observation bed on inpatient bed availability. Acad Emerg Med. 2001;8(5):576.
32. Ross MA, Amsterdam E, et al. Chest Pain center accreditation is associated with better performance of centers for Medicare and Medicaid services core measures for acute myocardial infarction. Am J Cardiol. 2008;102(2): 120–124.
33. Rusnack RA, Stair TO, Hansen K, et al. Litigation against the emergency physician: common features in cases of missed myocardial infarction. Ann Emerg Med. 1989;18: 1029–1032
34. Rydman R J, Zalenski RJ, Roberts RR, et al. Patient satisfaction with an Emergency Department Chest Pain Observation Unit. Ann Emerg Med. 1997;(29):109–115.
35. Sayre MR, Bender AL, Chayan C, et al. Evaluating chest pain patients in an emergency department rapid diagnostic and treatment center is cost effective. Acad EMerg Med. 1994;1:A45.

36. Selker HP, et al. Use of the Acute Cardiac Ischemia Time-Insensitive Predictive Instrument (ACI-TIPI) to assist with triage of patients with chest pain or other symptoms suggestive of acute cardiac ischemia. Ann Intern Med. 1998;129:845–855.
37. Stommel R, Grant R, Eagle KA. Lessons learned from a community hospital chest pain center. Am J Cardiol. 1999;83:1033–1037.
38. Tatum J, et al. Comprehensive strategy for the evaluation and triage of the chest pain patient. Ann Emerg Med. 1997;Jan(29):116–125.
39. Trappe K, Jackson RE, Ross M. A significant portion of patients admitted from a chest pain observation unit have cardiac pathology. Ann Emerg Med. 2003;42:S8.
40. Wilkinson K, Severance H. Identification of chest pain patients appropriate for an emergency department observation unit. Emerg Med Clin North Am. 2001;19(1):35–66.
41. Zalenski RJ, Rydman RJ, et al. A National Survey of Emergency Department Chest Pain centers in the United States. Am J Cardiol. 1998;(81):1305–1309.
42. PEPPER (Program for Evaluation Payment Patterns Electronic Report) Website:http://www.cfmc.org/review/review_pepper.htm
43. RAC (Recovery Audit Contractor) http://www.cms.hhs.gov/RAC/Downloads/RAC_Demonstration_Evaluation_Report.pdf
44. Society of Chest Pain Center website: www.scpcp.org

Chapter 4
Pathophysiology and Definition of the Acute Coronary Syndromes

Ezra A. Amsterdam, Deborah Diercks, and J. Douglas Kirk

Abstract The acute coronary syndromes include ST elevation myocardial infarction, non-ST elevation myocardial infarction, and unstable angina. The latter two conditions are distinguished by evidence of myocardial infarction based on the elevation of cardiac injury markers. The underlying pathophysiology in the great majority of patients with ACS is atherothrombosis, which encompasses chronic coronary atherosclerotic disease and superimposed acute thrombotic occlusion. Rupture of a coronary atherosclerotic plaque initiates platelet activation and thrombotic coronary occlusion as well as a cascade of clotting mechanisms and inflammatory agents that contribute to myocardial ischemia and necrosis. Patients typically present with chest discomfort but a variety of ischemic equivalents may also predominate (dyspnea, lightheadedness, and cardiac failure). Typically, total coronary occlusion is associated with ST-segment elevation and elevation of injury markers of necrosis. With partial occlusion, there are usually ST and/or T wave abnormalities. All ACS patients are treated with intensive antithrombotic and anticoagulation therapy, as well management of associated problems such as ischemia heart failure and arrhythmias. Optimal treatment of ST elevation infarction is urgent coronary reperfusion, preferably by percutaneous coronary intervention (PCI). Non-ST elevation ACS patients receive comprehensive medical therapy and the majority undergo invasive evaluation within 48 hours of admission to determine their suitability for revascularization by PCI ($\sim$90% of patients) or coronary bypass surgery ($\sim$10% of patients). Of importance is the finding that, although mortality and morbidity of ST elevation infarction are higher than with non-ST elevation ACS during the acute phase, long-term prognosis is worse with non-ST elevation ACS. Therefore, intensive, acute, and long-term management of all patients with ACS is crucial and includes antithrombotic therapy, management of coronary risk factors, and treatment of associated cardiac conditions.

E.A. Amsterdam (✉)
Division of Cardiovascular Medicine, Cardiology, Suite 2800, 4860 Y Street,
Sacramento, CA 95817, USA
e-mail: eaamsterdam@ucdavis.edu

W.F. Peacock and C.P. Cannon (eds.), *Short Stay Management of Chest Pain*,
DOI 10.1007/978-1-60327-948-2_4,
© Humana Press, a part of Springer Science+Business Media, LLC 2009

Keywords Acute coronary syndromes · Atherothrombosis · Plaque rupture · Platelet activation · Thrombosis · Coronary occlusion · Antithrombotic therapy · Percutaneous coronary intervention · Coronary bypass surgery

Optimal management of the acute coronary syndromes (ACSs) requires an understanding of their pathophysiology and classification, both of which have undergone major revision in the past decade [1, 2]. Patients with ACS are a high-risk group and the contemporary classification, based on the related but distinctive pathophysiologies of the syndromes, has provided a useful framework and rational therapeutic targets upon which to base the broad range of current management.

Spectrum of the Acute Coronary Syndromes

According to current concepts, ACS is viewed as a continuum of increasing severity, from unstable angina (UA) to non-ST-segment elevation myocardial infarction (NSTEMI) and ST-segment elevation MI (STEMI) [1, 2] (Fig. 4.1). UA and NSTEMI comprise the NSTE ACS. The continuity of the syndromes

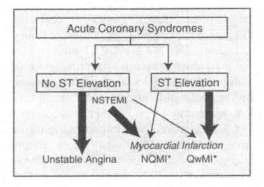

Fig. 4.1 Nomenclature of acute coronary syndromes (ACSs). Patients with ischemic discomfort may present with or without ST-segment elevation (STE) on the electrocardiogram (ECG). Most patients with STE (*large arrows*) ultimately develop a Q wave acute myocardial infarction (MI) (QwMI), whereas a minority (*small arrows*) develop a non-Q wave acute MI (NQMI). Patients who present without STE are experiencing either unstable angina (UA) or NSTEMI. The distinction between these two diagnoses is ultimately made based on the presence or the absence of a cardiac marker detected in the blood. Most patients with NSTEMI do not evolve a Q wave on the 12-lead ECG and are subsequently referred to as having sustained a NQMI; only a minority of NSTEMI patients develop a Q wave and are later diagnosed as having QwMI. Not shown is Prinzmetal's angina, which present with transient chest pain and STE but rarely MI. The spectrum of clinical conditions that ranges from UA to NQMI and QwMI is referred to as ACS. *Elevation of cardiac injury marker. Permission from Antman and Braunwald [18]

is emphasized by increasingly sensitive serum markers of cardiac injury such as the troponins, which have blurred the distinction between UA and NSTEMI [3].

ACS is typically characterized by prolonged chest pain compatible with myocardial ischemia/infarction, although patients may occasionally present with complaints such as dyspnea, epigastric pain, or fatigue. Definitive diagnosis of each form of ACS is based on the accompanying electrocardiogram (ECG) and serum markers of cardiac injury. STEMI is defined by ST-segment elevation indicative of acute injury; NSTEMI syndromes are typically associated with ischemic ST-segment and/or T wave abnormalities; uncommonly, however, there are no ECG alterations in NSTEMI.

Characteristic ECG alterations in ACS are depicted in Fig. 4.2. Both STEMI and NSTEMI are defined by increases in cardiac injury markers denoting myocardial necrosis. The most sensitive and specific cardiac injury markers are the cardiac troponins. The course of serum concentrations of troponin and that of older injury markers during MI is shown in Fig. 4.3. Whereas it was previously reported that a minority of patients with UA had mild elevations in injury makers, any characteristic rise and fall of these markers now confers a diagnosis of NSTEMI based on the recent universal definition of myocardial infarction [4]. NSTEMI and UA account for a large majority of ACS, a proportion that is likely to rise even further with the increasing sensitivity of diagnostic methods for cardiac necrosis.

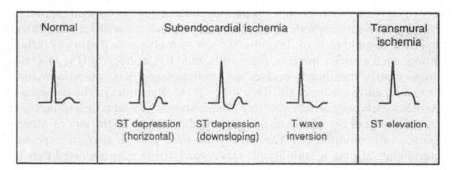

Fig. 4.2 Common transient electrocardiogram (ECG) abnormalities during ischemia. Subendocardial ischemia results in ST-segment depressions and/or T wave flattening or inversions. Severe transient transmural ischemia can result in STEs, similar to the early changes in acute MI. When transient ischemia resolves, so do the electrocardiographic changes. Permission from Sabatine et al. [19]

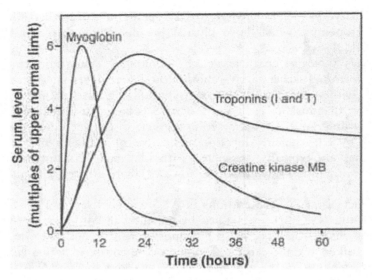

Fig. 4.3 Patterns of evolution of serum markers after the onset of myocardial necrosis. Permission from Amsterdam et al. [20]

Vulnerable Plaque and Plaque Rupture

Inflammation and Morphology

The central pathophysiologic event in the great majority of ACS is the rupture of a vulnerable or an unstable atherosclerotic plaque (Fig. 4.4) that induces coronary thrombosis and occlusion, which results in myocardial ischemia and/or injury [5] (Fig. 4.5), depending on the degree of coronary obstruction. According to current concepts, the plaque that ulcerates and sets in motion the cascade of thrombogenesis and coronary occlusion possesses a thin fibrous cap and a large lipid pool. It is also the site of multiple mediators of inflammation, such as macrophages, foam cells, and T lymphocytes (Fig. 4.4) that release matrix metalloproteinases and collagenases that promote erosion, ulceration, and rupture of the fibrous cap [5, 6]. By contrast, the presence of smooth muscle cells, which promote plaque stability by secreting collagen, an essential component of the fibrous cap, is diminished at the site of atherosclerotic inflammation [7]. The size of the lipid pool is also an important determinant of plaque stability. In this regard, it has been reported that the threshold for rupture conferred by this lesion is a lipid pool comprising 50% of plaque volume [8].

   The foregoing pathoanatomic factors establish a plaque characterized by a large lipid pool, an inflammatory milieu, and a thin fibrous cap, all of which render it prone to rupture. Rupture typically occurs at the margins of the plaque

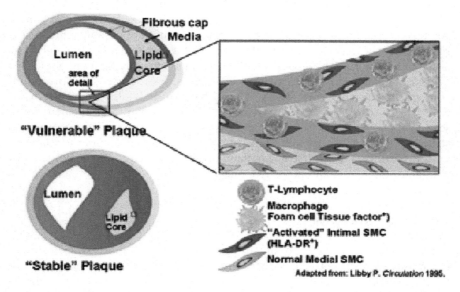

Fig. 4.4 Diagram demonstrating characteristics of "vulnerable" and "stable" atherosclerotic plaques. The vulnerable plaque usually has a substantial lipid core and a thin fibrous cap separating the thrombogenic macrophages (hearing tissue factor) from the blood. At sites of lesion disruption, smooth muscle cells are often activated. In contrast, the stable plaque has a thick fibrous cap protecting the lipid core from contact with the blood. Clinical data suggest that stable plaques more often show luminal narrowing detectable by angiography than do vulnerable plaques. Permission from Libby [21]

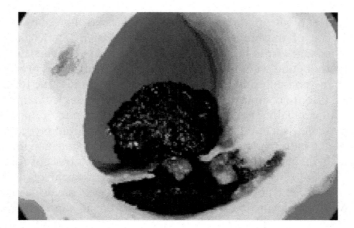

Fig. 4.5 Cross section of artery with ruptured plaque and partially occlusive thrombus protruding into the vessel lumen through the tear in the fibrous cap. Permission from Davies [5]

where it is thinnest, inflammatory cells are densely concentrated, and sheer stress is highest [9].Because of its susceptibility to disruption and rupture, it is referred to as a *vulnerable* plaque in contrast to a stable plaque (Fig. 4.4). The latter is characterized by a relatively thick fibrous cap, a smaller lipid pool, little evidence of inflammatory activity and is, thus, less subject to rupture and consequent coronary thrombosis. The stable plaque is also frequently associated with coronary collateral vessels, which may limit the incidence and severity of myocardial ischemia and injury. It should be noted that plaque structure is not static and may shift between the more stable and the relatively vulnerable during the course of a patient's disease, in relation to the influence of risk factors, therapy, and hemodynamic alterations.

Coronary Thrombosis

Plaque rupture, which can be catastrophic, initiates thrombosis by exposure of circulating platelets to tissue factor within the subendothelial collagen matrix of the plaque [10]. Tissue factor is derived from endothelial cells and macrophages within the plaque and is highly thrombogenic. It activates the coagulation cascade and induces surface aggregation of platelets and fibrin deposition, resulting in thrombogenesis at the site of plaque ulceration. Activated platelets intensely express the IIB/IIA receptor and release factors such as thromboxane A2 and serotonin that provoke vasospasm and augment platelet activity promoting further aggregation, hemostasis, and thrombogenesis [11]. ACS results when these pathogenic mechanisms overwhelm endogenous cardioprotective vasodilator and antithrombotic factors, whose production by abnormal endothelium of atherosclerotic arteries is deficient [12].

Thrombus forms on the surface of the plaque or can be initiated within the plaque after loss of integrity of the fibrous cap, which is followed by progression and protrusion of thrombus into the coronary lumen [5]. Thrombogenesis progresses in stages from partial to complete occlusion as platelets aggregate and finally are bound within a secondary fibrin network. This process can be arrested at any phase during its evolution, which determines the form of ACS that results. Prior to complete occlusion, platelet aggregates from the thrombus in the path of circulating blood can embolize downstream to occlude the distal coronary vascular bed and increase the extent of jeopardized myocardium.

Appreciation of the pathogenesis of ACS provides the foundation for treatment directed at the underlying physiologic derangements. The basis of thrombolytic therapy for STEMI is susceptibility of the fibrin component of thrombus to dissolution by fibrinolytic agents. By contrast, the platelet core, which is the basis of NSTEMI ACS, is not responsive to fibrinolytic therapy and requires specific antiplatelet agents for inhibition of its genesis. Of course, antiplatelet therapy also has an important role in STEMI treatment. Standard pharmacologic anti-ischemic therpy is important in the treatment of both STEMI and NSTEMI ACS. Further therapeutic targets include preventive therapy to reduce atherosclerosis and favorable modification of the adverse characteristics of unstable atherosclerotic plaques by decreasing inflammation, strengthening the fibrous cap, reducing the lipid pool, inhibiting matrix metalloproteinases, and improving endothelial function. The latter approaches are areas of current intensive investigation.

Degree of Coronary Stenosis

The vulnerable plaque is typically noncritical in its quiescent state in terms of degree of obstruction of coronary lumen diameter, which is usually less than 50% stenosis. Indeed, it has been established that the majority of myocardial infarctions are associated with coronary stenoses of less than 50% prior to the advent of thrombotic obstruction [13]. Symptoms of myocardial ischemia are unusual with this degree of stenosis, which does not significantly impair coronary blood flow at rest or ability to augment flow with increased myocardial oxygen demand. Reduction of coronary blood flow reserve is associated with stenosis greater than 70%, while impairment of resting coronary flow occurs when lumen diameter is reduced by more than 90% [14]. These relationships are depicted in Fig. 4.6.

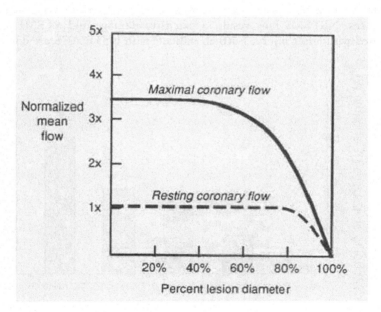

Fig. 4.6 Resting and maximal coronary blood flows are affected by the magnitude of proximal arterial stenosis (percent lesion diameter). The *dotted line* indicates resting blood flow, and the *solid line* represents maximal blood flow (i.e., when there is a full dilation of the distal resistance vessels). Compromise of maximal blood flow is evident when the proximal stenosis reduces the coronary lumen diameter by ≥70%. Resting flow may be compromised if the stenosis exceeds ~90%. Permission from Gould and Lipscomb [14]

The close correlation of ACS with modestly stenotic, unstable plaques appears inconsistent with the dependence of noninvasive diagnostic methods on the presence of severe lesions for identification of CAD and prediction of prognosis. However, this apparent paradox is resolved by findings from coronary angiography, indicating that critical lesions are associated with an abundance of less severe stenoses of the type that comprises unstable plaques [15]. Thus, the presence of a severe stenosis is a marker of an extensive atherosclerotic burden that includes numerous vulnerable lesions.

Clinicopathologic Correlations

As previously noted, the degree of thrombotic coronary obstruction typically determines the form of ACS that ensues after plaque ulceration and coronary thrombosis. The extent of ECG changes and the degree of elevation of cardiac injury markers generally correlate with the magnitude of myocardial damage and, thereby, morbidity and mortality (Fig. 4.7) [3]. Because NSTEMI usually involves less myocardial damage than STEMI, mortality and other serious complications, such as cardiogenic shock, congestive heart failure, and arrhythmias, are less frequent during the initial hospitalization in NSTEMI. However, in some cases, NSTEMI may result in extensive damage and STEMI may be associated with lesser injury. Further, patients with NSTE ACS are commonly

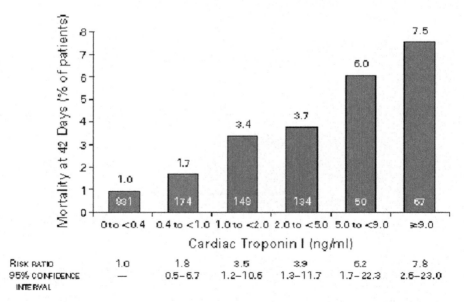

Fig. 4.7 Relationship between cardiac troponin I levels and risk of mortality in patients with ACS. Permission from Antman et al. [3]

older, have more extensive CAD, and more frequent recurrent events and, as seen in Fig. 4.8, posthospital mortality in the first year is higher than with STEMI [16].The basis for the latter finding may be related to delayed diagnosis and less aggressive therapy of NSTE ACS patients compared to those with STEMI. In general, because there is little or no evidence of acute myocardial necrosis in UA, early complications and mortality are lowest with this form of ACS.

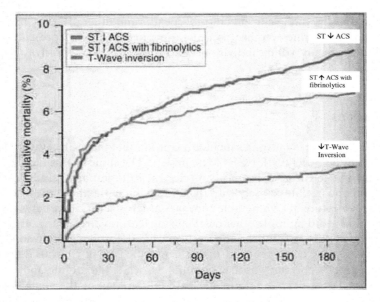

Fig. 4.8 Kaplan–Meier curves showing mortality in patients with acute coronary syndromes (ACSs) in the Global Use of Strategies of Open Occluded Coronary Arteries (GUSTO) IIb study, divided according to the electrocardiographic findings at presentation. Permission from Savonitto et al. [16]

Extent of ischemia and infarct size are also related to additional factors, such as the specific "culprit" coronary artery, the site of vessel occlusion, the presence of collateral coronary arteries, and hemodynamic factors influencing myocardial oxygen demand and supply during evolution of ACS.Thus, because it usually supplies the largest extent of myocardium, occlusion of the left anterior descending coronary artery generally results in more extensive ischemia/injury and greater morbidity and higher mortality than occlusion of the right or left circumflex arteries. Proximal coronary occlusion is associated with greater ischemia/injury than is distal occlusion; collateral coronaries can limit the extent of infarction as can factors favoring reduced myocardial oxygen demand (e.g., lower heart rate and blood pressure).Finally, the therapeutic background (beta blockers, antiplatelet agents, statins, and other cardioprotective drugs) at the onset of ACS can alter its evolution.

Nonatherosclerotic Causes of MI

Although uncommon, ACS can occur in the absence of obstructive CAD. Nonatherosclerotic etiologies include coronary vasospasm, coronary emboli, vasculitis, congenital coronary anomalies, trauma, and excessive myocardial oxygen demand in the presence of normal coronary arteries. The latter derangement can occur with cocaine abuse (which causes vasospasm as well as hypertension and tachycardia), severe aortic stenosis, and hypertrophic obstructive cardiomyopathy. In the current culture, cocaine and other drugs of abuse such as methamphetamines require consideration in all patients presenting with ACS but especially young individuals and those with no cardiovascular risk factors [17].

Conclusions

The acute coronary syndromes include a continuum of acute myocardial ischemia manifested by STEMI, NSETMI, and UA. The clinical classification of the syndromes, which is based primarily on electrocardiographic and cardiac injury marker data, correlates closely with the underlying pathoanatomy. The central event is the rupture of a vulnerable coronary atherosclerotic plaque. An inflammatory milieu and multiple other destabilizing features characterize the vulnerable plaque. Plaque rupture induces thrombotic coronary occlusion, which results in an acute coronary syndrome, the specific type of which is determined by the degree of coronary obstruction and associated anatomic and hemodynamic factors. Understanding of the pathophysiology of the acute coronary syndromes has provided a rational basis for current therapy and investigational approaches targeted at these derangements.

References

1. Braunwald E, Antman EM, Beasley JW, et al., ACC/AHA Guideline Update for the Management of Patients With Unstable Angina and Non-ST-Segment Elevation Myocardial Infarction – 2002: Summary Article: A Report of the American College of Cardiology/ American Heart Association Task Force on Practice Guidelines (Committee on the Management of Patients With Unstable Angina). Circulation 2002; 106:1893–1900.
2. Anderson JL, Adams CD, Antman EM, et al., ACC/AHA 2007 Guidelines for the Management of Patients With Unstable Angina/Non-ST-Elevation Myocardial Infarction – Executive Summary: A Report of the American College of Cardiology/American Heart Association Task Force on Practice Guidelines (Writing Committee to Revise the 2002 Guidelines for the Management of Patients With Unstable Angina/Non-ST-Elevation Myocardial Infarction) Developed in Collaboration with the American College of Emergency Physicians, the Society for Cardiovascular Angiography and Interventions, and the Society of Thoracic Surgeons Endorsed by the American Association of Cardiovascular and Pulmonary Rehabilitation and the Society for Academic Emergency Medicine. Journal of the American College of Cardiology 2007;50:652–726.

3. Antman EM, Tanasijevic MJ, Thompson B, et al., Cardiac-specific Troponin I levels to predict the risk of mortality in patients with acute coronary syndromes. N Engl J Med 1996;335:1342–1349.

4. Task Force M, Thygesen K, Alpert JS, et al., Universal definition of myocardial infarction: Kristian Thygesen, Joseph S. Alpert and Harvey D. White on behalf of the Joint ESC/ACCF/AHA/WHF Task Force for the Redefinition of Myocardial Infarction. Eur Heart J 2007; 28:2525–2538.

5. Davies MJ, Coronary disease: The pathophysiology of acute coronary syndromes. Heart 2000;83:361–366.

6. Libby P, Current concepts of the pathogenesis of the acute coronary syndromes. Circulation 2001;104:365–372.

7. Bennett MR, Apoptosis of vascular smooth muscle cells in vascular remodelling and atherosclerotic plaque rupture. Cardiovasc Res 1999;41:361–368.

8. Davies MJ, Richardson PD, Woolf N, et al., Risk of thrombosis in human atherosclerotic plaques: role of extracellular lipid, macrophage, and smooth muscle cell content. Br Heart J 1993;69:377–381.

9. Davies MJ, Stability and instability: Two faces of coronary atherosclerosis: The Paul Dudley White Lecture 1995. Circulation 1996;94:2013–2020.

10. Mallat Z, Benamer H, Hugel B, et al., Elevated levels of shed membrane microparticles with procoagulant potential in the peripheral circulating blood of patients with acute coronary syndromes. Circulation 2000;101:841–843.

11. Antithrombotic Therapy, Ch 37, in Theroux Acute Coronary Syndromes. 2003, Saunders: Philadelphia, PA. pp. 431–443.

12. Kinlay S, Libby P, and Ganz P, Endothelial function and coronary artery disease. Current Opinion in Lipidology 2001;12:383–389.

13. Ledru F, Reiber JC, Tuinenburg JC, et al., Coronary angiography and the culprit lesion in acute coronary syndromes, Ch 17, in Theroux Acute Coronary Syndromes. 2003, Saunders: Philadelphia, PA. pp. 226–249.

14. Gould KL and Lipscomb K, Effects of coronary stenoses on coronary flow reserve and resistance. The American Journal of Cardiology 1974;34:48–55.

15. Nakagomi A, Celemajer DS, Lumely T, et al. Angiographic severity of coronary narrowing is a surrogate marker for the extent of coronary atherosclerosis. American Journal of Cardiology 1996;78:516–519.

16. SavonittoS, Ardissino D, Granger CB, et al, Prognostic value of the admission electrocardiogram in acute coronary syndromes. JAMA 1999;281:707–713.

17. McCord J, Jneid H, and Hollander J, Management of cocaine-associated chest pain and myocardial infarction: A scientific st0tement from the American Heart Association Acute Cardiac Care Committee of the Council on Clinical Cardiology. Circulation 2008; 117:1897–1907.

18. Antman EM, Braunwald E, Acute myocardial infarction. In: Braunwald E, ed.: Heart Disease: A Textbook of Cardiovascular Medicine, 5th ed., vol. 2. Philadelphia, PA, WB Saunders CO, 1997, pp. 1184–1288.

19. Sabatine MS, O'Gara PT, Lilly LS, Ischemic heart disease. In: Lilly LS, ed.: Pathophysiology of Heart Disease, 2nd ed. Baltimore, MD, Lippincott Williams & Wilkins, 1998, p. 134.

20. Amsterdam EA, Lewis WR, Yadlapalli S, Evaluation of low-risk patients with chest pain in the emergency department: valve and limitations of recent methods. Cardiol Rev. 1999;7:17–26.

21. Libby P, Molecular bases of the acute coronary syndromes. Circulation 1995;91: 2844–2850.

Chapter 5
Emergency Department Presentation

Jeffrey A. Holmes and Sean Collins

Abstract Patients with acute coronary syndrome (ACS) may present to the emergency department (ED) via emergency medical services or self-transport. When they present via emergency medical services, a diagnostic-quality prehospital 12-lead EKG may enhance the sensitivity and specificity of ACS diagnosis and shorten time to treatment. The ED evaluation of the patient at risk for ACS includes a thorough history and physical assessment of major risk factors for coronary artery disease (diabetes mellitus, hyperlipidemia, hypertension, family history, smoking history), timely and repeated 12-lead EKG, and cardiac biomarkers (preferably point-of-care testing). When evaluating a patient for ACS, the emergency physician must be conscientious of the prevalence of atypical ACS symptoms such as dyspnea, nausea, diaphoresis syncope or pain in the arms, epigastrium, shoulder, or neck. These atypical presentations are most notably studied in the patients of older age, with diabetes mellitus, of female gender, and of nonwhite race. In addition to assessing for the presence of ACS, other life-threatening conditions must also be considered, the most important being aortic dissection, pulmonary embolism, pericarditis with pericardial tamponade, esophageal perforation (Boerhaave's syndrome), and spontaneous pneumothorax.

Keywords Acute coronary syndrome · Prehospital care · Presenting signs and symptoms · Biomarkers

Arrival to ED

Patients with acute coronary syndrome (ACS) may present to the emergency department (ED) via emergency medical services or self-transport. The prehospital care of patients with ACS who present via emergency medical services

J.A. Holmes (✉)
Department of Emergency Medicine, Maine Medical Center, Portland, ME, USA
e-mail: drjeffholmes@gmail.com

W.F. Peacock and C.P. Cannon (eds.), *Short Stay Management of Chest Pain*,
DOI 10.1007/978-1-60327-948-2_5,
© Humana Press, a part of Springer Science+Business Media, LLC 2009

(EMS) includes aspirin, sublingual nitrates if blood pressure allows, supplemental oxygen, continuous cardiac monitoring, and perhaps morphine. When available, EMS may obtain a prehospital 12-lead EKG and electronically transfer it to the appropriate receiving facility for immediate interpretation by an emergency physician. Previous studies have determined that diagnostic-quality prehospital 12-lead EKGs can be obtained with great success by paramedics [1], can enhance the sensitivity and specificity of ACS diagnosis [2], and can shorten time to treatment after hospital admission. Canto et al. have shown that a prehospital EKG may improve the in-hospital mortality of patients with acute myocardial infarction through wider, faster in-hospitalization utilization of reperfusion strategies and greater usage of invasive procedures, factors that may possibly reduce short-term mortality [3]. Patients with ST-segment myocardial infarction (STEMI) may also be identified earlier with prehospital EKGs, facilitating rapid transport to an appropriate interventional facility that can achieve the goal of a 'door-to-balloon time' of 60–90 min. [4]. Le May et al showed that proper training of paramedics in prehospital ECG interpretation resulted in an immediate referral to a cardiac catheterization laboratory and a door-to-balloon time of 69 min (versus 123 for interhospital transfer). Door-to-balloon times of less than 90 min were achieved in 79.7% of patients who were transferred from the field and in 11.9% of patients transferred from emergency departments ($p < 0.001$) [5].

Patients at high risk for complications (e.g., congestive heart failure, hypotension, tachycardia, or larger anterior wall infarction) may be better managed by specialists and facilities with cardiac interventional and surgical capabilities should be strongly considered. These patients, however, may be better served by being stabilized at an outside hospital prior to transfer to a specialty hospital by EMS. Specialized care for these patients may reduce mortality and improves care.

While there are possible dangers of self-transport to the emergency room for chest pain, no conclusive data exist to show that outcomes are improved in patients with ACS who are transported via ambulance versus private car. There are some data that suggest the sickest patients may self-select for severity, with those who are more ill initiating ambulance transport [6].

Classical Presentations of Acute Coronary Syndrome

The initial evaluation of the patient at risk for ACS includes assessing the presence of the major risk factors for coronary artery disease (diabetes mellitus, hyperlipidemia, hypertension, family history, smoking history). While these have been shown to be rather poor predictors of ACS [7], their presence, along with the history and physical, electrocardiogram, and cardiac markers form the basis for risk stratification. In patients with known coronary artery disease and anginal symptoms, the emergency physician must establish the pattern of symptoms to determine whether they indicate stable angina, unstable angina, or acute myocardial infarction. While stable angina is usually due to fixed atherosclerotic disease, unstable angina differs in that it is pathophysiologically a precursor of acute myocardial infarction (AMI) and should be treated aggressively.

Stable angina pectoris, or "exertional" *angina*, is defined as a transient, episodic chest discomfort that comes on with physical or psychological stress, lasts less than 20 min, and is relieved by rest or nitroglycerin (NTG) [8]. While the description of the pain depends on multiple patient factors, it is classically described as an ache, heaviness, or pressure that is retrosternal in location and radiates to the neck or the left arm. It follows a characteristic predictable and reproducible pattern that is constant in frequency. Associated symptoms may include dyspnea, diaphoresis, palpitations, nausea/vomiting, or dizziness. The symptoms of stable angina are most often due to myocardial ischemia from fixed atherosclerotic disease. The physical exam is usually unrevealing but if the pain is ongoing, the patient may appear anxious or diaphoretic.

Unstable angina is defined as angina that (1) is of new onset (less than 1–2 hours), (2) occurs at rest for prolonged periods (>20 min), or (3) is crescendo angina, represented by an increase in frequency, duration, or requiring less provocation of onset. The chest discomfort and associated symptoms of unstable angina are classically similar to that of stable angina with the exception of the unique qualifying features listed. These differences in anginal symptoms are a result of the pathophysiologic differences from stable angina (i.e., stable plaque versus ruptured plaque). The physical exam of the patient with unstable angina is usually entirely normal but may reveal dysrhythmias, shock, altered mental status, and signs of congestive heart failure (e.g., rales, a third heart sound, jugular venous distension, hepatojugular reflex, and peripheral edema). The recognition of unstable angina is extremely important because of the high risk for myocardial infarction associated with this condition.

Variant angina ("Prinzmetal's angina") is angina caused by coronary artery vasospasm at rest with minimal fixed coronary artery lesions. It commonly exhibits a circadian pattern, with most episodes occurring in the early hours of the morning. The pain commonly is severe and may be associated with palpitations, presyncope, or syncope secondary to arrhythmia. It may be relieved by rest or NTG. The cardiac examination findings in patients with variant angina typically are normal, although a third or fourth heart sound or mitral regurgitation may be heard during episodes. Tachycardia or bradycardia may accompany episodes of prolonged chest pain, particularly with marked ST-segment elevation. The ECG reveals ST-segment elevation that is impossible to discern electrocardiographically and, at times, clinically from AMI due to an occlusive thrombus.

AMI is usually persistent (>20 min), severe, and associated with symptoms of dyspnea, diaphoresis, or nausea. It is a visceral pain that is vague and often described as discomfort rather than pain. It classically radiates to the jaw or left arm. While both non-ST-segment elevation myocardial infarction (NSTEMI) and STEMI may have similar presentations, STEMI patients tend to be more ill appearing and more often reveal dysrhythmias, shock, altered mental status, and signs of congestive heart failure (e.g., rales, a third heart sound, jugular venous distension, hepatojugular reflex, and peripheral edema). It is typically not completely relieved by rest or nitroglycerin.

Confounders

While the classic teaching and presentation of ACS is that of crushing, substernal chest pain that radiates to the arm or the jaw and is associated with nausea, weakness, and diaphoresis, many patients present with atypical symptoms. It may be more accurate to say that "the typical presentation of acute coronary syndrome is atypical." Pain perception and descriptions vary widely among patients and are influenced by numerous factors; those most notably studied include older age, diabetes mellitus, female gender, and nonwhite race [9]. Atypical presentations of patients with ACS include symptoms such as dyspnea, nausea, diaphoresis, syncope, or pain in the arms, epigastrium, shoulder, or neck. When these symptoms are present without chest pain, they are known as "anginal equivalents." Others may have no symptoms at all of myocardial infarction [10]. A recent review suggests that approximately 50% of patients with AMI will not have chest pain as a chief complaint [9].

Unfortunately, patients with atypical presentations are more difficult to diagnose and have poorer outcomes. These patients are also less likely to receive adjunct therapies shown to reduce mortality (i.e., aspirin, β-adrenergic blockers, heparin, thrombolysis, and primary angioplasty). The Second National Registry of Myocardial Infarction (NRMI-2) study found that MI patients without chest pain had a higher in-hospital mortality (23% versus 9% for those without chest pain) [11].

The elderly are a patient population well known for their atypical presentations of ACS. In fact, findings from Bayer and colleagues suggest that a patient's age has a direct correlation with atypical presentations. In a review of over 700 patients with proven myocardial infarction (average age 76.0), chest pain was seen in only 66% of patients; 75% over the age of 70; and only 50% over the age of 80. Above the age of 85, chest pain was present in only 38%, making an "atypical" presentation in this age group the rule rather than the exception. Syncope, stroke, and acute confusion became more common with increasing age and may be the sole presenting symptom [12]. In the Framingham cohort, silent or unrecognized infarctions were more common in the elderly – up to 60% of AMIs in patients >85 years of age [13, 14]. These atypical presentations of ACS in the elderly have been shown to have a worse prognosis [a threefold higher risk of in-hospital death (12 versus 4%, P<0.0001)] in part because of delays in diagnosis and treatment [13, 15]. Because of this higher incidence of atypical symptoms and worse outcomes in the elderly, the physician should have a high index of suspicion for ACS in the elderly patient.

Coronary artery disease (CAD) is the leading cause of death in women and there are important gender differences to note in their presentations of coronary ischemia. On average, women are almost a decade older than men at the time of their MI, with greater than 55% of their AMIs at 70 years or older [16]. Patients and physicians may not have a high enough suspicion that symptoms at a younger age of presentation could be from coronary ischemia. Finnegan and colleagues' survey revealed that women describe myocardial infarction as a "male problem" and more often attributed the symptoms of MI to other chronic noncardiac symptoms [17]. This attitude is most likely largely responsible for their well-documented delay in presentation when symptoms of ACS start [18].

When women do present with symptoms, they are more likely to have an atypical presentation. A large medline review performed by Canto and colleagues revealed the absence of chest pain or discomfort with ACS more commonly in women than in men in both the cumulative summary from large cohort studies (37 versus 27%) and the single-center and small reports or interviews (30 versus 17%) [19]. Data from the Framingham study also indicate that the percentage of unrecognized infarcts was highest in women and older men [10]. The frequency of other associated symptoms of ACS differs between men and women. Generally, women are more likely to experience middle or upper back pain, neck pain, jaw pain, shortness of breath, paroxysmal nocturnal dyspnea, nausea or vomiting, indigestion, loss of appetite, weakness or fatigue, cough, dizziness, and palpitations compared to men [20–23].

Nonwhite patients represent another population with disturbingly higher rates of missed ACS. From a multicenter prospective trial, Pope and colleagues showed that nonwhite race patients were more likely not to be hospitalized if they presented with either acute cardiac ischemia (odds ratio 2.2; 95% confidence interval 1.1–4.3) or acute infarction (odd ratio for discharge 4.5; 95% confidence interval 1.8–11.8) [24]. In this study, 5.8% of the black patients with AMI were not hospitalized, as compared with 1.2% of the white patients with infarction. While atypical presentations may be to blame in other confounding patient populations, this has not been well substantiated in blacks. In fact, some studies suggest that nonwhite patients have equal or lower rates of atypical ACS presentation as whites [11, 9]. Why then do minorities have higher rates of missed diagnosis? It is not clear, especially that the presence of more CAD risk factors in blacks [25, 26] does not have a strong influence on the diagnostic impressions of the physicians [27, 28]. Contributing factors to the higher rates of missed ACS may be attributed to the fact that minority groups tend to be lower income groups, have limited access to primary care providers and medications, and have longer delays in their presentation [29, 30].

Studies of patients with diabetes have clearly shown that they have a higher incidence of coronary artery disease and mortality than their nondiabetic counterparts. Diabetes is an independent risk factor for coronary artery disease, with the prevalence found as high as 55% among adult patients with diabetes compared with 2–4% for the general population [31]. Coronary artherosclerosis is not only more prevalent, but also clearly more extensive in diabetic than nondiabetic patients. Numerous studies have shown that at coronary angiography or autopsy, diabetic patients have a higher incidence of double- and triple-vessel disease and a lower incidence of single-vessel disease than their nondiabetic counterparts. A large autopsy study also showed that 91% of patients with adult onset diabetes and no known coronary heart disease had severe narrowing of at least one major coronary artery and 83% had severe two or three vessel involvement [32, 33].

In addition to the increased incidence and mortality of coronary heart disease in diabetics, their higher incidence of atypical presentations requires the emergency physician to be ever more vigilant in evaluating the diabetic with possible ACS. Their atypical presentations are most commonly believed to be due to their blunted appreciation for ischemic pain. Histologic and physiologic evidence of damage to cardiac afferent nerve fibers has been shown in diabetic patients, suggesting that neuropathy in these fibers exists and may play a role in blunting the perception of ischemic pain [34–36]. This may lead to symptoms that are mild, atypical, or truly silent and therefore accurate diagnosis of ACS based on the history may be more difficult. Atypical symptoms such as confusion, dyspnea, fatigue or nausea and vomiting may be the presenting complaint in 32–42% of diabetic patients with myocardial infarction compared with 6–15% of nondiabetic patients [37]. Several studies have also found that diabetics have a higher incidence of stress-induced angina. During exercise or thallium tolerance tests, they found that the incidence of painless ST depression was almost double that seen in nondiabetic patients (69 versus 39%) [38, 39]. In the Framingham study, 12% of MIs were believed to be truly asymptomatic. They were more common in diabetic patients (39%) compared with their nondiabetic counterparts (22%) [40].

Differential Diagnosis

The emergency physician should use a thorough history and physical exam to not only help determine the risk of possible ACS but also recognize and distinguish anginal chest pain from other serious and life-threatening conditions. Along with a thorough history, a focused cardiac, pulmonary, and vascular examination should be performed to fully characterize the patient's symptoms. While the differential diagnosis for both "typical" and "atypical" anginal symptoms is broad, the most important alternative diagnosis include aortic dissection, pulmonary embolism, pericarditis with pericardial tamponade, esophageal perforation (Boerhaave's syndrome), and spontaneous pneumothorax.

Patients with aortic dissection classically have risk factors that may include known atherosclerosis, uncontrolled hypertension, coarctation of the aorta, bicuspid aortic valves, aortic stenosis, Marfan syndrome, or Ehlers–Danlos syndrome [41]. They complain of a ripping, searing. or tearing chest pain that radiates to the intrascapular area of the back. It is typically maximal at onset and may be felt both above and below the diaphragm. Their physical exam may reveal a diastolic murmur from aortic insufficiency and unequal blood pressures in their upper extremities. The chest radiograph may show numerous nonspecific findings, the most helpful being a widened mediastinum. In a meta-analysis involving 21 studies with 1848 patients, the pooled sensitivity of a widened mediastinum was 83% in patients with proven dissection [42]. Because no combination of clinical factors and chest radiography is adequate to exclude the diagnosis, specific imaging with CT, MRI, or echocardiography may be necessary.

Esophageal rupture (Boerhaave's syndrome) is a rare but deadly cause of chest pain and must be considered by the evaluating physician. Most cases occur after endoscopy or less commonly after forceful vomiting. The patient classically describes a history of substernal, sharp chest pain that is of sudden onset after emesis. They are usually ill-appearing, dyspneic, and diaphoretic. While the exam may be normal, it may reveal a pneumothorax or subcutaneous air. In a review at Rhode Island Hospital, 44 cases were identified (30 cases were after endoscopic procedures) [43]. Of those that did not undergo endoscopy, presenting signs and symptoms in this cohort included vomiting (50%), chest pain (43%), tachycardia (71%), and decreased breath sounds (36%). All but one of these 14 patients had an abnormal chest ray and the correct diagnosis was made in only three cases. Once again, the "classic" presentation is more "classic" than common. Swallow studies (barium or gastrograffin) are typically the initial study of choice, but may be normal in 25% of cases and should not be used to exclude the diagnosis.

Spontaneous pneumothorax is due to a sudden change in the barometric pressure in the lungs, most often in patients with obstructive lung disease (asthmatics and COPD). It is most typically described as a sharp, sudden pleuritic chest pain that is associated with dyspnea. Patients may be ill-appearing, dyspneic, and diaphoretic. The physical exam may be normal or reveal decreased breath sounds and hyperexpansion on the affected side. An upright inspiratory chest radiograph will usually reveal the diagnosis, although expiratory films may be performed to increase the contrast between the pleural space and the lung parenchyma when there is diagnostic uncertainty.

Pulmonary embolism (PE) is an often insidious and potentially lethal diagnosis. While the mortality of PE is traditionally estimated as high as 30%, it falls to 8% with timely diagnosis and treatment. Patients may present with any combination of chest pain, dyspnea, syncope, shock, or hypoxia but, like ACS, may also present with atypical symptoms. Classic risk factors that promote a state of thrombosis include but are not limited to malignancy, lower extremity trauma, prolonged inactivity (bed rest, hospitalization), and thrombophilic disease states (e.g., protein C deficiency). If chest pain is present, it is classically described as sharp and pleuritic. The physical exam may be asymptomatic or include leg pain and swelling, tachypnea, tachycardia, hypoxia, or hypotension. Numerous studies have been performed to help risk stratify patients. A meta-analysis by Brown et al. showed that an ELISA D-dimer has a sensitivity of 0.94 (95% confidence interval [CI] 0.88–0.97) and a specificity of 0.45 (95% CI 0.36–0.55) [44]. Used with a low and possibly moderate pretest probability as determined by a clinical decision aid (such as the Wells Criteria or Charlotte Rule), a high negative predictive value can be achieved. Although D-dimer testing may be adequate in low and possibly moderate-risk patients, those considered high risk require either a CT angiogram or a V/Q scan to more accurately exclude the diagnosis.

Guideline Recommendations

The ECG is the single most important diagnostic test in the evaluation of patients with chest pain. Obtaining the initial ECG as soon as possible will help identify patients with AMI who will benefit from early reperfusion therapy and is a valuable tool to help risk stratify patients. Emergency departments are strongly urged to establish a triage protocol that meets the American College of Cardiology and the American Heart Association guidelines for ECG acquisition within the first 10 min upon the presentation of a patient with chest discomfort or symptoms consistent with ACS [45]. Time to ECG acquisition has also been identified as one of the key components of the National Heart Attack Alert Program's initiative to shorten time to interventional therapy (time to ECG acquisition) [46]. While obtaining a 12-lead ECG may seem conceptually easy, only one-third of all patients in a large NSTEMI registry (CRUSADE) received an initial ECG within this time window. In fact, the average time between presentation and first ECG was 40 min. [15]. Diercks et al. found in a population of over 60,000 patients with NSTEMI, female gender was the most significant predictor of delayed ECG acquisition [47].

The National Heart Attack Alert Program identifies the process of obtaining an ECG in three distinct phases: deciding to obtain an ECG, taking the ECG, and presenting the ECG to the treating physician for interpretation. They suggest that a protocol be in place to allow nurses to obtain a 12-lead EKG without a physician's order and to do so with criteria liberal enough to include patients with atypical symptoms. Of note, in addition to 12-lead ECG technicians, EMTs and nurses should be trained and immediately available to obtain a 12-lead on a readily available 12-lead ECG machine. Lastly, ECGs must be immediately presented to a treating physician and a documented interpretation written on the chart or ECG itself.

It is also important to remember that an ECG is a "snapshot" of a dynamic disease process. While an isolated ECG may provide important initial information in the risk stratification of the patient, the trend or evolving nature of an ECG may be more important. Patients who present with anginal symptoms that resolved prior to presentation and are not symptom-free may have a nondiagnostic ECG that missed critical electrocardiographic disturbance. The ACC/AHA guidelines support obtaining serial 12-lead ECGs in the ED to improve sensitivity for detecting ACS if the initial ECG is nondiagnostic [4].

Cardiac Biomarkers

Cardiac biomarkers such as myoglobin, creatinine kinase-MB (CK-MB), and troponin are critical for risk stratification, initiating anti-ischemic therapy, and disposition of decision making. ACC/AHA consensus guidelines on Unstable Angina/Non-ST-segment Elevation Myocardial Infarction and the American Association of Clinical Biochemistry recommend that cardiac markers should be made available to the clinician within 30–60 min from the time of ED presentation [4]. Traditionally, central laboratory processing of blood samples was the method by which the treating physician obtained this data. However, it is complicated for laboratories to consistently deliver cardiac biomarker results within 60 min with laboratory-based serum or plasma assays. The lengthy process that starts with blood sampling and ends with marker results in the emergency physician's hands, termed "vein to brain" interval, is rather complex. This includes the lab draw, delivery of blood sample to the lab, centrifugation, assay time, data return to the emergency department, and finally data acquisition by the treating physician. Point-of-care testing has evolved to include cardiac biomarkers and offers a response to the process challenges in the central laboratory.

Point-of-care (POC) testing consists of laboratory testing that is performed close to the bedside with the advantage of having more rapid turnaround time (TAT) to the physician. The most common markers for cardiac risk stratification are CKMB, cardiac troponin (Tn) I or T, brain natriuretic peptide (BNP), and myoglobin. Cardiac troponins are quickly becoming the most preferred POC test for these patients because an abnormal troponin level not only identifies a higher risk patient but also drives guideline-based therapy [4]. Currently there are many different cardiac assays from which to choose. It is important to note that at present there is no standardization across the spectrum of the different TnI assays and they must be interpreted under their relative normal range.

Numerous studies have shown several assays to have excellent sensitivity, specificity, and ability to reduce TAT, time to therapeutic intervention, and ED length of stay. Apple and colleagues found the detection limit for the i-STAT whole-blood TnI POC assay to be 0.02 ng/L with a 99th percentile reference limit of 0.08 ng/L. This study suggested that the TnI assay was a sensitive and precise monitor of TnI and appropriate to use in the risk stratification of patients with possible ACS [48]. Numerous other studies have all suggested significant decreases in turnaround time and total ED length of stay [49–52, 53]. A recent randomized trial of the use of POC TnI versus central laboratory TnI in 860 patients suggested that time to anti-ischemic therapy was reduced when a POC assay was used [54]. The vein-to-brain time in the POC arm was 38 min, while in the central laboratory arm was 109 min ($p < 0.001$). Further, time to anti-ischemic therapy was reduced by 47 min in the POC arm ($p < 0.001$), suggesting that the use of POC assays impacts physician decision-making.

References

1. Aufderheide, T.P., et al., Feasibility of prehospital r-TPA therapy in chest pain patients. Ann Emerg Med, 1992. **21**(4): pp. 379–383.
2. Aufderheide, T.P., et al., The diagnostic impact of prehospital 12-lead electrocardiography. Ann Emerg Med, 1990. **19**(11): pp. 1280–1287.
3. Canto, J.G., et al., The prehospital electrocardiogram in acute myocardial infarction: Is its full potential being realized? National Registry of Myocardial Infarction 2 Investigators. J Am Coll Cardiol, 1997. **29**(3): pp. 498–505.
4. Anderson, J.L., et al., ACC/AHA 2007 guidelines for the management of patients with unstable angina/non ST-elevation myocardial infarction: A report of the American College of Cardiology/American Heart Association Task Force on Practice Guidelines (Writing Committee to Revise the 2002 Guidelines for the Management of Patients With Unstable Angina/Non ST-Elevation Myocardial Infarction): Developed in collaboration with the American College of Emergency Physicians, the Society for Cardiovascular Angiography and Interventions, and the Society of Thoracic Surgeons: Endorsed by the American Association of Cardiovascular and Pulmonary Rehabilitation and the Society for Academic Emergency Medicine. Circulation, 2007. **116**(7): pp. e148–e304.
5. Le May, M.R., et al., Comparison of early mortality of paramedic-diagnosed ST-segment elevation myocardial infarction with immediate transport to a designated primary percutaneous coronary intervention center to that of similar patients transported to the nearest hospital. Am J Cardiol, 2006. **98**(10): pp. 1329–1333.
6. Becker, L., M.P. Larsen, and M.S. Eisenberg, Incidence of cardiac arrest during self-transport for chest pain. Ann Emerg Med, 1996. **28**(6): pp. 612–616.
7. Jayes, R.L., Jr., et al., Do patients' coronary risk factor reports predict acute cardiac ischemia in the emergency department? A multicenter study. J Clin Epidemiol, 1992. **45**(6): pp. 621–626.
8. Marx, J.A., R. Hockberger, and R.M. Walls (eds.), *Rosen's Emergency Medicine, Concepts and Clinical Practice.* **Vol. 2, 6th ed.**, London: Mosby, 2006: pp. 1154–1198.
9. Gupta, M., J.A. Tabas, and M.A. Kohn, Presenting complaint among patients with myocardial infarction who present to an urban, public hospital emergency department. Ann Emerg Med, 2002. **40**(2): pp. 180–186.
10. Margolis, J.R., et al., Clinical features of unrecognized myocardial infarction – silent and symptomatic. Eighteen year follow-up: The Framingham study. Am J Cardiol, 1973. **32**(1): pp. 1–7.
11. Canto, J.G., et al., Prevalence, clinical characteristics, and mortality among patients with myocardial infarction presenting without chest pain. JAMA, 2000. **283**(24): pp. 3223–3229.
12. Bayer, A.J., Changing presentation of myocardial infarction with increasing old age. Am Geriatr Soc, 1986. **34**(4): pp. 263–266.
13. Brieger, D., et al., Acute coronary syndromes without chest pain, an underdiagnosed and undertreated high-risk group: Insights from the global registry of acute coronary events. Chest, 2004. **126**(2): pp. 461–469.
14. Kannel, W.B. and R.D. Abbott, Incidence and prognosis of unrecognized myocardial infarction. An update on the Framingham study. N Engl J Med, 1984. **311**(18): pp. 1144–1147.
15. Alexander, K.P., et al., Evolution in cardiovascular care for elderly patients with non-ST-segment elevation acute coronary syndromes: Results from the CRUSADE National Quality Improvement Initiative. J Am Coll Cardiol, 2005. **46**(8): pp. 1479–1487.
16. Chandra, N.C., et al., Observations of the treatment of women in the United States with myocardial infarction: A report from the National Registry of Myocardial Infarction-I. Arch Intern Med, 1998. **158**(9): pp. 981–988.

17. Finnegan, J.R., Jr., et al., Patient delay in seeking care for heart attack symptoms: Findings from focus groups conducted in five U.S. regions. Prev Med, 2000. **31**(3): pp. 205–213.
18. Gibler, W.B., et al., Persistence of delays in presentation and treatment for patients with acute myocardial infarction: The GUSTO-I and GUSTO-III experience. Ann Emerg Med, 2002. **39**(2): pp. 123–130.
19. Canto, J.G., et al., Symptom presentation of women with acute coronary syndromes: myth vs reality. Arch Intern Med, 2007. **167**(22): pp. 2405–2413.
20. Goldberg, R.J., et al., Sex differences in symptom presentation associated with acute myocardial infarction: A population-based perspective. Am Heart J, 1998. **136**(2): pp. 189–195.
21. Grundy, S.M., et al., AHA/ACC scientific statement: Assessment of cardiovascular risk by use of multiple-risk-factor assessment equations: A statement for healthcare professionals from the American Heart Association and the American College of Cardiology. J Am Coll Cardiol, 1999. **34**(4): pp. 1348–1359.
22. Everts, B., et al., Localization of pain in suspected acute myocardial infarction in relation to final diagnosis, age and sex, and site and type of infarction. Heart Lung, 1996. **25**(6): pp. 430–437.
23. Milner, K.A., et al., Gender differences in symptom presentation associated with coronary heart disease. Am J Cardiol, 1999. **84**(4): pp. 396–399.
24. Pope, J.H., et al., Missed diagnoses of acute cardiac ischemia in the emergency department. N Engl J Med, 2000. **342**(16): pp. 1163–1170.
25. Maynard, C., et al., Blacks in the Coronary Artery Surgery Study: Risk factors and coronary artery disease. Circulation, 1986. **74**(1): pp. 64–71.
26. Cooper, R.S. and E. Ford, Comparability of risk factors for coronary heart disease among blacks and whites in the NHANES-I Epidemiologic Follow-up Study. Ann Epidemiol, 1992. **2**(5): pp. 637–645.
27. Maynard, C., et al., Causes of chest pain and symptoms suggestive of acute cardiac ischemia in African-American patients presenting to the emergency department: A multi-center study. J Natl Med Assoc, 1997. **89**(10): pp. 665–671.
28. Venkat, A., et al., The impact of race on the acute management of chest pain. Acad Emerg Med, 2003. **10**(11): pp. 1199–1208.
29. Goldberg, R.J., J.H. Gurwitz, and J.M. Gore, Duration of, and temporal trends (1994–1997) in, prehospital delay in patients with acute myocardial infarction: The second National Registry of Myocardial Infarction. Arch Intern Med, 1999. **159**(18): pp. 2141–2147.
30. Gurwitz, J.H., et al., Delayed hospital presentation in patients who have had acute myocardial infarction. Ann Intern Med, 1997. **126**(8): pp. 593–599.
31. Fein, F.S. and J. Scheuer, *Heart Disease in Diabetes Mellitus: Theory and Practice*. In: Rifkin, H., Porte. D. Jr., eds. New York: Elsevier, 1990: pp. 812–823., 1990.
32. Hambly, R.I., et al., Reappraisal of the role of the diabetic state in coronary artery disease. Chest, 1976. **70**(2): pp. 251–257.
33. Waller, B.F., et al., Status of the coronary arteries at necropsy in diabetes mellitus with onset after age 30 years. Analysis of 229 diabetic patients with and without clinical evidence of coronary heart disease and comparison to 183 control subjects. Am J Med, 1980. **69**(4): pp. 498–506.
34. Watkins, P.J. and J.D. Mackay, Cardiac denervation in diabetic neuropathy. Ann Intern Med, 1980. **92**(2 Pt 2): pp. 304–307.
35. Faerman, I., et al., Autonomic neuropathy and painless myocardial infarction in diabetic patients. Histologic evidence of their relationship. Diabetes, 1977. **26**(12): pp. 1147–1158.
36. Lloyd-Mostyn, R.H. and P.J. Watkins, Defective innervation of heart in diabetic autonomic neuropathy. Br Med J, 1975. **3**(5974): pp. 15–17.

37. Nesto, R.W. and R.T. Phillips, Asymptomatic myocardial ischemia in diabetic patients. Am J Med, 1986. **80**(4C): pp. 40–47.
38. Murray, D.P., et al., Autonomic dysfunction and silent myocardial ischaemia on exercise testing in diabetes mellitus. Diabet Med, 1990. **7**(7): pp. 580–584.
39. Nesto, R.W., et al., Angina and exertional myocardial ischemia in diabetic and nondiabetic patients: Assessment by exercise thallium scintigraphy. Ann Intern Med, 1988. **108**(2): pp. 170–175.
40. Kannel, W.B. and D.L. McGee, Diabetes and cardiovascular disease. The Framingham study. JAMA, 1979. **241**(19): pp. 2035–2038.
41. Nienaber, C.A. and K.A. Eagle, Aortic dissection: New frontiers in diagnosis and management: Part I: From etiology to diagnostic strategies. Circulation, 2003. **108**(5): pp. 628–635.
42. Klompas, M., Does this patient have an acute thoracic aortic dissection? JAMA, 2002. **287**(17): pp. 2262–2272.
43. Lemke, T. and L. Jagminas, Spontaneous esophageal rupture: A frequently missed diagnosis. Am Surg, 1999. **65**(5): pp. 449–452.
44. Brown, M.D., et al., The accuracy of the enzyme-linked immunosorbent assay D-dimer test in the diagnosis of pulmonary embolism: A meta-analysis. Ann Emerg Med, 2002. **40**(2): pp. 133–144.
45. Braunwald, E., et al., ACC/AHA 2002 guideline update for the management of patients with unstable angina and non-ST-segment elevation myocardial infarction – summary article: A report of the American College of Cardiology/American Heart Association task force on practice guidelines (Committee on the Management of Patients With Unstable Angina). J Am Coll Cardiol, 2002. **40**(7): pp. 1366–1374.
46. Lusiani, L., et al., Prevalence, clinical features, and acute course of atypical myocardial infarction. Angiology, 1994. **45**(1): pp. 49–55.
47. Diercks, D.B., et al., Frequency and consequences of recording an electrocardiogram >10 minutes after arrival in an emergency room in non-ST-segment elevation acute coronary syndromes (from the CRUSADE Initiative). Am J Cardiol, 2006. **97**(4): pp. 437–442.
48. Apple, F.S., M.M. Murakami, and R.H. Christenson, et al., Analytical performance of the i-STAT cardiac troponin I assay. . Clin Chim Acta, 2004. **345**(1–2): pp. 123–127.
49. Lee-Lewandrowski, E., D. Corboy, et al., Implementation of a point-of-care satellite laboratory in the emergency department of an academic medical center. Arch Pathol Lab Med, 2004. **127**: pp. 456–460.
50. Kost, G.J. and N.K. Tran, Point-of-care testing and cardiac biomarkers: The standard of care and vision for chest pain centers. Cardiol Clin, 2005. **23**(vi): pp. 467–490.
51. Stubbs, P. and P.O. Collinson, Point-of-care testing: A cardiologist's view. Clin Chim Acta, 2001. **311**: pp. 57–61.
52. Yang, Z. and D. Min Zhou, Cardiac markers and their point-of-care testing for diagnosis of acute myocardial infarction. Clin Biochem 2006. **39**: pp. 771–780.
53. Storrow, A.B., C.J. Lindsell, S.P. Collins, G.J. Fermann, A.L. Blomkalns, J.M. Williams, et al., Emergency department multimarker point-of-care testing reduces time to cardiac marker results without loss of diagnostic accuracy. Point of Care, 2006. **5**: pp. 132–136.
54. Renaud, B., et al., Impact of point-of-care testing in the emergency department evaluation and treatment of patients with suspected acute coronary syndromes. Acad Emerg Med, 2008. **15**(3): pp. 216–224.
55. Heer, T., et al., Gender differences in acute non-ST-segment elevation myocardial infarction. Am J Cardiol, 2006. **98**(2): pp. 160–166.
56. Al-Mallah, M.H., R.N. Bazari, and S. Khanal, Delay in invasive risk stratification of women with acute coronary syndrome is associated with worse outcomes. J Thromb Thrombolysis, 2007. **23**(1): pp. 35–39.

Chapter 6
Risk Stratification: History, Physical, and EKG

Alan B. Storrow, Ian McClure, and Elizabeth Harbison

Abstract Chest pain annually accounts for over 5% of more than 110 million emergency department (ED) visits nationwide (PHS, PHS 2004;1250). Of these patients, approximately one-third will be diagnosed with acute coronary syndrome (ACS) (Storrow and Gibler, Ann Emerg Med 2000;35(5):449–61). ACS describes a continuum of conditions that ranges from unstable angina (UA) and non-ST-segment elevation myocardial infarction (NSTEMI) to ST-segment elevation myocardial infarction (STEMI), all due to varying degrees of coronary ischemia and cardiac cell death. The clinical presentation of a patient with UA can be insidious and presents challenges in diagnosis. Since each ACS component may potentially cause sudden cardiac death, it is prudent to use an individual's history, physical examination, and electrocardiogram to help determine degrees of risk for ACS. This risk stratification ultimately guides further evaluation, testing, and treatment.

Keywords Acute coronary syndrome · Electrocardiogram · Risk stratification · Physical examination · Chest pain

Introduction

Approximately eight million patients present annually to emergency departments with chest pain; five million are judged to have suspected ACS and less than half will ultimately have a cardiac diagnosis. Some three million patients with chest pain are discharged from the ED each year, and 40,000 of these will ultimately suffer acute myocardial infarction (AMI). This group unfortunately accounts for 20–39% of malpractice dollars awarded in emergency medicine [3–5].

A.B. Storrow (✉)
Department of Emergency Medicine, Vanderbilt University, 703 Oxford House, Nashville, TN 37232, USA
e-mail: alan.storrow@vanderbilt.edu

W.F. Peacock and C.P. Cannon (eds.), *Short Stay Management of Chest Pain*, DOI 10.1007/978-1-60327-948-2_6,
© Humana Press, a part of Springer Science+Business Media, LLC 2009

The evaluation and management of patients with chest pain or potential ACS is extremely challenging for the practicing emergency physician. Current diagnosis of ACS, including both AMI and UA, begins with a patient history, physical examination, and 12-lead ECG. Unfortunately, history is often variable in patients with ACS and nearly half of patients with AMI present to the ED with a nondiagnostic ECG.

Today, the chest pain center (CPC) serves as an integral component of many emergency departments. Their success and safety has largely been due to a focused protocol-driven approach directed at the ACS continuum. New therapies for ACS make this ED triage and risk stratification increasingly important. While different CPC protocols have been effective, all address the diagnosis and rapid treatment of *acute myocardial necrosis, rest ischemia,* and *exercise-induced ischemia.* These three concepts are the foundation for a successful CPC in the ED.

Triage of patients into appropriate risk categories, after obtaining a patient's initial history, physical, and ECG, is the most difficult part of acute chest pain evaluation. The CPC should be utilized for patients with a low to moderate risk for ACS, a low likelihood of complications, no contraindications to the protocol's tests, and no serious comorbidity, which may interfere with assessment or ED release at conclusion of the evaluation. In essence, CPC candidates can be broadly defined as hemodynamically stable patients with a history consistent with ACS and a nondiagnostic initial ECG. Inappropriate patient selection for a CPC will adversely impact patient response, outcomes, and costs. Patients with high pretest probability for ACS usually require further testing and treatment beyond what is traditionally offered in an ED CPC. Patients with a very low pretest probability of ACS will not benefit from CPC evaluation [2].

Classic presentations of AMI and UA, by initial history and ECG changes, do not present a diagnostic dilemma and should have protocol-driven care stressing reperfusion strategies, appropriate pharmacological therapy, and CCU admission. There is clear evidence that decreased time to treatment is beneficial for AMI, thus rapid therapy is a critical component of an ED's overall approach to potential ACS. For diagnostic purposes, these patients represent a minority of emergent chest pain presentations [2].

History and Risk Factors

Chest pain is the typical presentation of ischemic heart disease. It may be induced by activity or stress and typically resolves after several minutes of rest. Additional characteristics of this pain should be obtained, including location, severity, duration, radiation, and quality. It may be described as pressure, tightness, stabbing, burning, or sharp in nature. Other symptoms include nausea, vomiting, diaphoresis, dyspnea, palpitations, and fatigue. The most common anginal equivalent symptom is isolated new onset or worsening exertional dyspnea [6, 7]. Unfortunately, only 18% of coronary attacks are preceded by *long-standing* angina [5].

The classic presentation of an acute myocardial infarction, substernal chest pressure with radiation to the left arm or the jaw, is not always present. Typical symptoms may increase the likelihood of ACS, but atypical symptoms do not rule out ACS. In a multicenter chest pain study, 13% of patients with pleuritic chest pain and 7% of patients with pain reproducible with palpation ultimately received the diagnosis of ACS [8]. In 1,996 patients with AMI, 87% of men and 80% of women presented with chest pain [9, 10]. Women, the elderly, and diabetics were more likely to present with atypical symptomatology.

Traditional cardiac risk factors (family history, tobacco use, hypertension, diabetes mellitus, and hypercholesterolemia) are designed for the prediction of coronary artery disease, are limited to the prediction of ACS during an acute presentation [11–13], and should not be relied upon for disposition decisions in patients with possible ACS [7]. They are less predictive in a single-patient visit to the ED than when studied longitudinally in a population [8, 11, 14]. Cumulative risk factor burden is significant in patients under 40 years of age. As one increases in age, the total number of risk factors becomes less predictive of ACS [7, 15].

These issues notwithstanding, about 90% of coronary heart disease patients have prior exposure to at least one of the following risk factors: high total cholesterol, current treatment with cholesterol or high blood pressure-lowering drugs, hypertension, current cigarette use, and clinical report of diabetes [16]. According to a large international case–control study, nine easily modifiable risk factors account for over 90% of the risk of an initial AMI: cigarette smoking, abnormal blood lipid levels, hypertension, diabetes, abdominal obesity, lack of physical activity, low daily fruit and vegetable consumption, alcohol overconsumption, and psychosocial index [17]. Lastly, more than 90% of coronary heart disease event will occur in individuals with at least one risk factor and approximately 8% will occur in people with only borderline levels of multiple risk factors [18].

Physical Examination

Physical findings in patients with acute chest pain are somewhat limited in ACS diagnosis but may identify features that place a patient at higher risk for untoward outcome or provide clues to alternative problems. Abnormal vital signs, including hypotension, tachycardia, or bradycardia, increase a patient's risk of ACS, but are nonspecific. Bradycardic rhythms, in particular, may indicate inferior wall ischemia. Hypertension may be a result of baseline condition, pain, or anxiety. Hypotension occurs with volume depletion or cardiac contractility failure.

Cardiac failure, and thus suspicion of ACS, can be heralded by evidence of jugular venous distention, new murmurs, S3 gallops, rales, and peripheral edema. New murmurs are potentially indicative of papillary muscle dysfunction or mitral valve failure. One's physical examination should include examination of contraindications to antiplatelet and antithrombotic treatment such as hemoptysis or gross rectal bleeding [6, 7].

Electrocardiogram

The initial step in evaluating patients presenting to the ED with chest pain is obtaining a 12-lead electrocardiogram (EKG) within 10 min [6]. This quickly allows a physician to determine if there is an ST-segment elevation myocardial infarction (STEMI). If so, appropriate therapy is provided: percutaneous coronary intervention (PCI) in a cardiac catheterization laboratory or pharmacologic treatment with fibrinolytics. Its low sensitivity notwithstanding, the 12-lead EKG provides crucial information that drives such reperfusion strategies in STEMI and therefore is considered standard of care [2, 6]. It is those patients with potential ACS and without STEMI who benefit from further risk stratification. Unfortunately, most initial ECGs in patients with ACS are nondiagnostic for ischemia or infarction [19].

The principal advantages of an EKG are its low expense, wide availability, and noninvasive nature. It will provide a specific diagnosis in approximately 5% of ED patients with chest pain [20]. Despite this low sensitivity for diagnosing AMI and UA [21], ST-segment elevation remains the principal criterion for administering fibrinolytic therapy [22]. The ECG serves to detect ACS in a broad, diverse ED population. Its limitations include its static image of a single 10–12-second period of cardiac activity, lack of accurate detection for all areas of the myocardium [23, 24], and occasional waveform production that is difficult to interpret [25].

However, there are many findings on an initial EKG that carry prognostic significance and allow for risk stratification. In a retrospective 1999 study of over 12,000 patients, Savonitto et al. showed that specific findings on the initial EKG predicted an increased risk of 30-day death or reinfarction. These findings included isolated T wave inversions of more than 0.1 mV, ST-segment elevation of at least 0.05 mV in two contiguous leads, ST-segment depression of greater than 0.05 mV (alone or with concomitant T wave inversion), and combined ST-segment elevation or depression. ST-segment elevation correlated with higher rates of early morbidity and mortality, while ST depression was associated with later events [26] (Fig. 6.1).

The consequences of missing critical EKG findings in patients presenting with symptoms suggestive of ACS can be significant. A retrospective study analyzed a cohort of 2215 patients from five emergency departments who had ICD-9 discharge diagnoses of acute myocardial infarction (AMI) and assessed

Fig. 6.1 The initial EKG and Kaplan–Meier estimates of probability of death. *Top*, mortality rate up to 30 days; *bottom*, mortality rate up to 6 months. (used with permission from Savonitto et al. [26])

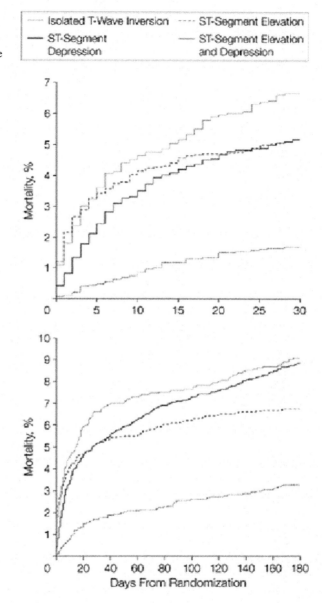

failure frequency of the treating provider to identify significant ST-segment depressions, ST-segment elevations, or T wave inversions on the presenting EKG. High-risk EKG findings were not documented in 12% of patients, and 8% of STEMI/ST elevations were missed. T wave inversions were missed 14% of the time, as were 18% of ST-segment depressions. Missed findings were more common in older patients with a history of congestive heart failure and other cardiovascular history as opposed to those patients who presented with chest pain alone and were associated with a lower likelihood of receiving appropriate treatment, including aspiring, beta-blockers, and reperfusion therapy [27].

Any ST-segment elevation, even subtle elevation of less than 1 mm, that occurs in two or more contiguous leads should prompt concern for ischemia. ST-segment elevation with anatomically reciprocal ST-segment depression improves the specificity of the ST elevation for diagnosis of acute coronary syndrome. The temptation to interpret ST-segment elevation as benign early repolarization, especially in patients older than 30, should be resisted. In addition, there are several conditions that can manifest themselves through ST-segment elevation, most commonly ventricular aneurysm, aortic dissection through coronary ostia, hyperkalemia, pericarditis, left ventricular hypertrophy, Wolff–Parkinson–White syndrome, and left bundle branch block.

ST-segment depression incurs a 10-fold greater risk of 1-year mortality than no ST depression [28]. ST-segment depression occurring in conjunction with ST-segment elevation in anatomically reciprocal leads (anterior/inferior, anterior/lateral) is highly suggestive of STEMI. Primary ST-segment depression is likely unstable angina or NSTEMI. Persistent ST-segment depression in the setting of ongoing chest pain despite maximal anti-ischemic therapy is an ominous sign and should be evaluated through cardiac catheterization.

While ST-segment depression alone is not an indication of thrombolytic therapy [26], ST-segment depression in leads V1–V4 may indicate a posterior wall MI due to the reciprocal electrical view of the infarct. This finding may be misinterpreted as anterior wall ischemia unless the diagnosis of a posterior MI is entertained. Anterior ST-segment depression should be considered a posterior wall infarct until proven otherwise, and the initial EKG displaying this finding can be followed by a posterior lead EKG.

Similarly, inferior ST-segment elevation should be evaluated with a right-sided EKG to look for right ventricle (RV) infarction. This is clinically important for management purposes, as patients with acute RV infarction are preload dependent in order to maintain adequate cardiac output. Nitrates should be used cautiously in these patients, as they can lead to hypotension and shock with little warning.

T wave inversion occurs in many conditions, but in the setting of chest pain may be an indication of cardiac ischemia. T wave inversion may also represent reperfusion of a completed infarct. Wellens' warning is a biphasic T wave with terminal T wave inversion in the anterior leads V2–V4 [29, 30]. This finding has a high specificity for proximal to mid-LAD occlusion and patients at high risk for reocclusion.

Pathologic Q waves, which are usually wider and deeper than the normal deflections that represent septal wall depolarization, often indicate ischemia or dead myocardium. Generally speaking, Q waves are considered significant if the amplitude is greater than one-third of the amplitude of the corresponding QRS complex. Preexisting Q waves from a previous myocardial infarction should not be ignored in patients presenting with chest pain, as they demonstrate strong evidence of coronary artery disease. It is also possible to see Q waves appear in the setting of STEMI/NSTEMI as the infarct evolves; these new Q waves indicate that an infarct is at least 12 hours old.

New LBBB should be considered a sign of ischemia or infarction and prompt an ischemic workup, especially when seen in the setting of acute chest pain. A set of clinical criteria that allow for EKG diagnosis of AMI in the setting of LBBB has been published [31, 32]. These criteria are (1) ST-segment elevation of 1 mm or more that is concordant with (in the same direction as) the QRS complex; (2) ST-segment depression of 1 mm or more in lead V1, V2, or V3; and (3) ST-segment elevation of 5 mm or more that is discordant with (in the opposite direction from) the QRS complex. Similar criteria were developed for the diagnosis of AMI in the setting of an internal pacemaker device, which produces an EKG pattern similar to that of an LBBB. In this setting, discordant ST-segment elevation greater than 5 mm was the most statistically significant criterion associated with AMI [33].

New rhythm disturbances in the setting of chest pain are disturbing and warrant investigation. Examples include second- or third-degree heart block, tachydysrhythmias, and bradyarrhythmias. Patients with chest pain due to ischemia or infarction may have disrupted intrinsic pacemaker function or conduction pathways; conversely, such arrhythmias may lead to poor diastolic coronary artery perfusion with further ischemia or infarct. These patients are at high risk and should be considered for coronary angiography; patients with active chest pain and arrhythmia should not be stress tested.

While serial EKGs are critical to look for dynamic ST-segment changes, they may miss acute changes due to intermittent occlusion and reperfusion. Investigation of continuous ST-segment trend monitoring found that high-risk patients were more likely to have their therapy altered to include intensive anti-ischemic and antithrombotic therapy as well as percutaneous coronary angioplasty [34–36]. Based on this and subsequent similar studies, the use of continuous ST-segment monitoring may allow for earlier detection of AMI and become more commonplace in the ED. The use of continuous ST monitoring presents challenges in lower risk groups and has not found wide acceptance.

Risk Prediction Tools

The Goldman criteria utilize history, exam, and ECG findings to predict low (<7%) or high (>7%) probability of AMI [21]. Because it is limited to AMI, it is less useful for patients with potential UA. The ACI-TIPI instrument predicts a probability of acute ischemia based on gender, age, chief complaint, and ECG findings [37]. It is a computerized ECG-based instrument that has utility for ACS triage but has not found wide use because of the difficulty in translating the predicted probability into disposition decisions. The AHCPR/NHLBI unstable angina guidelines predict the likelihood of coronary artery disease (CAD) and prognosis by utilizing many historical findings and the ECG. This guideline divides patients into high, moderate, and low likelihood of UA [38]. The moderate-likelihood category would contain some patients likely requiring hospital admission rather than CPC evaluation.

The TIMI risk score (Table 6.1) is a simple prognostication scheme that categorizes risk of death and ischemic events in patients with UA/NSTEMI [39]. It should not be used in isolation to determine ED disposition and has proven limited to discrete categorization in the ED [40]. However, the schema is well recognized and can predict outcome.

In 1997, The Medical College of Virginia detailed an elegant five-level approach to ACS risk stratification utilizing the initial ECG, chest pain characterization, and history [41] (Fig. 6.2). *Level 1* is defined as ECG criteria of ST-segment elevation AMI requiring immediate reperfusion, when appropriate, and ultimately CCU admission. *Level 2* patients have a high probability for UA and potential non-Q wave AMI, manifested by transient ST-segment elevation, ST-segment depression, T wave inversion, or known CAD with typical symptoms. These patients are considered for rapid antiplatelet, antithrombin, and vasoactive drugs and are admitted to the CCU for further evaluation and treatment. *Level 3* patients have a high probability of UA, but low probability of AMI. They are defined by >30 min of typical symptoms, a nondiagnostic ECG, and no prior history of CAD. Level 3 patients undergo a "fast-track" protocol to confirm myocardial necrosis after immediate rest myocardial perfusion imaging utilizing sestamibi. *Level 4* patients have a low to moderate probability of UA manifested by <30 min of typical symptoms or prolonged

Table 6.1 TIMI risk score

Score	Incidence of death, new or recurrent MI, recurrent ischemia requiring revascularization (%)
0/1	4.7
2	8.3
3	13.2
4	19.9
5	26.2
6/7	40.9

Scoring system: One point when risk factor present, zero point if absent (total seven points possible)
Age >65 years
Presence of more than three risk factors for coronary artery disease
Prior coronary stenosis ≥50%
Presence of ST-segment deviation on admission to EKG
More than two episodes of angina within past 24 hours
Prior use of ASA in past 7 days
Elevated cardiac markers

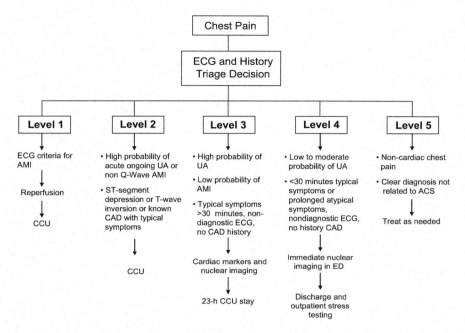

Fig. 6.2 Medical College of Virginia clinical pathways "Track" strategy

atypical symptoms, a nondiagnostic ECG, and no history of CAD. These patients receive immediate resting myocardial perfusion imaging in the ED and are considered for release from the ED and careful follow-up for stress radionuclide imaging if the initial evaluation is negative. *Level 5* implies noncardiac chest pain defined by a clear diagnosis not related to ACS. This strategy was reported to be a safe and effective method for rapid triage in 1,187 consecutive patients [41].

References

1. PHS. National hospital ambulatory medical care survey: 2002 emergency department summary. PHS 2004;1250.
2. Storrow AB, Gibler WB. Chest pain centers: diagnosis of acute coronary syndromes. Ann Emerg Med 2000;35(5):449–61.
3. Braunwald E, Jones RH, Mark DB, et al. Diagnosing and managing unstable angina. Agency for Health Care Policy and Research. Circulation 1994;90(1):613–22.
4. McCarthy BD, Beshansky JR, D'Agostino RB, Selker HP. Missed diagnoses of acute myocardial infarction in the emergency department: results from a multicenter study. Ann Emerg Med 1993;22(3):579–82.
5. Rosamond W, Flegal K, Furie K, et al. Heart disease and stroke statistics – 2008 update: a report from the American Heart Association Statistics Committee and Stroke Statistics Subcommittee. Circulation 2008;117(4):e25–146.

6. Anderson JL, Adams CD, Antman EM, et al. ACC/AHA 2007 guidelines for the management of patients with unstable angina/non ST-elevation myocardial infarction: a report of the American College of Cardiology/American Heart Association Task Force on Practice Guidelines (Writing Committee to Revise the 2002 Guidelines for the Management of Patients With Unstable Angina/Non ST-Elevation Myocardial Infarction): developed in collaboration with the American College of Emergency Physicians, the Society for Cardiovascular Angiography and Interventions, and the Society of Thoracic Surgeons: endorsed by the American Association of Cardiovascular and Pulmonary Rehabilitation and the Society for Academic Emergency Medicine. Circulation 2007;116(7):e148–304.

7. Brogan GX. Risk stratification for patients with non-ST-segment elevation acute coronary syndromes in the emergency department. In: Emergency Medicine Cardiac Research and Education Group; 2007:1–10.

8. Lee TH, Cook EF, Weisberg M, Sargent RK, Wilson C, Goldman L. Acute chest pain in the emergency room. Identification and examination of low-risk patients. Arch Intern Med 1985;145(1):65–9.

9. Goodacre S, Locker T, Morris F, Campbell S. How useful are clinical features in the diagnosis of acute, undifferentiated chest pain? Acad Emerg Med 2002;9(3):203–8.

10. Goodacre SW, Angelini K, Arnold J, Revill S, Morris F. Clinical predictors of acute coronary syndromes in patients with undifferentiated chest pain. QJM 2003;96(12): 893–8.

11. Jayes RL, Jr., Beshansky JR, D'Agostino RB, Selker HP. Do patients' coronary risk factor reports predict acute cardiac ischemia in the emergency department? A multicenter study. J Clin Epidemiol 1992;45(6):621–6.

12. Selker HP, Griffith JL, D'Agostino RB. A time-insensitive predictive instrument for acute myocardial infarction mortality: a multicenter study. Med Care 1991; 29(12):1196–211.

13. Selker HP, Griffith JL, D'Agostino RB. A tool for judging coronary care unit admission appropriateness, valid for both real-time and retrospective use. A time-insensitive predictive instrument (TIPI) for acute cardiac ischemia: a multicenter study. Med Care 1991;29(7):610–27.

14. Tintinalli JE, Kelen GD, Stapcyzynski JS. Emergency Medicine, a Comprehensive Study Guide. 6th ed: McGraw-Hill Companies, Inc., New York; 2004.

15. Han JH, Lindsell CJ, Storrow AB, et al. The role of cardiac risk factor burden in diagnosing acute coronary syndromes in the emergency department setting. Ann Emerg Med 2007;49(2):145–52, 52 e1.

16. Greenland P, Knoll MD, Stamler J, et al. Major risk factors as antecedents of fatal and nonfatal coronary heart disease events. JAMA 2003;290(7):891–7.

17. Yusuf S, Hawken S, Ounpuu S, et al. Effect of potentially modifiable risk factors associated with myocardial infarction in 52 countries (the INTERHEART study): case-control study. Lancet 2004;364(9438):937–52.

18. Vasan RS, Sullivan LM, Wilson PW, et al. Relative importance of borderline and elevated levels of coronary heart disease risk factors. Ann Intern Med 2005; 142(6):393–402.

19. Gibler WB, Lewis LM, Erb RE, et al. Early detection of acute myocardial infarction in patients presenting with chest pain and nondiagnostic ECGs: serial CK-MB sampling in the emergency department. Ann Emerg Med 1990;19(12):1359–66.

20. Lee TH, Rouan GW, Weisberg MC, et al. Sensitivity of routine clinical criteria for diagnosing myocardial infarction within 24 hours of hospitalization. Ann Intern Med 1987;106(2):181–6.

21. Goldman L, Cook EF, Brand DA, et al. A computer protocol to predict myocardial infarction in emergency department patients with chest pain. N Engl J Med 1988; 318(13):797–803.

22. Selker HP, Zalenski RJ, Antman EM, et al. An evaluation of technologies for identifying acute cardiac ischemia in the emergency department: a report from a National Heart Attack Alert Program Working Group. Ann Emerg Med 1997;29(1):13–87.

23. Rude RE, Poole WK, Muller JE, et al. Electrocardiographic and clinical criteria for recognition of acute myocardial infarction based on analysis of 3,697 patients. Am J Cardiol 1983;52(8):936–42.

24. Wrenn KD. Protocols in the emergency room evaluation of chest pain: do they fail to diagnose lateral wall myocardial infarction. J Gen Intern Med 1987;2(1):66–7.

25. Lee TH, Rouan GW, Weisberg MC, et al. Clinical characteristics and natural history of patients with acute myocardial infarction sent home from the emergency room. Am J Cardiol 1987;60(4):219–24.

26. Savonitto S, Ardissino D, Granger CB, et al. Prognostic value of the admission electro-cardiogram in acute coronary syndromes. JAMA 1999;281(8):707–13.

27. Masoudi FA, Foody JM, Havranek EP, et al. Trends in acute myocardial infarction in 4 US states between 1992 and 2001: clinical characteristics, quality of care, and outcomes. Circulation 2006;114(25):2806–14.

28. Kaul P, Fu Y, Chang WC, et al. Prognostic value of ST segment depression in acute coronary syndromes: insights from PARAGON-A applied to GUSTO-IIb. PARAGON-A and GUSTO IIb Investigators. Platelet IIb/IIIa Antagonism for the Reduction of Acute Global Organization Network. J Am Coll Cardiol 2001;38(1):64–71.

29. de Zwaan C, Bar FW, Janssen JH, et al. Angiographic and clinical characteristics of patients with unstable angina showing an ECG pattern indicating critical narrowing of the proximal LAD coronary artery. Am Heart J 1989;117(3):657–65.

30. Wellens HJ. Bishop lecture. The electrocardiogram 80 years after Einthoven. J Am Coll Cardiol 1986;7(3):484–91.

31. Sgarbossa EB. Recent advances in the electrocardiographic diagnosis of myocardial infarction: left bundle branch block and pacing. Pacing Clin Electrophysiol 1996;19(9):1370–9.

32. Sgarbossa EB, Pinski SL, Barbagelata A, et al. Electrocardiographic diagnosis of evol-ving acute myocardial infarction in the presence of left bundle-branch block. GUSTO-1 (Global Utilization of Streptokinase and Tissue Plasminogen Activator for Occluded Coronary Arteries) Investigators. N Engl J Med 1996;334(8):481–7.

33. Sgarbossa EB, Pinski SL, Gates KB, Wagner GS. Early electrocardiographic diagnosis of acute myocardial infarction in the presence of ventricular paced rhythm. GUSTO-I investigators. Am J Cardiol 1996;77(5):423–4.

34. Fesmire FM. A rapid protocol to identify and exclude acute myocardial infarction: continuous 12-lead ECG monitoring with 2-hour delta CK-MB. Am J Emerg Med 2000;18(6):698–702.

35. Fesmire FM, Decker WW, Diercks DB, et al. Clinical policy: Critical issues in the evaluation and management of adult patients with non-ST-segment elevation acute coronary syndromes. Ann Emerg Med 2006;48(3):270–301.

36. Fesmire FM, Hughes AD, Fody EP, et al. The Erlanger chest pain evaluation protocol: a one-year experience with serial 12-lead ECG monitoring, two-hour delta serum marker measurements, and selective nuclear stress testing to identify and exclude acute coronary syndromes. Ann Emerg Med 2002;40(6):584–94.

37. Selker HP, Beshansky JR, Griffith JL, et al. Use of the acute cardiac ischemia time-insensitive predictive instrument (ACI-TIPI) to assist with triage of patients with chest pain or other symptoms suggestive of acute cardiac ischemia. A multicenter, controlled clinical trial. Ann Intern Med 1998;129(11):845–55.

38. AHCPR. Unstable angina: diagnosis and management. Clin Pract Guide 1998;10.

39. Antman EM, Cohen M, Bernink PJ, et al. The TIMI risk score for unstable angina/ non-ST elevation MI: A method for prognostication and therapeutic decision making. JAMA 2000;284(7):835–42.

40. Chase M, Robey JL, Zogby KE, Sease KL, Shofer FS, Hollander JE. Prospective validation of the Thrombolysis in myocardial infarction risk score in the emergency department chest pain population. Ann Emerg Med 2006;48(3):252–9.
41. Tatum JL, Jesse RL, Kontos MC, et al. Comprehensive strategy for the evaluation and triage of the chest pain patient. Ann Emerg Med 1997;29(1):116–25.

Chapter 7
Cardiac Markers: A Chest Pain Center Focus

Robert H. Christenson

Abstract Use of cardiac biomarkers for care of patients presenting to the emergency department has a rich history beginning in the 1950s. Aspartate aminotransferase, lactate dehydrogenase isoenzymes, creatine kinase and its MB isoenzyme and myoglobin have all been utilized over the years. However a sentinel event occurred in the 1990s with the availability of assays for the myocardial specific biomarkers cardiac troponin T (cTnT) and cardiac troponin I (cTnI). Along with clinical features and the electrocardiogram, cTnI and cTnT measurements are now a cornerstone for early risk stratification, the diagnosis of myocardial infarction and clinical decision-making in the context of suspected acute coronary syndrome patients in the emergency department. Point-of-care measurements of cardiac troponin and other markers have been implemented at many institutions where the central laboratory is unable to provide results in one hour or less from the time of collection. Because cTnT and cTnI are believed to be released only upon myocardial necrosis, there has been substantial effort in identifying markers of myocardial ischemia that do not necessarily have irreversible cell death. Promising markers include ischemia modified albumin, C-reactive protein, myloperoxidase as well as B-type natriuretic peptide and its biologically inactive co-metabolite NT-proBNP. Also, attention has turned to measurement of very low troponin concentrations measured using assays that are able to measure troponin reliably at concentrations 10- to 100-fold lower than the best conventional troponin assays, with the idea of specifically detecting subtle cardiac injury associated with unstable angina. There are a number of clinical confounders for measurements including renal insufficiency, end stage renal disease, blunt chest trauma, pulmonary embolism, chemotherapy and recent cardiac procedures. Interpretation of cardiac marker results in these clinical circumstances can be complicated and the clinical course of the patient relative to temporal increase in biomarkers must be taken into account.

R.H. Christenson (✉)
University of Maryland Medical Center, Baltimore, MD, USA
e-mail: rchristenson@umm.edu

W.F. Peacock and C.P. Cannon (eds.), *Short Stay Management of Chest Pain*,
DOI 10.1007/978-1-60327-948-2_7,
© Humana Press, a part of Springer Science+Business Media, LLC 2009

Few tests have the clinical value and impact of cTnT and cTnI, and it is unlikely that these tests will be replaced for the diagnosis of MI in the foreseeable future. For risk stratification and patient management, however, other markers of inflammation, heart dysfunction or the coagulation process may provide complementary information. Some of these novel markers may come from the proteomic, metabolomic and molecular diagnostic studies. However, it is critical to note that the real value of any new or existing markers will hinge on evidence that their utilization can be shown to improve clinical and/or economic outcomes.

Keywords Cardiac troponin I · Cardiac troponin I · CK-MB · Myoglobin · Guidelines · Myocardial infarction redefinition · Timing of sample collection

Introduction

The discovery in the 1950s that the enzyme aspartate transaminase is released into circulation after cardiac injury was the first step in biomarkers becoming fundamental to diagnosis, risk stratification, and management of patients presenting with signs and symptoms of the acute coronary syndromes. The evolution of cardiac biomarkers continued through the 1970s with the routine measurement of lactate dehydrogenase and its LD1–LD5 isoenzymes and then later with the emergence of total creatine kinase (CK) activity and its CK-MB isoenzyme. In the 1980s, vastly improved CK-MB "mass" immunoassays became available that do not rely on enzymatic activity.

A development that shifted the diagnostic paradigm for acute coronary syndromes occurred during the 1990s. This shift can be termed the "*era of troponin*," and occurred with the development of cardiac troponin T (cTnT) and cardiac troponin I (cTnI) testing. Along with clinical features and the electrocardiogram (ECG), cardiac cTnI and cTnT measurements are now a cornerstone for the assessment of the suspected acute coronary syndrome patient. In fact, a Class I recommendation from guidelines of the National Academy of Clinical Biochemistry (NACB) is the following: "Biomarkers of myocardial necrosis should be measured in all patients who present with symptoms consistent with acute coronary syndromes" [1]. The evidence base for biomarkers, i.e., cardiac troponin, is so compelling that the very diagnostic criteria for MI have been redefined based on cardiac troponin measurements [2].

Although cardiac troponin values are important in the workup of the suspected acute coronary syndrome patients, the NACB guidelines remind us that the patient's clinical presentation (history, physical exam) and ECG must be used in conjunction with biomarkers in the diagnostic evaluation [1].

Cardiac Necrosis Markers

Cardiac Troponin T and Cardiac Troponin I

The troponin complex comprises three structural proteins termed troponin T, troponin C, and troponin I. The troponin complex is fundamental for the contraction of all striated muscles, both skeletal and cardiac. Because of the unique physiological demands on myocardium, cardiac-specific isoforms of the troponin T and troponin I proteins evolved. The cardiac isoforms of TnT and TnI have amino sequences that are different from their skeletal muscle counterparts and are virtually exclusive for myocardial tissue. Thus assays for cTnT and cTnI have exquisite cardiac specificity and is one important reason why cTnT and cTnI have become the preferred markers for the assessment of the acute coronary syndromes [1,2].

Laboratory tests are commonly used for one or more of the following applications: screening, diagnosis, prognostication, monitoring, and guidance of therapy and management. Although few laboratory tests are used for all of these applications, any diagnostic test (laboratory or otherwise) that does not independently impact patient management decisions and improves important outcomes is of modest clinical value. Based on the compelling evidence, cTnT and cTnI have been utilized for diagnosis of myocardial infarction (MI), risk stratification of suspected acute coronary syndrome patients, and for guidance of therapy and intervention.

Diagnosis of Myocardial Infarction

Cardiac troponin is the preferred marker for the diagnosis of MI in patients suspected of having an acute coronary syndrome [1,2]. One must keep in mind that troponin is a structural protein such that some hours are frequently required for release and detection in circulation. Thus a critically important point when utilizing cardiac troponin is timing of blood sample collection. In general, blood should be obtained at hospital presentation, followed by serial sampling based on the clinical circumstances. For most patients this includes sampling upon presentation and then 6–9 hours later. Further samples should be collected if the suspicion of acute coronary syndrome remains a clinical possibility. With serial sampling in the presence of a clinical history suggestive of acute coronary syndrome, guidance is that a cardiac troponin value on at least one occasion during the first 24 hours after the acute event above the maximal concentration exceeding the 99th percentile of values for reference control group is indicative of myocardial necrosis consistent with MI [1,2]. Observation of a rise and fall in values indicates an acute event and may be helpful in determining the timing of myocardial injury.

The use of the 99th percentile of a reference control (normal) population as a cutpoint for cTnT or cTnI can be a source of confusion and some variability. This is because manufacturers of cardiac troponin assays have not used a common set of samples for establishing the characteristics of control populations. Currently the best approach is for clinicians and laboratory medicine staff to jointly decide what the 99th percentile cutpoint concentration should be using information provided by the manufacturers, characteristics of the local population, their own studies, and experience with the specific cardiac troponin assay.

Although cTnT and cTnI are found only in myocardium, troponin elevations are not a diagnostic sine qua non for acute coronary syndrome. In other words, cTnT and cTnI measurements are heart specific but not disease specific. Rather, cardiac troponin can be elevated in a whole host of conditions, some of which are listed in Table 7.1. Analytical false-positive elevations in cTnT and cTnI have also been reported [3]; however, these appear to be relatively rare with improved assays. When elevated cTnT or cTnI results are observed in patients, as a general rule one should think heart, but not exclusively acute coronary syndromes until further evidence is available.

Table 7.1 Elevations of cardiac troponin without overt ischemic heart disease

- Trauma (including contusion, ablation, pacing, ICD firings including atrial defibrillators, cardioversion, endomyocardial biopsy, cardiac surgery, after interventional closure of ASDs)
- Congestive heart failure – acute and chronic
- Aortic valve disease and HOCM with significant LVH
- Hypertension
- Hypotension, often with arrhythmias
- Postoperative noncardiac surgery patients who seem to do well
- Renal failure
- Critically ill patients, especially with diabetes, respiratory failure, gastrointestinal bleeding, sepsis
- Drug toxicity, e.g., adriamycin, 5-fluorouracil, herceptin, snake venoms, carbon monoxide poisoning
- Hypothyroidism
- Abnormalities in coronary vasomotion, including coronary vasospasm
- Apical ballooning syndrome
- Inflammatory diseases, e.g., myocarditis, parvovirus B19, Kawasaki disease, sarcoid, smallpox vaccination, or myocardial extension of BE
- Post-PCI patients who appear to be uncomplicated
- Pulmonary embolism, severe pulmonary hypertension
- Sepsis
- Burns, especially if total surface burn area (TBSA) > 30%
- Infiltrative diseases including amyloidosis, hemochromatosis, sarcoidosis, and scleroderma
- Acute neurological disease, including cerebrovascular accident, subarachnoid bleeds
- Rhabdomyolysis with cardiac injury
- Transplant vasculopathy
- Vital exhaustion

Table from "Troponin: the biomarker of choice for the detection of cardiac injury." – Reprinted from *CMAJ* 08-Nov-05; 173 (10), Pages 1191–1202 by permission of the publisher. © 2005 Canadian Medical Association.

The technical characteristics of cardiac troponin assays are an important consideration for both clinicians and laboratorians. These groups should collaborate to fully understand the cardiac troponin assay(s) run at local institution(s). One important factor is the precision of the test at the diagnostic cutpoint, i.e., the 99th percentile of the reference control population. In accordance with guidelines, cardiac troponin assays have been moving toward a total imprecision, represented by the total coefficient of variation (%CV) of ≤10% at the 99th percentile normal reference limit [4]. Another point is that troponin and other biomarker assays must be characterized with respect to potential interferences that may cause either false-positive or false-negative results. Potential interferences include rheumatoid factor(s), human anti-mouse antibodies, heterophile antibodies, and other related proteins that can interfere with immunoassays [4]. Preanalytical assay characteristics that should be established include acceptable specimen type and stability of the measurements over time and across temperature ranges. Identification of antibody/epitope/recognition sites for each biomarker is also important; assays should target certain epitopes on the troponin molecule, such as the stable 41–49 amino acid region of troponin I that is less susceptible to interferences. The International Federation for Clinical Chemistry's Committee for the Standardization of Markers Cardiac Damage recently published updated specifications for cardiac markers [6]. Clinicians should work with laboratory medicine staff to assure that performance of their cardiac troponin assay remains stable over time. One strategy for helping to assure stability is performing routine quality control in the relevant measurement concentration range; this includes routine quality control at low troponin concentrations where clinical decisions are made.

Early Risk Stratification

A cTnT or cTnI level is also the preferred marker for risk stratification and should be measured in all patients with suspected acute coronary syndrome [1]. A large body of evidence clearly indicates that cardiac troponin increases indicate a high-risk profile in patients with clinical characteristics consistent with acute coronary syndrome. Patients with elevated troponin levels are about threefold higher compared to similarly presenting patients without elevated troponin [1]. Importantly, the prognostic information obtained from cardiac troponin measurement is independent of and complementary to other important clinical indicators of risk including patient age, ST deviation, and presence of heart failure [1,5–10]. Also, a meta-analysis demonstrated that patients presenting with normal concentrations of CK-MB but increased troponin were at increased risk [11]; this evidence further demonstrated the superiority of cardiac troponin as a biomarker in acute coronary syndromes. cTnT and cTnI appear to have similar value for risk assessment in acute coronary syndromes [12].

The troponin concentration that confers increased risk of death and recurrent ischemic risk among patients with a compelling clinical history suggesting acute coronary syndromes was determined to be very low, near the upper limit of the normal or detectable range [10,13–15]. These data, in part, provided strong justification for setting the MI cutpoint at the 99th percentile of the reference control population. Like recommendations for MI diagnosis, the cutpoint for designating a high-risk profile is a maximal (peak) concentration exceeding the 99th percentile of values for a reference control group [1]. Also, blood for testing should be collected on hospital presentation followed by serial specimens with timing of sampling based on the clinical circumstances. For most patients, blood should be obtained for testing at hospital presentation and at 6–9 hours, but later samples should be obtained if concern remains [1].

Clinical Decision Making

Several therapies have been shown to improve outcomes in patients who have positive cTnT or cTnI values, whereas treated patients who are cardiac troponin negative do not show improved outcomes. Thus an increased concentration of cardiac troponin should prompt consideration of management guidelines for patients with indicators of high risk and a clinical history consistent with acute coronary syndromes [16].

An early invasive management strategy has demonstrated benefit in patients who are cardiac troponin positive at presentation. Evidence showed a ~55% reduction in the odds of death or MI when a strategy of early angiography (within 4–48 hours) and revascularization (when appropriate) was used in cardiac troponin-positive acute coronary syndrome patients compared with a conservative management strategy [17]. Thus patient outcomes can be improved when an elevated concentration of troponin at presentation is used to guide utilization of early angiography and revascularization if appropriate [1,17].

Glycoprotein IIb/IIIa (GP IIb/IIIa) receptor inhibition has also shown to be an effective therapy when administered in the 24 hours before percutaneous intervention in troponin-positive acute coronary syndrome patients [18]. Various GPIIb/IIIa receptor antagonists all appear to demonstrate similar results: a 70% relative reduction in the risk of death or MI compared to troponin-positive patients treated with placebo [18]. On the other hand, troponin-negative patients treated with GPIIb/IIIa receptor antagonists showed no improved outcome compared with placebo therapy [18]. Using positive cardiac troponin results as an aid in guiding initiation of GPIIb/IIIa therapy in the 24 hours before intervention can improve patient outcomes.

Anti-thrombotic therapy with low-molecular weight heparin therapy has also been shown to benefit patients with a positive cardiac troponin level [1,19]. Patients with an increased serum concentration of cTnI at presentation showed a 50% reduction in death, MI, or recurrent ischemia when treated with enoxaparin compared to unfractionated heparin [1]. In contrast, for patients who were cardiac troponin negative at presentation, enoxaparin showed no demonstrable advantage compared to unfractionated heparin [1]. Thus positive cardiac troponin results can help effectively guide continuation of low-molecular weight heparin therapy in acute coronary syndrome patients.

CK-MB Measurement

Prior to the era of troponin, CK-MB isoenzyme measurement was considered the "gold standard" biomarker for MI diagnosis. In the 1970s and early 1980s, CK-MB was predominantly performed by electrophoresis and other "activity" assays that were based on measuring the enzymatic ability of CK-MB to function in converting substrate to product. These enzyme activity assays were relatively insensitive, imprecise, and depended on CK-MB maintaining its functional ability to convert substrate to product. In the mid-1980s, improved CK-MB "mass" assays became widely available that had superior performance and stability characteristics. The term "mass" is used because these assays measure the CK-MB isoenzyme as a protein by immunoassay, rather than depending on the isoenzyme's functional activity. Recent guidelines state that CK-MB activity assays are an anachronism and should not be used as a biomarker for the diagnosis of MI [1]. These same guidelines state that CK-MB "mass" measurements are an acceptable alternative when cardiac troponin is not available [1]. On occasions when CK-MB mass is measured, serial sampling is necessary with measurement at patient presentation and then sample timing based on the clinical circumstances. For most patients, blood should be obtained for testing at hospital presentation and at 6–9 hours. The cutpoint for CK-MB is the 99th percentile of values for a sex-specific reference control group on two successive samples, with a rise and/or fall in levels of the marker necessary to make the MI diagnosis [1].

As a practical matter, the same technology is used to measure CK-MB mass as is used to measure cardiac troponin. Thus virtually all platforms that measure CK-MB mass also measure cardiac troponin; for this reason, cTnT or cTnI is always available and should be used instead of CK-MB mass as the preferred marker for MI diagnosis, risk stratification, and guiding management.

It is noteworthy that measurement of more than one specific biomarker of myocardial necrosis (e.g., cardiac troponin and CK-MB) is not necessary for establishing the diagnosis of MI and is not recommended. As stated above, a meta-analysis demonstrated that patients presenting with normal concentrations of CK-MB but increased troponin were at increased risk [11], demonstrating the superiority of cardiac troponin as a biomarker in acute coronary syndromes. CK-MB mass measurements in the emergency department have been steadily decreasing in the past few years and will continue to do so with increased utilization of cTnT or cTnI.

Myoglobin

In the 1980s and 1990s, myoglobin measurements were put forward as a valuable diagnostic tool for the early diagnosis or rule out of MI because its release was earlier than CK-MB and first-generation cardiac troponin assays. There has always been a fundamental problem with myoglobin measurements because the protein is present in high concentrations in both skeletal muscle and myocardial tissue. Therefore, blood increases of the protein are not cardiac specific. However, because of its small molecular size and consequent rapid rise after myocardial necrosis, myoglobin retained value mainly as an early rule-out marker of MI, and the combined use of myoglobin and more specific markers of myocardial necrosis (cardiac troponin or CK-MB) was claimed to be useful for the early exclusion of MI [20]. With improvements in the precision and detection limits of cardiac troponin assays, utilization of myoglobin has fallen out of favor. Recent guidelines address myoglobin's possible use along with a cardiac troponin as an early marker in patients who present within 6 hours of the onset of symptoms; the NACB includes a weak Class IIb recommendation for considering measurement [1]. Even this weak recommendation probably overstates the diagnostic value of myoglobin in the context of acute coronary syndrome. As a result, the protein is rarely measured except as a compulsory part of a panel with cardiac troponin. With the improvement of cardiac troponin assays and recommended use of the 99th percentile as the cutpoint for MI diagnosis and risk stratification, myoglobin measurement is now an anachronism.

Ischemia and Risk Stratification Markers

Although cardiac troponin is a cornerstone of biomarker testing and should be measured in all patients suspected of having an acute coronary syndrome, it is a marker of necrosis and can only indicate an increased risk profile in patients for whom cardiac tissue has undergone irreversible injury. It is well documented that patients with acute coronary syndromes who are troponin negative are still at about $\sim$7% increased risk of adverse events in the 6 months after initial presentation [10,21]. Markers of cardiac ischemia or other mechanisms are of potential value because about 40–60% of the acute coronary syndrome continua do not have necrosis [22], so other indicators of increased risk may add information to cardiac troponin and the ECG. Markers of cardiac ischemia or other mechanisms have been an area of intense investigation and a litany of biochemical markers have been suggested as ischemia markers and risk stratification tools. Various candidate markers have been reviewed recently [23], and a few promising markers will be specifically discussed here.

Ischemia-Modified Albumin

Oxidative stress and other physiological processes that occur during myocardial ischemia reportedly cause modifications in circulating albumin; the resulting modified albumin form has been coined "ischemia-modified albumin" (IMA) and has diminished capacity for binding cobalt and other metals [24]. This observation led to the development of an albumin cobalt binding test for the measurement of IMA, and therefore the presence (or absence) of myocardial ischemia. The albumin cobalt binding test for IMA was FDA cleared as a serum biomarker of cardiac ischemia and risk stratification tool in suspected acute coronary syndrome patients. One proposed use is for consideration of discharge patients for whom the ECG is nondiagnostic for ischemia, cardiac troponin is negative, and the IMA test is also negative.

A meta-analysis was conducted that included all studies evaluating the sensitivity and negative predictive value (NPV) of IMA in suspected acute coronary syndromes patients evaluated in an ED [25]. This analysis showed that using three indicators together – an ECG that is nondiagnostic for ischemia, a negative cardiac troponin, and a negative IMA test – yielded a sensitivity of 94.4% and an NPV of 97.1% for diagnosis of acute coronary syndrome [25]. The respective sensitivity and NPV for longer term outcomes were 89.2 and 94.5% [25].

Although the clinical evidence for IMA indicates promise for use in ruling out acute coronary syndromes and early risk stratification in the ED, a number of issues regarding utilization remain. For example, positive IMA results have not been demonstrated to discriminate between unstable angina and cardiac necrosis. Thus how to interpret a positive IMA is incompletely elucidated. A study designed to evaluate the test in a decision-making algorithm would add insight into its clinical use. Despite these limitations, it has been suggested that IMA may be considered for use in conjunction with the ECG and cardiac troponin for the exclusion of suspected acute coronary syndromes in patients with a low clinical probability [1].

Myeloperoxidase

Myeloperoxidase (MPO) is an enzyme that catalyzes the in vivo production of hypochlorite (bleach) from chloride and hydrogen peroxide; MPO is stored in abundant quantities in the azurophilic granules of polymorphonuclear neutrophils and macrophages. The hypochlorite product of MPO must be viewed as both a physiological friend and a foe. MPO is a friend because the enzyme is released during the inflammatory response, presumably because hypochlorite's highly caustic properties are essential for resolving infections and in clearing damaged tissue after injury. MPO is viewed as a foe because its hypochlorite product is involved in oxidizing LDL and may be an active player in destabilizing coronary plaque by degrading collagen, which is particularly troublesome when it occurs at the vulnerable plaque shoulder. This degradation can lead to plaque erosion and increased susceptibility for rupture, an important root cause of acute coronary syndromes.

Several studies have demonstrated that acute coronary syndrome patients having increased MPO in their blood are at increased risk [23,26,27]. One study conducted in the ED environment showed that the odds of major adverse events at 30 days and 6 months increased with each quartile increase in MPO blood concentration. Importantly, this increase in risk was 4.4-fold higher in patients who had elevated MPO but were persistently negative for cardiac troponin [27].

There is currently one MPO assay that has achieved FDA clearance as an aid for risk stratification in suspected acute coronary syndrome patients. Caution is advised because MPO assays for measurement are not standardized; some measure the functional enzymatic activity, while others utilize immunoassay technology to measure MPO as a protein. MPO increases are not necessarily indicative of ischemia, but are also increased in infectious, inflammatory, and infiltrative disease processes. Nonetheless, in light of the promising data that have been published of MPO, it may be anticipated that several manufacturers will have assays available on automated platforms in the near future.

High-Sensitivity C-Reactive Protein

Atherosclerosis is an inflammatory process and the inflammatory response is believed to represent an important contributor to plaque instability [28]. Perturbation of the vascular endothelium, as well as the maturation of atheromatous plaque, clearly involves inflammatory processes that can ultimately compromise the protective fibrous cap that separates the procoagulant contents of the plaque's core and circulating platelets and coagulation proteins. Although other proteins involved in the inflammatory response, including MPO, serum amyloid A, IL-6 and other cytokines, and cellular adhesion molecules, have been examined as risk indicators for acute coronary syndrome, the robust acute-phase protein CRP has been the focus of clinical investigation [29].

CRP has been shown to rise in patients presenting with acute coronary syndrome as a consequence of the inflammatory response to myocardial necrosis [30]. However, elevated levels of CRP are also frequent in a large proportion of ED patients without myocardial necrosis, and the precise basis for the relationship between inflammatory markers and increased risk in acute coronary syndrome patients has not been conclusively established [1]. Numerous studies have indicated that hs-CRP is an independent predictor of short- and/or long-term outcome among patients with acute coronary syndrome [1]. Specifically, measurement of hs-CRP appears to contribute additional prognostic value in patients who are cardiac troponin negative [31,32]. Of interest, studies indicate that the relationship between hs-CRP and outcome is most robust with respect to mortality with a weaker relationship to recurrent MI [1,32].

Measurement of hs-CRP may be useful, in addition to a cardiac troponin, for risk assessment in patients with suspected acute coronary syndrome [1]. However, the benefits of therapy based on hs-CRP remain uncertain and guidance of management should not be based solely upon measurement of CRP [1].

B-Type Natriuretic Peptide and N-Terminal proBNP

BNP is a heart hormone that has powerful physiological effects including natriuresis, vasodilatation, and inhibition of the renin–angiotensin–aldosterone system [33]. Ischemia appears to be an important stimulus for B-type natriuretic peptide (BNP) synthesis and release [34]. BNP and its inert cometabolite amino-terminal proBNP (NT-proBNP) are released from cardiac myocytes in response to hemodynamic stress and specifically increased wall stress in the ventricles of the heart [35]. Impairment of ventricular relaxation and resulting nonsystolic ventricular dysfunction is one of the earliest consequences of myocardial ischemia, preceding angina and ST-segment deviation. This pathophysiology and a strong association between BNP and NT-proBNP with mortality in patients with unstable angina support the idea that cardiac ischemia can stimulate release of BNP in the absence of necrosis [36].

A strong relationship between BNP or NT-proBNP and outcomes in patients with acute coronary syndrome in the absence of necrosis has been shown in numerous studies [1,37]. In patients with acute MI, elevated levels of BNP and NT-proBNP have been shown to predict a greater likelihood of death or heart failure, independent of other prognostic variables [1,38,39]. In general, plasma concentrations rise rapidly and peak at approximately 24 hours after infarction. When measured ∼40 hours after presentation, a highly significant relationship between BNP and subsequent risk of mortality was observed [40], where the rate of death ranged from <1% among patients with BNP concentrations in the lowest quartile to 15% in those with a BNP concentration in the highest quartile ($p<0.0001$) [40]. This finding has been confirmed in multiple studies of both BNP and NT-proBNP [1] including substudies of clinical trials and observational data from community-based cohorts. It is noteworthy that BNP and NT-proBNP can help identify patients without systolic dysfunction or signs of heart failure who are at higher risk of death and heart failure and provide prognostic information that is complementary to cardiac troponin [1].

Measurement of BNP or NT-proBNP may be a useful addition to a cardiac troponin for risk assessment in patients with a clinical syndrome consistent with acute coronary syndromes [1]. However, the benefits of therapy based on BNP and NT-proBNP measurements remain uncertain, so application of management guidelines for acute coronary syndromes should not be based solely upon BNP or NT-proBNP values [1].

Future Development

It is be viewed as disappointing to many in the cardiac marker field that no ischemia marker that is specific for heart tissue has yet been identified. Many biomarkers discussed in a recent review have been associated with increased risk of adverse events [23], rather than indicators of myocardial ischemia. Many of these markers have good NPV; high NPV can be a valuable characteristic, for example, in the wayD-dimer is used for ruling out pulmonary embolism in low-risk ED patients [41]. However, the most important use of any biomarker is for the guidance of patient management, an issue that none of the ischemia markers adequately address at the current time. Perhaps the most promising use of these rather nonspecific markers is in combinations, focusing on various pathophysiological mechanisms of the acute coronary syndromes. The use of any biomarker combinations must be carefully validated to assure that they actually add useful information to what is available with cardiac troponin, the ECG, and clinical characteristics.

Because no biomarker of ischemia or risk stratification is cardiac specific, attention has turned to the measurement of very low troponin concentrations, i.e., assays that are able to measure troponin reliably at concentrations 10- to 100-fold lower than the best conventional troponin assays. These very low troponin assays can detect an increasing pattern in cardiac troponin that is well below the 99th percentile of the reference control population. This may allow identification of small amounts of myocardial injury that may be associated with cardiac ischemia and unstable angina. Thus more effective risk stratification and perhaps even diagnosis of unstable angina could be possible. There are a couple of companies that have focused on the development of "hypersensitive" cardiac troponin assays; these companies are Singulex (Alameda, CA) and Nanosphere (Northbrook, IL). More activity in the developing hypersensitive troponin assays can be expected.

Point-of-Care Testing for Cardiac Biomarkers

Point-of-care testing (POCT) involves measurement of cardiac biomarkers at or near the patient bedside. Implementation of POCT for any clinical application is always driven by a "need for speed" that exceeds a central laboratory's ability to deliver information in time to improve either clinical or economic outcomes. POCT testing is invariably more costly than central lab testing and is encumbered by regulatory requirements. POCT is typically considered an option of last resort because virtually all organizations would prefer to measure cardiac markers within the infrastructure of the central laboratory, rather than going through all the trouble and expense of implementing POCT. Although the need for a rapid turnaround time for cardiac troponin has not been linked to improve clinical outcomes [42], faster results have been shown to facilitate patient flow and expedite decision making [43]. Current guidelines strongly recommend that cardiac marker results be available within 1 hour and optimally within 30 minutes of collection for care of patients in the ED [44]. The turnaround time should be measured from sample collection to reporting of the result to a responsible caregiver. Furthermore, institutions that are unable to consistently deliver cardiac marker results within 1 hour should implement POCT [44].

The following discussion is based directly on recommendations relating to POCT that are specified in recent guidelines from the NACB (http://www. aacc.org/SiteCollectionDocuments/NACB/LMPG/acute_heart/ACS_PDF_ chapter5.pdf, accessed June 14, 2008). To decide if implementing POCT is necessary, stakeholders in the ED, hospital administrators, and the clinical laboratory should work together to develop an accelerated protocol for the provision of biochemical markers in the evaluation of patients with possible acute coronary syndromes. In most institutions, the laboratory will have the responsibility for POCT or satellite testing in the ED area; therefore, laboratory personnel must be involved in the selection and maintenance of testing devices, assuring the competency of testing individuals, and the ongoing documentation of monitoring compliance with regulatory requirements.

Although turnaround time is frequently the focus for cardiac marker testing, the quality of these tests themselves, in particular troponin, must not be compromised by performance outside the central lab. Thus the specifications and characteristics of POCT and central laboratory testing must be the same and should yield similar results. In situations where the POCT system and central laboratory results differ substantially, these data should be listed separately in the patient record with different interpretive information to minimize the possibility of medical error when patients change locations. While it is recognized that qualitative systems can provide useful information, quantitative results are strongly preferred at POC.

Establishing and maintaining a strong multidisciplinary collaboration between ED staff, laboratory medicine, cardiology, primary care physicians, and hospital administration is important for the use of quality assurance measures, implantation of evidence-based guidelines and measures to reduce medical error and improve the treatment of patients with possible acute coronary syndromes. An important part of this collaboration is assuring provision of cardiac troponin and other biomarker information that is both timely and accurate. A most effective means for accomplishing this goal is focused interaction between clinicians and the clinical laboratory for understanding the details of local cardiac troponin testing.

Clinical Confounders for Biomarker Testing

There are numerous clinical conditions that can confound, modulate, or limit the use of cardiac biomarkers for the assessment of suspected acute coronary syndrome patients. As stated earlier, there is no evidence that cTnT or cTnI is released from tissues other than myocardium. Therefore, cardiac troponin concentrations exceeding the 99th percentile of a reference population should be considered reflective of myocardial damage. As discussed below, not all increases in cardiac troponin are due to an ischemic etiology nor do they all reflect an acute coronary event. Prevalent conditions that may be confounders are discussed in this section. It is important to remember that whenever biomarker results are incongruous with the clinical scenario, clinicians should contact laboratory medicine staff.

Renal Insufficiency and End-Stage Renal Disease

Many end-stage renal disease (ESRD) patients have increases in cardiac troponin. Rather than a benign confounder, these cardiac troponin increases represent myocardial damage that may be acute, chronic, or have components of both. Discriminating between chronic and acute injury in the ED is important because each confers a different risk profile. A key difference between the patterns is that acute damage is associated with a dynamic change in cTnT or cTnI and is consistent with a diagnosis of MI [45]. Acute cardiac troponin increases can be discriminated from chronic elevations by the presence of the $\geq 20\%$ rising pattern in the 6–9 hours after presentation [46,47]. Such an increase represents a significant (three standard deviation) change in troponin based on the typical 5–7% analytical CV within the MI concentration range for most assays. ESRD patients who have a dynamic increase in cardiac troponin are a high-risk cohort, having about a threefold increase in mortality compared to similar patients without renal failure [48]. Given the prognostic importance of acute troponin increases, it has been suggested that the use of acute pharmacologic or invasive interventions in standard clinical guidelines is appropriate for ESRD patients with evidence of cardiac ischemia and increased cardiac troponin [49].

Chronically increased cardiac troponin in ESRD patients has also been identified as a predictor of worse prognosis. Of interest, the incidence of abnormal values in ESRD cohorts is considerably higher for cTnT (82%) than for cTnI (5–15%) depending on the assay [50]. Both cTnT and cTnI are predictive of risk in ESRD; however, cTnI is less useful on a routine basis because of the lower frequency of events in patients with increased values and the risk conferred by these results [51]. On the other hand, increased concentrations of cTnT are strongly associated with diffuse coronary artery disease and an independent predictor of death [50,51]. The FDA has recently cleared cTnT as a biomarker for risk stratification of all-cause mortality in ESRD patients. This use of cTnT is endorsed by the Kidney Disease Outcomes Quality Initiative [46]; however in the absence of myocardial ischemia, there are no specific therapeutic interventions known to reduce cardiovascular risk in these ESRD patients.

Recent NACB guidelines state that in renal failure patients with symptoms (e.g., acute chest pain), ECG or other clinical evidence suggesting myocardial ischemia, measurement of cardiac troponin is warranted for the evaluation of MI [52]. Also, as for all patients, ESRD patients who may have baseline elevations of cardiac troponin, who present with possible acute coronary syndrome, relying on dynamic changes in the cTn values of 20% or more should be used to define those with acute MI [52]. cTnT has been cleared by the FDA as an aid for defining the risk of mortality in ESRD patients [51].

Blunt Chest Trauma

Cardiac troponin appears to be a sensitive indicator of myocardial damage due to blunt chest trauma. A recent meta-analysis addressed the question of whether cardiac troponin can be used as a good indicator of underlying cardiac damage after chest trauma [53]. The meta-analysis included six studies of blunt chest trauma in which myocardial contusion was suspected. Unfortunately there is no gold standard for the diagnosis of myocardial contusion, so it was difficult to assess cardiac troponin and more modern methods for detecting cardiac injury. Nonetheless, the authors state that the diagnostic window for myocardial contusion appears to be smaller and occurs earlier in blunt chest trauma compared to that seen in MI [53]. It was suggested that samples for cardiac troponin measurement should be collected at presentation and then at 4–6 hours. Overall, an abnormal troponin concentration seems to be a good indicator of cardiac damage [53].

Pulmonary Embolism

Patients with the diagnosis of pulmonary emboli (PE) and increased cardiac troponin have a worse prognosis. It was demonstrated that when cTnI was ≤ 0.6 µg/L in PE patients, mortality was 4.8% versus 36% for cTnI>0.6 µg/L [54]. For cTnT, in-hospital mortality was 44% among PE patients who had levels >0.1 µg/L versus 3% among those who had the level >0.1 µg/L [55]. The therapeutic strategy for treating PE patients with increased troponin is not clear. However, it is important to recognize the diagnosis of PE, since mortality among troponin-positive PE patients is substantially higher than that among acute MI patients, except those in cardiogenic shock [52].

Chemotherapy

Cardiac troponin can be increased in patients undergoing chemotherapy that is known to damage heart tissue; one such therapy is the anthracyclines. Evidence shows that troponin-positive results in chemotherapy patients confer increased risk for developing heart failure [56]. Recent studies suggest that treatment with angiotensin-converting enzyme inhibitors dramatically reduces the frequency of heart failure in patients with an increased cardiac troponin [57]. Although it is recognized that troponin is released during chemotherapy and that positive individuals are at increased risk for the development of congestive heart failure, routine troponin measurements are not recommended for patients undergoing chemotherapies that are toxic to the heart, with the exception of patients receiving adriamycin [52].

Recent Cardiac Procedures

The occurrence of periprocedural myocardial damage has been the subject of debate since the inception of coronary intervention over 30 years ago. The reported incidence of cardiac troponin release, i.e., periprocedural damage, following percutaneous intervention varies widely, from 14 to 48% [52]. Contributors to this variation include the troponin assay used and corresponding cutoffs, the underlying indication for the revascularization procedure, the type of procedure performed, as well as other factors in individual patients. Studies have consistently shown that postprocedural increases in troponin and/or CK-MB are associated with major adverse clinical events and that even minor increases in CK-MB are associated with increased 6-month mortality [58]. While the exact mechanism remains to be elucidated, decreased tissue perfusion may be responsible in patients with high postprocedural cardiac troponin value, and may be the explanation for the increased incidence of adverse cardiac events [52].

There is controversy and doubt regarding the interpretation of periprocedural cardiac injury, mainly because many studies did not measure the baseline troponin values before procedures. Recent data suggest that it may actually be the preprocedure troponin value that defines risk rather than the interventional procedure itself. Evidence for this point is shown by analyses that demonstrate that the prognostic significance of postprocedure troponin values disappears after correcting for the preprocedure (baseline) troponin level [52].

In the absence of an acute myocardial event, a valid means for assessing periprocedural injury includes measurement of cTnT and cTnI before and after percutaneous coronary intervention to determine the presence of ischemic cardiac damage. This holds so long as the baseline preprocedural value is less than the established 99th percentile [52]. Although any increase should be considered as indicating cardiac damage, the specific cardiac troponin cutoff concentrations indicating increased risk have not been established.

Similar principles should be applied for CK-MB, whose rise may not be detected due to its lower sensitivity. The baseline CK-MB value predicts subsequent risk. Although earlier guidance was to use a threefold increase [59], the European Society of Cardiology (ESC) Task Force on Invasive Cardiology recommends a CK-MB cutoff concentration of five times the upper limit of normal [60].

Reinfarction

Serial measurements of biomarkers are important for demonstrating the characteristic rise and fall that aids in the diagnosis of MI. After the diagnosis of acute MI is confirmed, serial measures can also be useful for identifying ongoing or recurrent myocardial ischemia that causes reinfarction. In patients where recurrent MI is suspected from clinical signs and symptoms, immediate sample for biomarker measurement should be collected [1].

According to NACB guidelines, CK-MB is the preferred marker for the detection of reinfarction early after the index event when the concentration of cardiac troponin is still increasing [1]. Clearly, rises in cardiac troponin are demonstrable in cases of early reinfarction and recent data suggest that troponin values may provide similar information to CK-MB [2]. However, the scope of available evidence is significantly limited compared with that of CK-MB [1]. In addition, differences among cTnI methods have not been studied and could be substantial; also, cTnT is known to exhibit a bimodal distribution in its kinetics. Serial testing is typically necessary to discriminate a new increasing pattern of troponin if the concentration is not known to have returned to normal. Because CK-MB falls to the normal range by 48–72 hours after uncomplicated MI, it may aid in the rapid discrimination of reinfarction when symptoms recur between 72 hours and 2 weeks after the index MI, whereas troponin may still be elevated from the initial cardiac event. Measurement of CK-MB in conjunction with troponin may also be useful in determining the timing of recent MI [1,2]. Further investigation on troponin kinetics, with concurrent evaluation of troponin and CK-MB for the diagnosis of early reinfarction, is warranted. Data directly comparing these biomarkers for detection of reinfarction are few, and future studies may help guide deliberation as to whether CK-MB should continue to have a role in the routine care of patients with acute MI. A recurrent infarction is diagnosed if there is a greater than 20% increase in the second sample, which is equivalent to exceeding three SDs for most troponin assays; the value must also exceed the 99th percentile for indicating reinfarction.

The value of necrosis biomarkers for discriminating very early reinfarction (e.g., <18 hours) is limited, because the concentration of these markers is typically still increasing [52]. Routine serial acquisition of "surveillance" sampling for biomarkers of necrosis after they have returned to the normal range from the index event is not recommended [52].

Panels

In the past, frequent early testing of cardiac troponin and/or CK-MB, particularly in combination with myoglobin, was examined and forwarded as a valid approach for the early detection MI and to facilitate rapid initiation of treatment. This strategy has also shown value in some studies for expedited exclusion of MI [61], as was the use of the change in necrosis markers repeated over an interval of 2 hours [61,62,63]. Although some authors have advocated a rapid "rule-in" protocol with frequent early sampling using cardiac troponin and other markers of myocardial necrosis, this approach is not favored in guidelines but may be appropriate if tied to therapeutic strategies [1]. In light of the redefinition of MI, the accumulation of evidence for risk stratification, and the development of more sensitive assays for cardiac troponin, the use of panels that include myoglobin and CK-MB must be revisited to examine their actual added value. It is suspected that this added value will be modest at best.

A new era of multimarker panels that include biomarkers that reflect the pathogenesis and consequences of acute coronary syndromes may be of use for classification and individualization of treatment [64]. Accumulating evidence indicates that a multimarker strategy that includes a pathobiologically diverse set of biomarkers adds to biomarkers of necrosis for risk assessment [65]. To date, the majority of evidence regarding this strategy entails newer markers paired with troponin, and hs-CRP and BNP or NT-proBNP are the most extensively studied. As new markers and therapies are discovered, a multimarker paradigm employing a combination of biomarkers for risk assessment and clinical decision making has the potential to improve outcomes for patients with acute coronary syndromes [65].

Future Developments

In the context of cardiac necrosis and MI, few analytes in laboratory medicine have the clinical value and impact of cTnT and cTnI. After all, cardiac troponin was mainly responsible for the redefinition of MI [2]. For this reason it is difficult to conceive of a marker to replace cardiac troponin for the diagnosis of MI.

For risk stratification, cardiac troponin, BNP or NT-proBNP, and other markers appear to provide independent and complementary information. Strategies for utilizing these markers clinically require further prospective validation. However, recommendations indicate that these markers may be of value. It is important to note that the real value of these markers will be when (if) their use can be shown to influence patient management and improve clinical and/or economic outcomes.

The quest for a cardiac-specific ischemia marker continues. Very high-sensitivity cardiac troponin assays that are capable of reliable 10- to 100-fold lower detection compared to current assays may be the path forward. Demonstrating that an acute rise in cardiac troponin is significantly higher than the sum of biological and analytical variation could lead to detection of very subtle cardiac injury and may be possible. Of course demonstrating that this rise has value in terms of outcomes will be necessary.

There has been a great deal of work in the fields of proteomics, metabolomics, and molecular diagnostics in the past few years. The products of these efforts have not yet impacted the services available to clinicians, but may do so in the near future. The acute coronary syndromes impact society from both humanistic and economic perspectives perhaps more than any other disease process and will remain a central focus for future diagnostic testing.

References

1. Morrow DA, Cannon CP, Jesse RL, Newby LK, Ravkilde J, Storrow AB, Wu AH, Christenson RH. National Academy of Clinical Biochemistry Laboratory Medicine Practice Guidelines: Clinical characteristics and utilization of biochemical markers in acute coronary syndromes. Circulation 2007;115:e356–75.
2. Thygesen K, Alpert JS, White HD. Universal definition of myocardial infarction. Circulation. 2007;116:2634–53.
3. Fleming SM, O'Byrne L, Finn J, Grimes H, Daly KM. False-positive cardiac troponin I in a routine clinical population. Am J Cardiol 2002;89:1212–5.
4. Apple FS, Jesse RL, Newby LK, Wu AH, Christenson RH. National Academy of Clinical Biochemistry and IFCC Committee for Standardization of Markers of Cardiac Damage Laboratory Medicine Practice Guidelines: Analytical issues for biochemical markers of acute coronary syndromes. Circulation 2007;115:e352–5.
5. Antman EM, Tanasijevic MJ, Thompson B, Schactman M, McCabe CH, Cannon CP, et al. Cardiac-specific troponin I levels to predict the risk of mortality in patients with acute coronary syndromes. N Engl J Med 1996;335:1342–9.
6. Mair J, Jaffe AS, Christenson RH, Wu AHB, Panteghini M, Ordonez J, Apple FS. Quality Specifications for Cardiac Troponin. Clin Chem 2008 (in press).
7. Ohman EM, Armstrong PW, Christenson RH, Granger CB, Katus HA, Hamm CW, et al. Cardiac troponin T levels for risk stratification in acute myocardial ischemia. GUSTO IIA Investigators. N Engl J Med 1996;335:1333–41.
8. Lindahl B, Venge P, Wallentin L. Relation between troponin T and the risk of subsequent cardiac events in unstable coronary artery disease. The FRISC study group. Circulation 1996;93:1651–7.
9. Morrow DA, Rifai N, Tanasijevic MJ, Wybenga DR, de Lemos JA, Antman EM. Clinical Efficacy of Three Assays for Cardiac Troponin I for Risk Stratification in Acute Coronary Syndromes: A Thrombolysis In Myocardial Infarction (TIMI) 11B Substudy. Clin Chem 2000;46:453–460.
10. Kaul P, Newby LK, Fu Y, Hasselblad V, Mahaffey KW, Christenson RH, et al. Troponin T and quantitative ST-segment depression offer complementary prognostic information in the risk stratification of acute coronary syndrome patients. J Am Coll Cardiol 2003;41:371–80.
11. Heidenreich PA, Alloggiamento T, Melsop K, McDonald KM, Go AS, Hlatky MA. The prognostic value of troponin in patients with non-ST elevation acute coronary syndromes: a meta-analysis. J Am Coll Cardiol 2001;38:478–85.
12. Morrow DA, Cannon CP, Rifai N, Frey MJ, Vicari R, Lakkis N, et al. Ability of minor elevations of troponin I and T to identify patients with unstable angina and non-ST

elevation myocardial infarction who benefit from an early invasive strategy: Results from a prospective, randomized trial. JAMA 2001;286:2405–2412.

13. Morrow DA, Antman EM, Tanasijevic M, Rifai N, de Lemos JA, McCabe CH, et al. Cardiac troponin I for stratification of early outcomes and the efficacy of enoxaparin in unstable angina: a TIMI 11B substudy. J Am Coll Cardiol 2000;36:1812–7.

14. Morrow DA, Cannon CP, Rifai N, Frey MJ, Vicari R, Lakkis N, et al. Ability of minor elevations of troponin I and T to identify patients with unstable angina and non-ST elevation myocardial infarction who benefit from an early invasive strategy: Results from a prospective, randomized trial. JAMA 2001;286:2405–2412.

15. Venge P, Lagerqvist B, Diderholm E, Lindahl B, Wallentin L. Clinical performance of three cardiac troponin assays in patients with unstable coronary artery disease (a FRISC II substudy). Am J Cardiol 2002;89:1035–41.

16. Braunwald E, Antman EM, Beasley JW, Califf RM, Cheitlin MD, Hochman JS, et al. ACC/AHA 2002 guideline update for the management of patients with unstable angina and non-ST-segment elevation myocardial infarction– summary article: a report of the American College of Cardiology/American Heart Association task force on practice guidelines (Committee on the Management of Patients With Unstable Angina). J Am Coll Cardiol 2002;40:1366–74.

17. Morrow DA, Cannon CP, Rifai N, Frey MJ, Vicari R, Lakkis N, et al. Ability of minor elevations of troponin I and T to identify patients with unstable angina and non-ST elevation myocardial infarction who benefit from an early invasive strategy: Results from a prospective, randomized trial. JAMA 2001;286:2405–2412

18. Kong DF, Califf RM, Miller DP, Moliterno DJ, White HD, Harrington RA et al. Clinical outcomes of therapeutic agents that block the platelet glycoprotein IIb/IIIa integrin in ischemic heart disease. Circulation 1998;98:2829–35.

19. Lindahl B, Venge P, Wallentin L. Troponin T identifies patients with unstable coronary artery disease who benefit from long-term antithrombotic protection. Fragmin in Unstable Coronary Artery Disease (FRISC) Study Group. J Am Coll Cardiol 1997;29:43–8.

20. Kontos MC, Anderson FP, Hanbury CM, Roberts CS, Miller WG, Jesse RL. Use of the combination of myoglobin and CK-MB mass for the rapid diagnosis of acute myocardial infarction. Am J Emerg Med 1997;15:14–9.

21. Morrow DA, de Lemos JA, Sabatine MS, Murphy SA, Demopoulos L, DiBattiste P, et al. Evaluation of B-type natriuretic peptide for risk assessment in unstable angina/ non-ST elevation MI: BNP and prognosis in TACTICS-TIMI 18. J Am Coll Cardiol 2003;41:1264–1272.

22. Morrow DA, Rifai N, Tanasijevic MJ, Wybenga DR, de Lemos JA, Antman EM. Clinical Efficacy of Three Assays for Cardiac Troponin I for Risk Stratification in Acute Coronary Syndromes: A Thrombolysis In Myocardial Infarction (TIMI) 11B Substudy. Clin Chem 2000;46:453–460.

23. Apple FS, Wu AH, Mair J, Ravkilde J, Panteghini M, Tate J et al. Future biomarkers for detection of ischemia and risk stratification in acute coronary syndrome. Clin Chem 2005;51:810–24.

24. Bar-Or D, Lau E, Winkler JV. A novel assay for cobalt-albumin binding and its potential as a marker for myocardial ischemia-a preliminary report. J Emerg Med 2000;19:311–5.

25. Peacock F, Morris DL, Anwaruddin S, Christenson RH, Collinson PO, Goodacre SW, et al. Meta-analysis of ischemia-modified albumin to rule out acute coronary syndromes in the emergency department. Am Heart J. 2006;152:253–62.

26. Baldus S, Heeschen C, Meinertz T, Zeiher AM, Eiserich JP, Münzel T et al. Myeloperoxidase serum levels predict risk in patients with acute coronary syndromes. Circulation 2003; 108:1440–5.

27. Brennan ML, Penn MS, Van Lente F, Nambi V, Shishehbor MH, Aviles RJ et al. Prognostic value of myeloperoxidase in patients with chest pain. N Engl J Med 2003;349: 1595–604.

28. Libby P, Ridker PM, Maseri A. Inflammation and atherosclerosis. Circulation 2002;105: 1135–43.
29. Liuzzo G, Biasucci LM, Gallimore JR, Grillo RL, Rebuzzi AG, Pepys MB, et al. The prognostic value of C-reactive protein and serum amyloid a protein in severe unstable angina. N Engl J Med 1994;331:417–24.
30. Pietila K, Hermens WT, Harmoinen A, Baardman T, Pasternack A, Topol EJ, et al. Comparison of peak serum C-reactive protein and hydroxybutyrate dehydrogenase levels in patients with acute myocardial infarction treated with alteplase and streptokinase. Am J Cardiol 1997;80:1075–7.
31. Lindahl B, Toss H, Siegbahn A, Venge P, Wallentin L. Markers of myocardial damage and inflammation in relation to long-term mortality in unstable coronary artery disease. FRISC Study Group. Fragmin during Instability in Coronary Artery Disease. N Engl J Med 2000;343:1139–47.
32. Morrow DA, Rifai N, Antman EM, Weiner DL, McCabe CH, Cannon CP, et al. C-reactive protein is a potent predictor of mortality independently of and in combination with troponin T in acute coronary syndromes: a TIMI 11A substudy. Thrombolysis in Myocardial Infarction. J Am Coll Cardiol 1998;31:1460–5.
33. Azzazy HM, Christenson RH. B-type natriuretic peptide: physiologic role and assay characteristics. Heart Fail Rev 2003;8:315–20.
34. Tateishi J, Masutani M, Ohyanagi M, Iwasaki T. Transient increase in plasma brain (B-type) natriuretic peptide after percutaneous transluminal coronary angioplasty. Clin Cardiol 2000;23:776–80.
35. de Lemos JA, McGuire DK, Drazner MH. B-type natriuretic peptide in cardiovascular disease. Lancet 2003;362:316–22.
36. e Lemos JA, Morrow DA. Brain natriuretic peptide measurement in acute coronary syndromes: ready for clinical application? Circulation 2002;106:2868–70.
37. Omland T, de Lemos JA, Morrow DA, Antman EM, Cannon CP, Hall C, et al. Prognostic Value of N-terminal Pro-Atrial and Pro-Brain Natriuretic Peptide in Patients with Acute Coronary Syndromes: A TIMI 11B substudy. Am J Cardiol 2002;89:463–465.
38. Arakawa N, Nakamura M, Aoki H, Hiramori K. Plasma brain natriuretic peptide concentrations predict survival after acute myocardial infarction. J Am Coll Cardiol 1996;27:1656–61.
39. Richards AM, Nicholls MG, Yandle TG, Frampton C, Espiner EA, Turner JG, et al. Plasma N-terminal pro-brain natriuretic peptide and adrenomedullin: new neurohormonal predictors of left ventricular function and prognosis after myocardial infarction. Circulation 1998;97:1921–9.
40. de Lemos JA, Morrow DA, Bentley JH, Omland T, Sabatine MS, McCabe CH, et al. The prognostic value of B-type natriuretic peptide in patients with acute coronary syndromes. N Engl J Med 2001;345:1014–21.
41. Stein PD, Hull RD, Patel KC, Olson RE, Ghali WA, Brant R, Biel RK, Bharadia V, Kalra NK. D-dimer for the exclusion of acute venous thrombosis and pulmonary embolism: a systematic review Ann Intern Med 2004;20;140:589–602.
42. Roe MT, Christenson RH, Ohman EM, Bahr R, Fesmire FM, Storrow A et al. A randomized, placebo-controlled trial of early eptifibatide for non-ST-segment elevation acute coronary syndromes. Am Heart J 2003;146:993–8.
43. Lee-Lewandrowski E, Corboy D, Lewandrowski K, Sinclair J, McDermot S, Benzer TI. Implementation of a point-of-care satellite laboratory in the emergency department of an academic medical center. Impact on test turnaround time and patient emergency department length of stay. Arch Pathol Lab Med 2003;127:456–60.
44. Nichols JH, Christenson RH, Clarke W, Gronowski A, Hammett-Stabler CA, Jacobs E et al. Executive summary. The National Academy of Clinical Biochemistry Laboratory Medicine Practice Guideline: evidence-based practice for point-of-care testing. Clin Chim Acta 2007;379:14–28.

45. McCullough PA, Nowack RM, Foreback C, Tokarski G, Tomianovich MC, Khoury KR, et al. Performance of multiple cardiac biomarkers measured in the emergency department in patients with chronic kidney disease and chest pain. Acad Emerg Med 2002;9:1389–96.
46. Kidney Disease Outcomes Quality Initiative. Clinical practice guidelines for cardiovascular disease in dialysis patients. Am J Kidney Dis 2005;45 (suppl 3): S1–S154.
47 Jaffe AS. Chasing troponin. How low can you go if you can see the rise? J Am Coll Cardiol 2006;48:1763–4.
48. Aviles RJ, Askari AT, Lindahl B, Wallentin L, Jia G, Ohman EM, et al. Troponin T levels in patients with acute coronary syndromes, with and without renal dysfunction. N Engl J Med 2002;346:2047–52.
49. Scirica BM, Morrow DA. Troponins in acute coronary syndromes. Prog Cardiovasc Dis 2004;47:177–88.
50. Apple FS, Murakami MM, Pearce LA, Herzog CA. Predictive value of cardiac troponin I and T for subsequent death in end-stage renal disease. Circulation 2002;106:941–5. 11.
51. deFilippi C, Wasserman S, Rosanio S, Tiblier E, Sperger H, Tocchi M, Christenson R, et al. Cardiac troponin T and C-reactive protein for predicting prognosis, coronary atherosclerosis, and cardiomyopathy in patients undergoing long-term hemodialysis. JAMA 2003;290:353–9.
52. Wu AH, Jaffe AS, Apple FS, Jesse RL, Francis GL, Morrow DA et al. National Academy of Clinical Biochemistry laboratory medicine practice guidelines: use of cardiac troponin and B-type natriuretic peptide or N-terminal proB-type natriuretic peptide for etiologies other than acute coronary syndromes and heart failure. Clin Chem 2007;53:2086–96.
53. Jackson L, Stewart A. Best evidence topic report. Use of troponin for the diagnosis of myocardial contusion after blunt chest trauma. Emerg Med J 2005;22:193–5.
54. La Vecchia L, Ottani F, Favero L, Spadaro GL, Rubboli A, Boanno C, et al. Increased cardiac troponin I on admission predicts in-hospital mortality in acute pulmonary embolism. Heart 2004;90:633–7.
55. Scridon T, Scridon C, Skali H, Alverez A, Goldhaber SZ, Solomon SD. Prognostic significance of troponin elevation and right ventricular enlargement in acute pulmonary embolism. Am J Cardiol 2005;96:303–5.
56. Akkerhuis KM, Alexander JH, Tardiff Be, Boersma E, Harrington RA, Lincoll AM, Simoons ML. Minor myocardial damage and prognosis. Are spontaneous and percutaneous coronary intervention-related events different? Circulation 2002;105:554–6.
57. Cardinale D, Sandri MGT, Martinoni A, Tricca A, Civelli M, Lamantgia G, et al. Left ventricular dysfunction predicted by early troponin I release after high-dose chemotherapy. J Am Coll Cardiol 2000;36:517–22.
58. Cardinale D, Colombo A, Sandri MT, Lamantia G, Colombo N, Civilli M, et al. Prevention of high-dose chemotherapy-induced cardiotoxicity in high-risk patients by angiotensin-converting enzyme inhibition. Circulation 2006;114:2474–81.
59. Califf RM, Abdelmeguid AE, Kuntz RE, Popma JJ, Davidson CJ, Cohen EA, et al. Myonecrosis after revascularization procedures. J Am Coll Cardiol 1998;31:241–51.
60. Silber S, Albertsson P, Aviles FF, Camici P, Colombo A, Hamm C, et al. for The Task Force for Percutaneous Coronary Interventions of the European Society of Cardiology. Guidelines for percutaneous coronary interventions. Eur Heart J 2005;226:804–47.
61. McCord J, Nowak RM, McCullough PA, Foreback C, Borzak S, Tokarski G, et al. Ninety-minute exclusion of acute myocardial infarction by use of quantitative point-of-care testing of myoglobin and troponin I. Circulation 2001;104:1483–8.
62 Fesmire FM, Fesmire CE. Improved identification of acute coronary syndromes with second generation cardiac troponin I assay: utility of 2-hour delta cTnI > or = +0.02 ng/mL. J Emerg Med 2002;22:147–52.
63. Fesmire FM, Christenson RH, Fody EP, Feintuch TA. Delta creatine kinase-MB outperforms myoglobin at two hours during the emergency department identification and

exclusion of troponin positive non-ST-segment elevation acute coronary syndromes. Ann Emerg Med 2004;44:12–9.
64. Sabatine MS, Morrow DA, de Lemos JA, Gibson CM, Murphy SA, Rifai N, et al. Multimarker approach to risk stratification in non-ST elevation acute coronary syndromes: simultaneous assessment of troponin I, C-reactive protein, and B-type natriuretic peptide. Circulation 2002;105:1760–3.
65. Morrow DA, Braunwald E. Future of biomarkers in acute coronary syndromes: moving toward a multimarker strategy. Circulation, 2003:250–2.

Chapter 8
Risk Stratification Using Scoring Systems

Judd E. Hollander and Anna Marie Chang

Abstract Several risk stratification scoring systems have been developed that incorporate information from the history, physical examination, electrocardiogram, and occasionally the initial cardiac marker results. The Goldman algorithm, ACI-TIPI, neural networks, and the TIMI risk score can all help risk stratify patients with potential acute coronary syndrome but none of them is able to identify a cohort of patients at less than 1% risk who may be safe for discharge from the ED. The GRACE and PURSUIT risk scores all help stratify patients with unstable angina but have no proven benefit in cohorts of patients with undifferentiated chest pain. This chapter reviews the various scoring systems and the evidence basis for their use in the appropriate patient population.

Keywords Chest pain · Risk stratification · Acute coronary syndrome

There are several risk stratification algorithms that have incorporated information from the history, physical examination, electrocardiogram, and occasionally the initial cardiac marker results. Details of the most commonly used scoring systems are described below.

Goldman Risk Score

The Goldman risk score was originally derived retrospectively through the analysis of a large cohort of patients presenting to the ED with chest pain. It has been prospectively validated and is useful as an initial risk stratification tool [1]. It is important to note that the final algorithm is heavily based on electrocardiographic findings and chest pain characteristics (Fig. 8.1). The Goldman algorithm

J.E. Hollander (✉)
Department of Emergency Medicine, University of Pennsylvania, Philadelphia, PA, USA
e-mail: hollandj@uphs.upenn.edu

W.F. Peacock, C.P. Cannon (eds.), *Short Stay Management of Chest Pain*,
DOI 10.1007/978-1-60327-948-2_8,
© Humana Press, a part of Springer Science+Business Media, LLC 2009

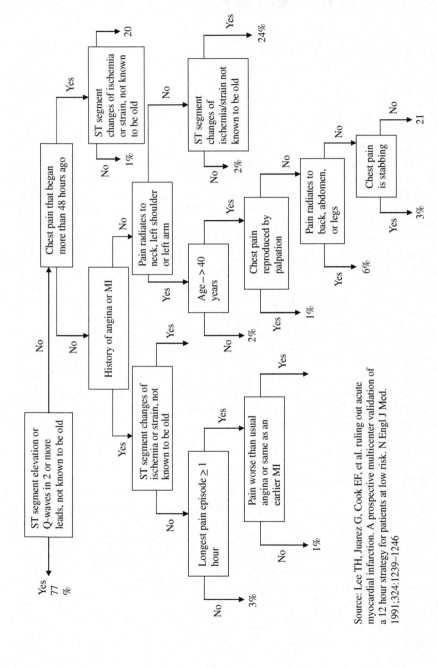

Source: Lee TH, Juarez G, Cook EF, et al. ruling out acute myocardial infarction. A prospective multicenter validation of a 12 hour strategy for patients at low risk. N Engl J Med. 1991;324:1239–1246

Fig. 8.1 The Goldman risk stratification algorithm for prediction of acute myocardial infarction (source Lee et al. [1])

stratifies patients into subcategories at risk of AMI ranging from 1 to 77%. The sensitivity of the algorithm for predicting AMI varies from 88 to 91%. The specificity varies from 78 to 92% [2]. Unfortunately, the Goldman risk score does identify a group of patients with less than 1% risk for AMI. Therefore, it cannot be used to identify ED patients that could potentially be discharged without a "rule out." Cardiac marker results were not incorporated into the algorithm; however, even the addition of a negative first cardiac troponin I to the low-risk groups is still associated with a 5% rate of 30-day adverse outcomes, preventing the use of the algorithm in conjunction with a single marker to allow ED discharge [3]. On the other hand, the Goldman algorithm is quite useful to predict the need for intensive care unit admission, development of cardiovascular complications, and outcome and therefore can be used to facilitate disposition decision making such as admission to a cardiac care unit or an observation unit [4].

ST-segment elevation or Q waves on the ECG, other ST T wave changes suggesting myocardial ischemia, low systolic blood pressure, pulmonary rales above the bases, or an exacerbation of known ischemic heart disease all predicted complications [5]. Although this algorithm does not prospectively identify patients safe for discharge, it has been independently validated and strict adherence to it would reduce intensive care unit admission by 16%, resulting in potentially large cost savings [5].

ACI-TIPI

The ACI-TIPI (acute cardiac ischemia time-insensitive predictive instrument) is a computer-generated tool embedded within an electrocardiogram machine that can be used to determine the likelihood of ACS at the time of initial clinical evaluation. It incorporates age, sex, presence of chest or left arm pain, a chief symptom of chest or left arm pain, along with elements of the electrocardiogram such as pathologic Q waves, and the presence and degree of ST-segment elevation or depression and T wave elevation or inversion. The electrocardiogram is printed along with a percent likelihood of "acute cardiac ischemia." Four studies including 5,496 patients have found that when combined with physician impression, it has a sensitivity of 86–95% and a specificity of 78–92% for prediction of ACS [2]. When nonemergency medicine house staff used the ACI-TIPI, it accelerated the time until the disposition decision [6]. In a study of over 10,000 patients with potential ACS, in the subset of patients ultimately not felt to have cardiac ischemia, the use of ACI-TIPI was associated with a small reduction in CCU admissions from 15 to 12% and a slight increase in emergency department discharges to home from 49 to 52% [7]. ACI-TIPI has not been widely incorporated into clinical practice in EDs. It has not been shown to make a clinically relevant difference in diagnostic accuracy compared with contemporary emergency physician judgment.

Artificial Neural Networks

The artificial neural network is a nonlinear statistical paradigm that recognizes complex patterns and can maintain accuracy even when some input data are missing. It is thought that the network's ability to allow variable weighting to input information as opposed to the fixed weighting of other statistical approaches allows it to perform more accurately than other approaches.

The artificial neural network can accurately identify the presence of myo-cardial infarction in patients with chest pain [8–10]. Unlike the Goldman algorithm and the ACI-TIPI, the neural network incorporates initial cardiac marker determinations. When cardiac troponin I and CK-MB determinations are added to the network, it has a sensitivity of 95% and a specificity of 96%. One advantage of the neural network is that it maintains accuracy despite missing up to 5% of the input data [9]. For prediction of AMI, the neural network has better sensitivity and specificity than the Goldman and ACI-TIPI scores. In the same data set, a Goldman risk of ≥7% had a sensitivity of 74% and specificity of 68%. An ACI-TIPI score ≥25% had a sensitivity of 62% and specificity of 73% [10]. The artificial neural network incorporates more clinical information than either the Goldman score or the ACI-TIPI (Table 8.1). Despite the improved performance, clinicians did not incorporate this "black box" feedback into their clinical decision making [11].

Table 8.1 Clinical criteria included in several ED risk stratification schemes

Goldman score	ACI-TIPI	Baxt neural network
Demographics		
Age ≥ 40 years	Age	Age
	Gender	Gender
		Race
Presentation characteristics		
Chest pain duration ≥48 hours	Presence of chest or left arm pain	Left anterior chest pain
Longest pain episode >1 hour	Chief symptom of chest or left arm pain	Left arm pain
History of angina or MI		History of prior coronary disease, AMI, angina, or CHF
Pain worse than usual angina or same as prior MI		Pain pressing in nature
Pain radiates to neck, left shoulder, or left arm		Pain crushing in nature
Pain radiates to back, abdomen, or legs		Pain radiating to neck
Chest pain reproduced by palpation		Pain radiating to left arm
Chest pain is stabbing		

Table 8.1 (continued)

Goldman score	ACI-TIPI	Baxt neural network
		Shortness of breath
		Diaphoresis
		Nausea and vomiting
Past history		
		Hypertension
		Diabetes mellitus
		Elevated cholesterol
		Family history of coronary artery disease
Electrocardiographic criteria		
ST-segment elevation or Q waves in two or more leads, not known to be old	Pathologic Q waves	Q waves old
		Q waves not known to be old
ST-segment changes of ischemia or strain, not known to be old	Presence and degree of ST-segment elevation or depression	ST-segment elevation old
		ST-segment elevation not known to be old
	T wave elevation or inversion	T wave inversion old
		T wave inversion not known to be old
		ST-segment depression old
		ST-segment depression not known to be old
		Left bundle branch block old
		Left bundle branch block not known to be old
		Hyperacute T waves old
		Hyperacute T waves old not known to be old
Cardiac marker determination		
		Including presentation CK, CK-MB, and troponin I

TIMI Risk Score

The TIMI (thrombolysis in myocardial infarction) risk score is composed of seven items (Table 8.2), which when combined into a score of 0–7 allows the emergency physician to risk stratify patients whether or not they have ACS. It was derived in an unstable angina/NSTEMI patient population, where 14-day event rates increased significantly as the TIMI risk score increases: 4.7% for a score of 0/1; 8.3% for 2; 13.2% for 3; 19.9% for 4; 26.2% for 5; and 40.9% for

Table 8.2 Elements of the TIMI score for unstable angina

Age 65 years or older
Three or more traditional risk factors for coronary artery disease
Prior coronary stenosis of 50% or more
ST-segment deviation on presenting electrocardiogram
Two or more anginal events prior 24 hours
Aspirin use within 7 days prior to presentation
Elevated cardiac markers

The presence of each of the above is assigned 1 point. The maximal possible score is 7.

6/7 [12]. When applied to a broad-based chest pain patient population, it performed similarly and was able to risk stratify the patients with respect to 30-day death, AMI, and revascularization [13, 14]. Chase et al. [14] found that higher TIMI scores were associated with an incidence of 30-day death, AMI, and revascularization [TIMI 0, 1.7% (95% confidence interval, 0.42–2.95); TIMI 1, 8.2% (5.27–11.04); TIMI 2, 8.6% (5.02–12.08); TIMI 3, 16.8% (10.91–22.62); TIMI 4, 24.6% (16.38–32.77); TIMI 5, 37.5% (21.25–53.75); TIMI 6, 33.3% (0–100)].

The TIMI score performs well in both males and females [15]. A TIMI risk score calculator can be downloaded from www.timi.org. A separate TIMI risk score exists for STEMI patients, but it is generally not used in emergency medicine practice, because STEMI patients require revascularization, regardless of the TIMI score. As expected, not all the individual items in the TIMI score have the same predictive value (Table 8.3). Electrocardiographic changes and elevated markers have the greatest predictive value [13, 14]. A simplified four-item version of the TIMI risk score that includes only age, ST-segment deviation, elevated troponin I, and known coronary stenosis may perform as well as the standard seven-item score [16].

Table 8.3 Relative risk of composite outcome for each TIMI risk score component

TIMI variable	Relative risk	95% confidence interval
Age ≥ 65	1.3	0.92–1.88
Prior CAD	3.1	2.26–4.24
≥3 cardiac risk factors	2.1	1.54–2.92
ST-segment deviation	5.3	3.81–7.23
Aspirin use	2.3	1.64–3.10
≥2 anginal events in 24 hours	1.7	1.22–2.30
Elevated cardiac biomarkers	6.3	4.64–8.45

PURSUIT Risk Score

The PURSUIT (Platelet Glycoprotein IIb-IIIa in Unstable Angina: Receptor Suppression Using Integrilin Therapy) risk model [17] was developed based on patients enrolled in the PURSUIT trial, which evaluated the role of glycoprotein IIb/IIIa inhibitors in unstable angina/NSTEMI patients. It was derived to help guide the clinical decision-making process for admitted patients. In the PURSUIT risk model, critical clinical features associated with an increased 30-day incidence of death and the composite of death or myocardial (re)infarction were age, heart rate, systolic blood pressure, ST-segment depression, signs of heart failure, and cardiac enzymes [17]. Calculating the risk score is a bit complicated; hence, it is not really used in clinical practice. The model has never been validated in the ED setting with a broad cohort of chest pain patients, but the items included in the model all have face validity and are known to be associated with worse outcomes. It does not appear likely that the lack of these items could allow discharge of patients from the ED. It cannot be recommended for help with the admit or discharge decision.

GRACE Risk Score

The GRACE (Global Registry of Acute Coronary Events) risk model was derived from registry data of patients with an acute coronary syndrome. The GRACE risk tool was developed on the basis of 11,389 patients, validated in subsequent GRACE and GUSTO IIb cohorts, and predicts in-hospital death in patients with STEMI, NSTEMI, or unstable angina [18]. The variables in the model are age, Killip class, systolic blood pressure, ST-segment deviation, cardiac arrest during presentation, serum creatinine level, positive initial cardiac markers, and heart rate. The sum of scores is applied to a reference monogram to determine the corresponding all-cause mortality from hospital discharge to 6 months later. The GRACE clinical application tool can be accessed at http://www.outcomes-umassmed.org/GRACE/acs_risk.cfm. The model has never been validated in the ED setting with a broad cohort of chest pain patients, but the items included in the model all have face validity and are known to be associated with worse outcomes. It does not appear likely that the lack of these items could allow discharge of patients from the ED. Thus, its utility would lie only in identifying patients who might benefit from aggressive therapy including revascularization. An analysis comparing the TIMI, GRACE, and PURSUIT risk scores concluded that all three demonstrated good predictive accuracy for death and MI at 1 year. They might have a role identifying patients who might benefit from aggressive therapy, including early myocardial revascularization [19].

Clinical Impression

The reason clinical algorithms have been developed is because it has long been known that clinical judgment is not adequate to rule out an acute coronary syndrome with sufficient accuracy to allow early discharge from the emergency department. Most of these studies were done in the era prior to board-certified emergency physicians staffing the ED; however, contemporary data still suggest that clinical judgment alone is not sufficient. Miller et al. studied whether a physician's impression of noncardiac chest pain was adequate to exclude an acute coronary syndrome [20]. In 17,737 patients, they found that 6.8% of patients who were felt to have noncardiac disease at the conclusion of the ED evaluation had possible and 2.8% had definite 30-day adverse cardiovascular events.

A theoretical reason why clinical and computer algorithms cannot identify patients that do *not* have ACS is that they have focused on symptoms consistent with a diagnosis of an ACS [10, 12, 13, 21, 22] and have not incorporated information about noncardiac conditions [23]. Disla et al. examined patients given an ED diagnosis of costochondritis and found that 6% sustained an AMI [24]. Hollander et al., in a study of 1995 ED patients with potential acute coronary syndromes, found that the presence of a clear-cut alternative noncardiac diagnosis was associated with a reduced risk of an in-hospital, triple-composite end point (death/MI/revascularization) with a risk ratio of 0.32 (95% CI, 0.19–0.55) and a 30-day, triple-composite end point with a risk ratio of 0.45 (95% CI, 0.29–0.69) [24]. However, patients with a clear-cut alternative noncardiac diagnosis still had a 4% event rate at 30 days (95% confidence interval, 2.4–5.6%) [24]. Thus, the use of this criterion alone for safe and immediate release of ED patients that present with potential ACS is also not possible.

Although clinical and computer algorithms can successfully risk stratify patients, they are not able to reliably identify a group of patients at such low risk of an ACS that they could be safely and immediately released from the emergency department [4, 7, 9, 10, 13, 14, 20, 21, 25, 26]. The best use of clinical judgment or a risk stratification tool is to assist with disposition location (observation unit, cardiac care unit, etc.) and to guide further testing or intervention. The Medical College of Virginia Hospital has developed a model program using a risk stratification-based pathway to guide further diagnostic testing [25, 27]. In their institution, they stratify patients into five risk categories and have a tailored approach to the patients within each category. Unfortunately, the risk stratification into these five risk categories is based upon clinical judgment and not a specific risk stratification algorithm that can be incorporated by other institutions. Nonetheless, they have demonstrated that initial assessment of cardiovascular risk followed by a tailored diagnostic strategy can be quite successful. Only a small number of patients are STEMI (level 1), and nearly half are low risk (level 4). The rate of MI and revascularization decreases as the risk level decreases. Level 3 patients had an intermediate risk with 4% sustaining AMI and 13% had either AMI or revascularization. The incidence of AMI in the level 4 patients was only 0.9% consistent with their low risk; however, they accounted for 6% of all MIs, again supporting the well-known fact that clinical judgment alone is not sufficient to allow safe discharge from the ED with objective testing for most patients. The MCV algorithm incorporates objective testing to help "rule in" or rule out myocardial ischemia. They use sestamibi imaging for the low-risk patients. Data suggest that coronary CT angiography can also identify low-risk patients rapidly (see Chapter 13) [28–30].

References

1. Lee TH, Juarez G, Cook EF, et al. Ruling out myocardial infarction: a prospective multicenter validation of a 12-hour strategy for patients at low risk. N Engl J Med 1991;324:1239–1246.
2. Lau J, Ioannidis JPA, Balk EM, et al. Diagnosing acute cardiac ischemia in the Emergency Department: A systematic review of the accuracy and clinical effect of current technologies. Ann Emerg Med. 2001;37:453–460.
3. Limkakeng A Jr., Gibler WB, Pollack C, et al. Combination of Goldman risk and initial cardiac troponin I for Emergency Department chest pain patient risk stratification. Acad Emerg Med, 2001;8:696–702.
4. Goldman L, Cook EF, Johnson PA, Brand DA, Rouan GW, Lee TH: Prediction of the need for intensive care in patients who come to emergency departments with acute chest pain. N Engl J Med 1996;334:1498–1504.
5. Qamar A, McPherson C, Babb J, Bernstein L, Werdmann M, Yasick D, Zarich S. The Goldman algorithm revisited: prospective evaluation of a computer-derived algorithm versus unaided physician judgment in suspected acute myocardial infarction. Am Heart J. 1999;138:705–9.
6. Sarasin FP, Reymond JM, Griffith JL, et al. Impact of the acute cardiac ischemia time insensitive predictive instrument (ACI-TIPI) on the speed of triage decision making for emergency department patients presenting with chest pain: a controlled clinical trial. J Gen Intern Med., 1994;9:187–194.
7. Selker HP, Beshanski JR, Griffith JL, et al. Use of the acute cardiac ischemia time-insensitive predictive instrument (ACI-TIPI) to assist with triage of patients with chest pain or other symptoms suggestive of acute cardiac ischemia: a multicenter, controlled clinical trial. Ann Intern Med., 1998;129:845–855.
8. Kennedy RL, Harrison RF, Burton AM, et al. An artificial neural network system for diagnosis of acute myocardial infarction (AMI) in the accident and emergency department: evaluation and comparison with serum myoglobin measurements. Computer Methods & Programs in Biomedicine 1997;52:93–103.
9. Baxt WG, Shofer FS, Sites FD, Hollander JE. A neural computational aid to the diagnosis of acute myocardial infarction. Ann Emerg Med. 2002;39:366–373.
10. Baxt WG, Shofer FS, Sites FD, Hollander JE. A neural network for the prediction of cardiac ischemia in patients presenting to the Emergency Department with chest pain. Ann Emerg Med. 2002;40:575–583.
11. Hollander JE, Sease KL, Sparano DM, Sites FD, Shofer FS, Baxt WG. Effects of neural network feedback to physicians on admit/discharge decision for emergency department patients with chest pain. Ann Emerg Med. 2004;44:199–205.

12. Antman EM, Cohen M, Bernink PJ, et al. The TIMI risk score for unstable angina/ non-ST elevation MI: A method for prognostication and therapeutic decision making. JAMA. 2000:284:835–4.
13. Pollack CV Jr., Sites FD, Shofer FS, Sease KL, Hollander JE. Application of the TIMI risk score for unstable angina and non-ST elevation acute coronary syndrome to an unselected Emergency Department chest pain population. Acad Emerg Med., 2006;13:13–18.
14. Chase M, Robey JL, Zogby KE, Sease KL, Shofer FS, Hollander JE. Prospective validation of the TIMI risk score in the Emergency Department chest pain patient population. Ann Emerg Med., 2006;48:252–259.
15. Karounos M, Chang AM, Robey JL et al. TIMI risk score: does it work equally well in both males and females. Emerg Med J 2007;24:471–474.
16. Jaffery Z, Hudson MP, Jacobsen G, Nowak R, McCord J. Modified thrombolysis in myocardial infarcation (TIMI) risk score to stratify patients in the emergency department with possible acute coronary syndrome. J Thromb Thrombolysis 2007;24:137–144.
17. Boersma E, Pieper KS, Steyerberg EW, et al. Predictors of outcome in patients with acute coronary syndromes without persistent ST-segment elevation. Results from an international trial of 9461 patients. The PURSUIT Investigators. Circulation 2000; 101:2557–67.
18. Granger CB, Goldberg RJ, Dabbous O, et al. Predictors of hospital mortality in the global registry of acute coronary events. Arch Intern Med 2003; 163:2345–53.
19. Giugliano RP, Braunwald E. The year in non-ST-segment elevation acute coronary syndromes. J Am Coll Cardiol 2005; 46:906–19.
20. Miller CD, Lindsell CJ, Khandelwal S, et al. Is the initial diagnostic impression of "noncardiac chest pain" adequate to exclude cardiac disease? Ann Emerg Med 2004; 44:565–574.
21. Goldman, L, Weinberg M, Weisberg M, et al. A computer-derived protocol to aid in the diagnosis of emergency room patients with acute chest pain. N Engl J Med 1982; 307:588–96.
22. Goldman L, Cook EF, Brand DA, et al: A computer protocol to predict myocardial infarction in emergency department patients with chest pain. N Engl J Med 1988; 318:797–803.
23. Hollander JE, Robey JL, Chase M, Brown AM, Zogby KE, Shofer FS. Relationship between a clear-cut alternative noncardiac diagnosis and 30 day outcome in Emergency Department patients with chest pain. Acad Emerg Med., 2007;14:210–215.
24. Disla E, Rhim HR, Reddy A, Karten I, Tarana A. Costochondritis: a prospective analysis in an emergency department setting. Arch Intern Med., 1994;154:2466–2469.
25. Tatum JL, Jesse RL, Kontos MC, et al: Comprehensive strategy for the evaluation and triage of the chest pain patient. Ann Emerg Med 1997;29:116–125
26. Selker HP, Zalenski RJ, Antman EM, et al. An evaluation of technologies for identification of acute cardiac ischemia in the emergency department: a report from a National Heart Attack Alert Program Working Group. Ann Emerg Med. 1997;29:13–87.
27. Kontos MC, Jesse RL. Evaluation of the emergency department chest pain patient. Am J Cardiol., 2000;85:32B–39B.
28. Gallagher MJ, Ross MA, Raff GL, Goldstein JA, O'Neill WW, O'Neil B. The Diagnostic Accuracy of 64-Slice CT Coronary Angiography Compared with Stress Nuclear Imaging in Emergency Department Low Risk Chest Pain Patients. Ann Emerg Med. 2007; 49:125–136.
29. Goldstein JA, Gallagher MJ, O"Neill WW et al. A randomized controlled trial of multi-slice coronary computed tomography for evaluation of acute chest pain. J Am Coll Cardiol 2007;49;863–871.
30. Hollander JE, Litt HI, Chase M, Brown AM, Kim W, Baxt WG. Computed tomography coronary angiography for rapid disposition of low risk emergency department patients with chest pain syndromes. Acad Emerg Med., 2007;14:112–116.

Chapter 9
Emergency Department Disposition of Patients Presenting with Chest Pain

Kelly Owen and Deborah B. Diercks

Abstract The disposition of patients with chest pain, concerning for acute coronary syndrome, presenting to the emergency department, is a challenge for emergency physicians. The creation of chest pain observation units had added another option, other than discharge or admission, for further evaluation of patients with chest pain. The key to rapid and safe evaluation and treatment is risk stratification. Most patients can be classified into high risk, intermediate risk, and low risk. High-risk patients are usually appropriate for admission to an inpatient cardiology service. Intermediate-risk patients can be admitted either to observation unit or inpatient service, but should receive further risk stratification during their hospital visit. Low-risk patients can be sent to an observation unit and should receive stress testing within 72 hours of presentation.

Keywords Chest pain · Observation unit · ST elevation myocardial infarction (STEMI) · Unstable angina (UA) · Non-ST elevation myocardial infarction (NSTEMI) · Acute coronary syndrome (ACS)

Introduction

Each year approximately 6 million patients present to the emergency department (ED) with chest pain concerning for an acute coronary syndrome (ACS) [1]. This accounts for nearly 5% of total ED visits. Despite advances in technology and biochemical testing, 2–5% of patients with ACS are still discharged from the ED, resulting in increased mortality [2]. The challenge for the emergency physician is effectively risk stratifying patients with chest pain, and selecting an appropriate disposition. Possible dispositions include, immediate percutaneous coronary intervention (PCI) or thrombolysis, hospital admission, observation, or discharge.

D.B. Diercks (✉)
Department of Emergency Medicine, University of California, Davis Medical Center,
2315 Stockton Boulevard, PSSB 2100, Sacramento, CA 95661, USA
e-mail: dbdiercks@ucdavis.edu

W.F. Peacock, C.P. Cannon (eds.), *Short Stay Management of Chest Pain*,
DOI 10.1007/978-1-60327-948-2_9,
© Humana Press, a part of Springer Science+Business Media, LLC 2009

Risk Stratification

Patients presenting with chest pain and STEMI, or new LBBB in the setting of symptoms concerning for myocardial infarction, have straightforward dispositions. The more challenging patients are those without these findings. After an initial EKG is negative for STEMI, there are two important questions that must be addressed. First, Are symptoms due to ACS from coronary artery disease (CAD)? Second, What is the likelihood that the patient will experience an adverse event during this episode? There are multiple systems that have been developed to aid in the evaluation of both short- and long-term risk assessments.

The Thrombolysis in Myocardial Infarction (TIMI) risk score for unstable angina/non-ST elevation myocardial infarction (UA/NSTEMI) has been prospectively validated in emergency department patients with chest pain [3, 4]. The TIMI risk calculator can be downloaded at www.timi.org. The TIMI score consists of seven variables (See Table 9.1) each worth one point. Therefore, scores can range from 0 to 7. Studies have shown an increased risk of adverse events (defined as death, MI, or revascularization) with higher score. Events ranged from 2 to 5% with a score of 0/1, to over 30–40% for a score of 6/7. Jaffery et al. have proposed that a modified TIMI score using only four data points (age ≥65 years, ST-segment deviation ≥ 0.5 mm, elevated troponin and coronary artery stenosis ≥ 50%) has similar prognostic value. However, this remains to be validated [5]. The ability of the TIMI score to identify a low-risk cohort suitable for discharge home from the hospital has been evaluated in undifferentiated chest pain patients in emergency department settings [4]. Unfortunately, the low-risk group had a rate of adverse events that exceeded thresholds for a safe discharge home. Therefore, the TIMI risk score should not be used in isolation for the identification of patients appropriate for discharge home.

Table 9.1 TIMI risk score

Factors	Points
Age >65	1
>3 CAD risk factors	1
Known CAD	1
Aspirin use in past 7 days	1
Recent (<24 hours) severe angina	1
Elevated cardiac markers	1
ST deviation ≥ 0.5 mm	1
Total	**0–7**

TIMI, Thrombolysis in Myocardial Infarction; CAD, coronary artery disease.

There are other systems that can further aid assessment of risk. A model based on data from The Global Registry of Acute Coronary Events (GRACE) database has been developed and validated, for both in-hospital and 6-month outcomes. GRACE uses age, heart rate, blood pressure, renal function, and Killip class to predict risk of death alone, as well as a combined endpoint of MI and death. It also takes into account ECG changes, cardiac arrest at admission, and elevated cardiac markers [6]. It can be accessed, with an automatic risk calculator, online at www.outcomes-umassmed.org.

There have been multiple studies comparing the efficacy of TIMI and GRACE. Lyon et al. found that both models had similar accuracy in risk stratification; however, a GRACE score could only be calculated in 76% of patients [7]. Ramsay et al. compared TIMI and GRACE to clinical judgment. They found that GRACE was superior to TIMI in predicting risk. However, both were better than clinical evaluation [8].

The PURSUIT model was developed for patients with UA/NSTEMI. It is based on the relationship between patient's baseline characteristics and the occurrence of death or non-fatal MI at 30 days [9].

These models are useful in the decision of the intensity of the level of care needed for patients as they allow the identification of patients at high risk for adverse events. It is important to remember that these models were derived in patients diagnosed with UA/NSTEMI, therefore all patients were already admitted to the hospital. Although not studied in a clinical setting, it is reasonable to assume that patients with high scores on either registry may warrant a higher level of care such as an intensive care unit or admission to a cardiology service.

There is hope that with time and further studies, an ideal model of risk stratification will be developed. Until that time, the current systems should be combined with elements from the history, physical, ECG, and laboratory data, to determine overall risk.

Who Warrants Immediate PCI or Thrombolysis?

According to the AHA/ACC guidelines for patients with chest pain, an initial screening ECG should be performed within 10 min of arrival to the ED [10]. ST elevation myocardial infarction (STEMI) is defined as an ECG showing ST-segment elevation greater than or equal to 1 mm (0.1 mV) in at least two contiguous leads. In the setting of chest pain, either STEMI or new left bundle branch block (LBBB) is an indication for immediate revascularization (PCI or thrombolysis). Regardless of the mode of reperfusion, the goal of therapy is to decrease the time of cardiac ischemia. This is defined as the time from onset of symptoms to the time of reperfusion [11].

The other indication for acute PCI or thrombolysis is a true posterior MI. This is defined as ST-segment depression in two contiguous anterior precordial leads and/or isolated ST-segment elevation in a posterior chest lead. Multiple studies have demonstrated the value of ECG changes in the posterior (V7–V9) leads [12–14].

Another EKG change that should raise suspicion for acute ischemia requiring PCI is marked (greater than or equal to 2 mm [0.2 mV]) symmetrical precordial T-wave inversion. These findings are consistent with a lesion in the left anterior descending artery (LAD). These patients often have anterior wall hypokinesis on echocardiogram and are at high risk if treated with only medical therapy [15]. It has been demonstrated that there is reversal of T-wave inversion and hypokinesis with revascularization [16].

There are two types of facilities that currently treat patients with STEMI, those with the availability and ability to perform PCI, and those without. In multiple trials, PCI was shown to be superior to thrombolysis in acute myocardial infarction. Grines et al. reviewed individual patient data from 11 randomized controlled trials directly comparing PCI to thrombolysis and found decreased rates of death, reinfarction, and hemorrhagic stroke in the PCI group. This difference was still evident 6 months post therapy [17].

AHA/ACC guidelines state that PCI should be performed within 90 min of the arrival at the first medical facility, and Table 9.2 shows the indications for immediate PCI. Thrombolytic therapy should be started within 30 min of presentation to the hospital [11]. Dalby et al. performed a meta-analysis evaluating transfer for PCI versus thrombolysis and concluded that transfer for PCI was beneficial [18]. Thus, if transfer can be accomplished within the 90-minute window, transfer for PCI is the preferred method of treatment. If this is not an attainable goal, thrombolysis should be initiated.

Table 9.2 Indications for immediate PCI

Type of MI	EKG changes
Anterior MI	ST elevation
Posterior MI	ST depression in two contiguous posterior leads
	ST elevation in a single posterior lead
LAD lesion	Marked T-wave inversion: ≥ 2 mm symmetrical precordial inversion

PCI, percutaneous coronary intervention; MI, myocardial infarction; LAD, left anterior descending artery.

Thrombolytic therapy is not always universally successful in restoring blood flow to occluded coronary arteries. In these cases, initial thrombolytic therapy, with the intent to perform PCI, or rescue PCI is an acceptable strategy. Patients who develop cardiogenic shock (especially those less than 75 years old), have severe congestive heart failure/pulmonary edema, or have a hemodynamically compromising ventricular arrhythmia, are candidates for PCI. Multiple studies have shown a survival benefit of early PCI in patients with cardiogenic shock [19, 20]. For patients without this clinical instability, failure of thrombolytic therapy is defined as less the 50% resolution of ST elevation at 90 min.

Pre-hospital ECG performed by ACLS-trained emergency medical service (EMS) providers can help to direct patients with STEMI to hospitals with the capacity to perform PCI, thus decreasing the need for thrombolysis or transfer.

Which Patients Require Hospitalization?

The first branch point in diagnosis and treatment in chest pain is the initial ECG. Once the diagnosis of STEMI is excluded, more information must be gathered through history, physical, laboratory studies, and serial ECGs. This data can assist in classifying patients as high, intermediate, or low risk. High-risk patients are generally appropriate for hospital admission (see Table 9.3).

Table 9.3 Characteristics of high-risk patients

High-risk patients: Appropriate for hospital admission
Known history of CAD, including MI
Prolonged chest pain (>20 min) typical for ischemia
Accelerating tempo if ischemic pain or other symptoms in past 48 hours
Hypotension
Pulmonary edema or rales
New S3 or MR murmur
New ST-segment deviation ($\geq$ 1 mm)
T-wave inversion in multiple precordial leads
Elevated cardiac TnI, TnT, or CK-MB

CAD, coronary artery disease; MI, myocardial infarction; MR, mitral regurgitation; TnI, troponin I; TnT, troponin T; CK-MB, creatinine kinase MB segment.

The initial ECG can offer other important clues to the diagnosis of ACS. ST depressions greater than 0.5 mm (0.05 mV), or inverted T-waves, during a symptomatic episode are strongly suggestive of chest pain due to coronary artery disease (CAD) [21]. These changes can either be due to UA or NSTEMI, the determination being based on the results of laboratory markers of cardiac necrosis. Pitta et al. found that patients with ST-segment depression have a similar risk of in-hospital mortality (15.8%) compared to patients with ST-segment elevation or new LBBB (15.5%) [22]. Despite the prognostic value of the initial ECG, a normal ECG does not completely rule out the diagnosis of ACS. Slater et al. evaluated 775 consecutive patients with symptoms suggestive of ACS. One hundred and seven had a normal ECG and 73 had minimal changes. Of these patients 10% with a normal ECG developed AMI, and 6% with minimal changes had AMI [23].

Other elements of the history, physical, and laboratory data can help determine the need for admission to the hospital. Patients with elevated troponin should be admitted to an inpatient unit. In patients with chest pain, isolated elevation of troponin is a predictor of increased mortality and future adverse events [24]. Furthermore, studies have shown that patients with elevated troponin, admitted for chronic obstructive pulmonary disease (COPD) exacerbation or admitted to the medical intensive care unit (MICU), have a higher mortality rate both in hospital and after discharge [25, 26]. Thus these patients are at too high of risk to be admitted to an observation unit.

The history is also important in determining risk. The five most important historical factors in the prediction of acute ischemia are: the nature of anginal symptoms, prior history of CAD, male sex, older age, and an increasing number of traditional risk factors [21]. Patients with an increasing frequency or severity of chest pain over the previous 48 hours should be considered high risk for CAD. Though traditional risk factors are not themselves predictive, diabetes and diseases other than CAD are predictive of worse outcomes.

Physical exam findings can also increase the likelihood that chest pain is from coronary ischemia. Shock, as evidenced by inadequate end organ perfusion, can occur in both STEMI and NSEMI. As discussed above, these patients benefit from PCI. Other physical exam findings that indicate high risk are pulmonary edema or rales, a new S3, new MR murmur, hypotension, sustained VT, bradycardia, and tachycardia. Patients with these findings should be considered for hospital admission.

Patients Who May Warrant Early Intervention?

Although patients with UA/NSTEMI clearly warrant admission to the hospital, another critical decision is ensuring these patients are admitted to the appropriate service, and at institutions that can provide adequate care. The determination of the provider for these patients once admitted is often based on local practices. However, data from the Can Rapid Risk Stratification of Unstable Angina Patients Suppress Adverse Outcomes with Early Implementation (CRUSADE) trial suggest that patients with UA/NSTEMI have more guideline-based care when admitted to a cardiology service. Roe et al. reported that 63.2% of patients in the CRUSADE registry were admitted to a cardiology service. These patients were more likely to receive guideline-based care within the first 24 hours, undergo invasive management, and receive appropriate discharge medications. In addition, those patients admitted to a cardiology service had a lower adjusted risk of in-hospital mortality (adjusted odds ratio 0.80, 95% confidence interval 0.73–0.88). This difference was less robust after adjustment for differences in the use of acute medications and invasive procedures (adjusted odds ratio 0.92, 95% confidence interval 0.83–1.02) [27]. This suggests that admission to a cardiology service may be the preferred disposition in these patients.

Multiple trials have been done on the treatment of NSTEMI. There are two possibilities for treatment. The first option is early invasive therapy, which consists of diagnostic or therapeutic catheterization, followed by coronary artery bypass grafting (CABG) if needed. Second is the initial conservative strategy, which optimizes medical management prior to invasive treatment. Evidence from the CRUSADE trial suggests that earlier catheterization and intervention for NSTEMI result in better hospital outcomes [28].

Despite clear recommendations in the AHA/ACC guidelines for who warrants invasive management it appears that those at lowest risk are preferentially receiving this intervention [21]. Zia et al. reported that data from two large registries show that patients with lower risk were more likely to undergo invasive procedures. Data from the CRUSADE registry reported that 53% of patients classified as high risk versus 76% as low risk underwent cardiac catheterization [29]. As the current AHA/ACC guidelines recommend early cardiac intervention in high-risk patients, physicians must ensure that patients have the opportunity to undergo early intervention. As not every hospital has the capability to offer this care, patients may need to be transferred to another institution.

Which Patients Require Hospitalization or an Observation Unit?

Patients at high risk for coronary artery disease require hospitalization and benefit from early invasive therapy. Patients at intermediate risk (See Table 9.4) could be appropriate for either hospitalization, or an observation unit, depending on the facilities available. Intermediate-risk patients lack any high-risk features of the history, physical, and ECG, however, they do not meet low-risk criteria.

Table 9.4 Characteristics of intermediate-risk patients

Intermediate-risk patients: Appropriate for hospital or observation
No high-risk features
Diabetes or ≥ 2 other CAD risk factors
Known other atherosclerotic disease elsewhere the CAD
Age >70
Fixed Q-waves on ECG
ST depression 0.5–1 mm or T-wave inversion >1 mm
Normal cardiac biomarkers

CAD, coronary artery disease; ECG, electrocardiogram.

The ECG findings in patients at intermediate risk for ACS include fixed Q-waves, or ST depression 0.5–1 mm or T-wave inversion >1 mm. Cannon et al. retrospectively reviewed the admission ECG of patients with UA or NSTEMI. They found that the initial ECG had prognostic value for one-year mortality or MI. At one-year follow-up death or MI occurred in 8.2% of patients without ECG changes, 11% with ≥1 mm ST-segment deviation, and 16.3% of patients with only 0.5 mm ST-segment elevation [30].

Elements of the history that are important include age, male sex, diabetes, and vascular disease other than CAD. Though traditional risk factors for CAD do not independently predict risk, when taken together, patients with an increased number of risk factors have an increased risk of CAD.

The decision to admit to the hospital, versus monitoring in an observation unit, depends on the type of observation unit and functional testing available. It has been shown in multiple studies that observation units are safe, cost-effective and reduce the number of admissions [31, 32]. In a randomized clinical trail, Farkouh et al. showed that it was safe, effective, and cost saving for intermediate-risk patients with unstable angina to be sent to an observation unit based in the ED. These patients all met criteria for unstable angina, and were classified as intermediate risk by the Agency for Health Care Policy and Research guidelines for unstable angina. Patients were randomized to usual care or observation unit management. After entry into the observation unit patients underwent serial biomarker testing (0, 2, and 4 hours). After this period of observation patients underwent an exercise treadmill, nuclear scintigraphy, or stress echocardiography. Using this protocol there was no difference in the rate of cardiac events between those admitted to the observation unit or hospital [33].

The goal of an observation unit for intermediate-risk patients is to reclassify them into high or low risk. Intermediate-risk patients should have an evaluation of cardiac function performed during their hospital stay. The evaluation can be by exercise treadmill, nuclear medicine study, or cardiac catheterization. High-risk patients are determined either by biomarkers that become elevated during the observation unit time course, acute ECG changes, or a positive functional study. These patients should then be admitted to the hospital for further evaluation. Low-risk patients are subsequently defined as those who do not develop positive biomarkers or ECG changes and have a negative functional study. Low-risk patients can be safely discharged. Aroney et al. used a similar clinical pathway. They demonstrated that at 6-month follow-up, MI was not missed in any patient re-classified as low risk. About 1% of the patients did have cardiac events; however, these were all elective revascularization procedures. In contrast, at 6-month follow-up, 19% of patients re-classified as high-risk patients had cardiac events (mostly revascularizations) [34].

There are differences between hospital systems on the availability of functional studies. In order to qualify for an observation unit, a patient must be able to have the test of choice performed in an expedient manner. For example, if an institution can only perform treadmill testing, then patients who are unable to exercise will need hospitalization. It is imperative that intermediate-risk patients are not sent home prior to further risk stratification. Thus, if an institution is unable to perform studies 7 days a week, patients should be hospitalized until the evaluation is completed.

Patients Appropriate for an Observation Unit

Low-risk patients are appropriate for an observation unit (See Table 9.5). Low-risk patients do not have any high- or intermediate-risk features. They have a normal exam with normal vital signs, a normal ECG and the absence of diabetes. Chest pain is often brief or atypical. Atypical chest pain includes pleuritic pain (sharp pain brought on by respiration or cough); primary or sole location in the middle or lower abdominal region; pain localized to a fingertip; pain reproduced with movement or palpation; very brief episodes (a few seconds or less); and radiation to the lower extremities [21]. Though these features make chest pain from a cardiac cause less likely, there are patients with ACS who will have these symptoms. Pain relieved by nitroglycerin or pain relieved by a "GI" cocktail does not have prognostic value [35, 36].

Table 9.5 Characteristics of low-risk patients

Low-risk patients: Appropriate for observation unit
No high- or intermediate-risk factors
Normal ECG
Normal exam, including vital signs
Negative cardiac biomarkers
Absence of diabetes
Recent cocaine use

ECG, electrocardiogram.

Patients with low-risk chest pain should be evaluated for non-cardiac causes of pain. If, after further evaluation, an alternate cause of chest pain is not found, these patients are appropriate for an observation unit. If, after observation, the low-risk patient has negative cardiac biomarkers and no ECG changes, there are two options. If functional testing is available, they should receive a functional study. The type of study utilized in the low-risk patient should be selected based on local institution protocols. However, an acceptable alternative option is discharge with follow-up and further out-patient work-up within 72 hours [21].

Multiple studies have shown that outpatient exercise treadmill testing (ETT) is safe and cost-effective. Chan et al. demonstrated that there is no difference in 30-day cardiac death, MI, CABG, or PCI in low-risk patients who received inpatient, outpatient, or no ETT [37]. Meyer et al. evaluated a pathway in which low-risk patients were scheduled for outpatient ETT within 72 hours. At 6-month follow-up, 2% of patients required coronary intervention, and less than 1% had AMI [38].

An alternative approach to low-risk patients is early stress testing. Amsterdam et al. have shown that risk stratification in low-risk patients can be achieved with early exercise stress testing after one negative set of cardiac biomarkers [39]. If this is not possible, and the decision is made for outpatient stress testing, the follow-up appointment should be made for the patient while in the ED. Richards et al. have shown that patients are more likely to follow-up and receive outpatient stress testing if the appointment is made in the ED [40].

Patients Appropriate for Discharge

The most difficult decision for the emergency physician is determining the patients appropriate for discharge home. The AHA/ACC has not given guidelines or descriptions of what constitutes very-low-risk patient. Often patients are admitted to an observation unit because of worry about missing ACS and lack of guidelines. This results in increased utilization of resources and increased cost of patient care. The other consequence of testing very-low-risk patients is the risk of false positive test results. False positive test results may result in unnecessary cardiac catheterization, which carries a 1% risk of serious morbidity [41].

It would seem intuitive that patients with a clear-cut alternative non-cardiac diagnosis would be safe for discharge (or admission as the condition required). However, Hollander et al. found that patients with a clear-cut alternative non-cardiac diagnosis still had a 4% cardiac event rate at 30 days [42]. These patients did have a lower in-hospital risk of death, MI, and revascularization. Thus, a clear-cut non-cardiac diagnosis alone is not enough to exclude very-low-risk patients from needing cardiac evaluation.

Miller et al. looked at the initial clinical impression of the treating physician on outcome in patients with chest pain [43]. They noted in patients that were identified as having non-cardiac chest pain the rate of adverse events was 2.8%. Importantly, age, history of diabetes, and a history of heart failure were associated with the occurrence of adverse events in the group of non-cardiac chest pain. The investigators concluded that when the initial impression is non-cardiac chest pain, high-risk features, such as traditional cardiovascular risk factors, were associated with adverse cardiac events and should be considered prior to disposition [43].

The problem remains that missing CAD, which could result in ACS, is considered unacceptable. Though many groups have attempted to evaluate decision rules in the very-low-risk population, no one has been successful in creating a rule that finds 100% of patients that will have an event in the next 30 days. Currently Hess et al. are attempting to derive a clinical decision rule for the triage of emergency department patients with chest pain [44]. It remains to be seen if they will be successful and if this rule will be able to be prospectively validated. Until that time, clinicians will have to use the available diagnostic aids coupled with clinical judgment to make the most informed decision possible.

Special Considerations

Women

Women account for a significant proportion of UA/NSTEMI. They tend to be older and have an increasing number of co-morbidities (hypertension, diabetes, and heart failure) [21]. Giannoglou et al. investigated the difference between men and women undergoing coronary angioplasty. They found that significant stenosis was less common in women, and when found was more likely to be in older patients. [45].

Women are more likely to present with atypical symptoms. Men with ACS often report chest pain radiating down the left arm, which is associated with diaphoresis. Studies have shown that women are more likely to present with back and jaw pain, nausea and/or vomiting, dyspnea, indigestion, and palpitations [46, 47]. These atypical characteristics should be considered when evaluating women with chest pain.

Women with NSTEMI/UA, and chest pain, are more likely than men to be discharged from the ED. However, this did not translate into an increased mortality at 1-year follow-up [48]. The indications for stress testing are the same in women as in men. Since the prevalence of CAD is significantly lower in women, the exercise ECG is less predictive. Perfusion studies with sestamibi have good sensitivity and specificity in women [21]. Careful attention to appropriate selection of the type of functional study is required. Based on the treating physicians assessment of the likelihood that the patients chest pain is from a cardiac etiology, disposition may depend on the type of functional study available in the outpatient setting, observation unit, and inpatient setting. Despite the overall poor performance of the exercise treadmill test in women, in those classified as low risk it has been shown to be a viable alternative [49].

Diabetes Mellitus

Patients with diabetes mellitus and unstable angina have a higher mortality than non-diabetic patients [50]. Diabetes is associated with older age, female gender, and a more prevalent history of coronary artery disease, hypertension, and renal failure. Pitsavos et al. found that diabetics with ACS sought care later than non-diabetics, and had higher in-hospital mortality [51]. Due to the increased morbidity and mortality of diabetics with chest pain, all diabetic patients should be considered intermediate risk at baseline. This may alter disposition decisions, as these patients should have risk stratification prior to discharge from the hospital if cardiac disease is suspected.

Elderly

The disposition of the elderly patient with chest pain presents a unique challenge to the emergency physician. "Elderly" is commonly used to describe patients aged 70 or older. By nature of age, elderly patients tend to have an increased number of co-morbidities, worse functional status, and a higher number of baseline ECG changes, than younger patients [21]. The use of diagnostic testing can be problematic in this group of patients due to inability to exercise and high rate of prior coronary artery disease.

Data from 2004 show that 35% of deaths in people older than 65 were from CAD. Even more telling is that 85% of deaths from CAD were in people older than 65 [52]. Despite the high morbidity and mortality of ACS in the elderly, studies have shown that evidence-based cardiac therapies are utilized less in this population [53]. Data from the GRACE registry have shown that high-risk elderly patients benefit from an early invasive strategy. They performed a subgroup analysis of young (<70), elderly (70–80), and very elderly (>80) patients with NSTEMI. Primary endpoints were stoke, death, and MI. Revascularization was beneficial in all groups for all primary outcomes and 6-month mortality [54].

Elderly patients should be considered intermediate risk at baseline. Although in most institutions these patients are often admitted to the hospital, depending on the type of diagnostic imaging modality available these patients may be evaluated in an observation unit when the symptoms are atypical and no objective findings are present. In those patients in whom the treating physician has a higher suspicion for acute coronary syndrome, consideration should be made for early admission to an inpatient service and possible early invasive strategy.

Cocaine and Methamphetamine-Induced Chest Pain

In younger patients with chest pain, consideration must be made for either cocaine or methamphetamine use. A urine toxicology screen should be obtained in this patient population. Weber et al. prospectively validated the use of a 9- to 12-hour observation period for patients with cocaine-associated chest pain, who did not have evidence of ischemia or cardiac complications [55]. Though cocaine has the potential to cause UA/NSTEMI, most of these patients are safe to go to an observation unit if the initial evaluation shows no high-risk features.

Methamphetamine has not been as widely studied as cocaine as a cause for chest pain. In a small study, Turnipseed et al. found that ACS was common in patients with methamphetamine use hospitalized for chest pain [56]. In this cohort 8% had significant cardiac complications. Patients with methamphetamine-induced chest pain are most likely appropriate for an observation unit with a monitored bed. However, the index of suspicion for significant CAD and ACS should be high.

Diercks et al. retrospectively reviewed charts of patients, with urine toxicology screens positive for either methamphetamine or cocaine, who were admitted to a chest pain observation unit [57]. They compared them to patients admitted for chest pain during the same time period, with negative urine toxicology screens. Neither group had evidence of ACS on ECG or cardiac biomarkers during initial ED evaluation. They found an equal rate of cardiac-related chest pain, defined as a positive stress test, in both groups. Thus, for patients with either cocaine- or methamphetamine-induced chest pain and risk factors symptoms concerning for a possible cardiac etiology, a low threshold for diagnostic testing should be used.

Conclusions

Chest pain remains a common presenting symptom for ED visits. As the age of the population increases, the number of visits will only increase. This will make evidence-based evaluation and disposition of chest pain patients even more essential. In summary, high-risk patients are generally appropriate for admission to an inpatient cardiology service. Intermediate-risk patients can be evaluated in an observation unit, but should have definitive testing done during their current hospital visit. Low-risk patients can be sent to an observation unit, and should have stress testing done within 72 hours of presentation.

References

1. Graff LG, Dallara J, Ross MA, Joseph AJ, Itzcovitz J, Andelman RP, Emerman C, Turbiner S, Espinosa JA, and Severance H. (1997) Impact on the Care of the Emergency Department Chest Pain Patient from the Chest Pain Evaluation Registry (CHEPER) study. *Am J Cardiol* **80**, 563–568.
2. Pope JH, Aufderheide TP, Ruthazer R, Woolard RH, Feldman JA, Beshansky JR, Griffith JL, and Selker HP. (2000) Missed Diagnoses of Acute Cardiac Ischemia in the Emergency Department. *N Engl J Med* **342**, 1163–1170.
3. Chase M, Robey JL, Zogby KE, Sease KL, Shofer FS, Hollander JE. (2006) Prospective Validation of the Thrombolysis in Myocardial Infarction Risk Score in the Emergency Department Chest Pain Population. *Ann Emerg Med* **48**, 252–259.
4. Pollack CV Jr, Sites FD, Shofer FS, Sease KL, Hollander JE. (2006) Application of the TIMI Risk Score for Unstable Angina and non-ST Elevation Acute Coronary Syndrome to an Unselected Emergency Department Chest Pain Population. *Acad Emerg Med* **13**, 12–18.
5. Jaffery Z, Hudson MP, Jacobsen G, Nowak R, McCord J. (2007) Modified Thrombolysis in Myocardial Infarction (TIMI) Risk Score to Risk Stratify Patients in the Emergency Department with Possible Acute Coronary Syndrome. *J Thromb Thrombolysis* **24**, 137–144.
6. Eagle KA, Lim MJ, Dabbous OH, Pieper KS, Goldberg RJ, Van de Werf F, Goodman SG, Granger CB, Steg PG, Gore JM, Budaj A, Avezum A, Flater MD, Fox KA; GRACE Investigators. (2004) A Validated Prediction Model for all Forms of Acute Coronary Syndrome: Estimating the Risk of 6-month Postdischarge Death in an International Registry. *JAMA* **291**, 2727–2733.

7. Lyon R, Morris AC, Caesar D, Gray S, Gray A. (2007) Chest Pain Presenting to the Emergency Department—to stratify risk with GRACE or TIMI. *Resuscitation* **74**, 90–93.

8. Ramsay G, Podogrodzka M, McClure C, Fox KA. (2007) Risk Prediction in Patients Presenting with Suspected Cardiac Pain: The GRACE and TIMI Risk Scores Versus Clinical Evaluation. *QJM* **100**, 11–18.

9. Boersma E, Pieper KS, Steyerberg EW, Wilcox RG, Chang WC, Lee KL, Akkerhuis KM, Harrington RA, Deckers JW, Armstrong PW, Lincoff AM, Califf RM, Topol EJ, Simoons ML. (2000) Predictors of Outcome in Patients with Acute Coronary Syndromes Without Persistent ST-Segment Elevation. Results from an International Trial of 9461 Patients. The PURSUIT Investigators. *Circulation* **101**, 2557–2567.

10. King SB et al. (2008) 2007 focused Update of the ACC/AHA/SCAI 2005 Guideline Update for Percutaneous Coronary Intervention: A Report of the American College of Cardiology/American Heart Association Task Force on Practice Guidelines: 2007 Writing Group to Review New Evidence and Update the ACC/AHA/SCAI 2005 Guideline Update for Percutaneous Coronary Intervention, Writing on Behalf of the 2005 Writing Committee. *Circulation* **117**, 261–295.

11. Antman EM et al. (2008) 2007 Focused Update of the ACC/AHA 2004 Guidelines for the Management of Patients With ST-Elevation Myocardial Infarction: A Report of the American College of Cardiology/American Heart Association Task Force on Practice Guidelines: Developed in Collaboration With the Canadian Cardiovascular Society Endorsed by the American Academy of Family Physicians : 2007 Writing Group to Review New Evidence and Update the ACC/AHA 2004 Guidelines for the Management of Patients with ST-Elevation Myocardial Infarction, Writing on Behalf of the 2004 Writing Committee. *Circulation* **117**, 296–329.

12. Zalenski RJ, Rydman RJ, Sloan EP, Hahn KH, Cooke D, Fagan J, Fligner DJ, Hessions W, Justis D, Kampe LM, Shah S, Tucker J, Zwicke D. (1997) Value of Posterior and Right Ventricular Leads in Comparison to the Standard 12-Lead Electrocardiogram in Evaluation of ST-Segment Elevation in Suspected Acute Myocardial Infarction. *Am J Cardiol* **79**, 1579–1585.

13. Matetzky S, Freimark D, Chouraqui P, Rabinowitz B, Rath S, Kaplinsky E, Hod H. (1998) Significance of ST Segment Elevations in Posterior Chest Leads (V7–V9) in Patients with Acute Inferior Myocardial Infarction; Application for Thrombolytic Therapy. *J Am Coll Cardiol* **31**, 506–511.

14. Matetzky S, Freimark D, Feinberg MS, Novikov I, Rath S, Rabinowitz B, Kaplinsky E, Hod H. (1999) Acute Myocardial Infarction with Isolated ST-Segment Elevation in Posterior Chest Leads V7–V9: "Hidden" ST-Segment Elevations Revealing Acute Posterior Infarction. *J Am Coll Cardiol* **34**, 748–753.

15. Haines DE, Raabe DS, Gundel WD, Wackers FJ. (1983) Anatomic and Prognostic Significance of New T-Wave Inversion in Unstable Angina. *Am J Cardiol* **52**, 14–18.

16. Renkin J, Wijns W, Ladha Z, Col J. (1990) Reversal of Segmental Hypokinesis by Coronary Angioplasty in Patients with Unstable Angina, Persistent T Wave Inversion, and Left Anterior Descending Coronary Artery Stenosis. Additional Evidence for Myocardial Stunning in Humans. *Circulation* **82**, 913–921.

17. Grines C, Patel A, Zijlstra F, Weaver WD, Granger C, Simes RJ; PCAT Collaborators. (2003) Primary Coronary Angioplasty Compared with Intravenous Thrombolytic Therapy for Acute Myocardial Infarction: Six-Month Follow UP and Analysis of Individual Patient Data from Randomized Trials. *Am Heart J* **145**, 47–57.

18. Dalby M, Bouzamondo A, Lechat P, and Montalescot G. (2003) Transfer for Primary Angioplasty Versus Immediate Thrombolysis in Acute Myocardial Infarction: A Meta-Analysis. *Circulation* **108**, 1809–1814.

19. Hochman JS, Sleeper LA, Webb JG, Dzavik V, Buller CE, Aylward P, Col J, White HD. (2006) Early Revascularization and Long-Term Survival in Cardiogenic Shock Complicating Acute Myocardial Infarction. *JAMA* **295**, 2522–2525.

20. Hochman JS, Sleeper LA, White HD, Dzavik V, Wong SC, Menon V, Webb JG, Steingart R, Picard MH, Menegus MA, Boland J, Sanborn T, Buller CE, Modur S, Forman R, Desvigne-Nickens P, Jacobs AK, Slater JN, LeJemtel TH. (2001) One-Year Survival Following Early Revascularization for Cardiogenic Shock. *JAMA* **285**, 190–192.
21. Anderson JL et al. (2007) ACC/AHA 2007 Guidelines for the Management of Patients With Unstable Angina/Non ST-Elevation Myocardial Infarction: Executive Summary: A Report of the American College of Cardiology/American Heart Association Task Force of on Practice Guidelines (Writing Committee to Revise the 2002 Guidelines for the Management of Patients With Unstable Angina/Non ST-Elevation Myocardial Infarction): Developed in Collaboration with the American College of Emergency Physicians, the Society for Cardiovascular Angiography and Interventions, and the Society of Thoracic Surgeons: Endorsed by the American Association of Cardiovascular and Pulmonary Rehabilitation and the Society for Academic Emergency Medicine. *Circulation* **116**, 803–877.
22. Pitta SR, Grzybowski M, Welch RD, Frederick PD, Wahl R, Zalenski RJ. (2005) ST-Segment Depression on the Initial Electrocardiogram in Acute Myocardial Infarction-Prognostic Significance and it's Effect on Short-Term Mortality: A report from the National Registry of Myocardial Infarction (NRMI-2, 3, 4). *Am J Cardiol* **95**, 843–848.
23. Slater DK, Hlatky MA, Mark DB, Harrell FE Jr, Pryor DB, Califf RM. (1987) Outcome in Suspected Acute Myocardial Infarction with Normal or Minimally Abnormal Admission Electrocardiographic Findings. *Am J Cardiol* **60**, 766–770.
24. Rao SV, Ohman EM, Granger CB, Armstrong PW, Gibler WB, Christenson RH, Hasselblad V, Stebbins A, McNulty S, Newby LK. (2003) Prognostic Value of Isolated Troponin Elevation Across the Spectrum of Chest Pain Syndromes. *Am J Cardiol* **91**, 936–940.
25. Babuin L, Vasile VC, Rio Perez JA, Alegria JR, Chai HS, Afessa B, Jaffe AS. (2008) Elevated Cardiac Troponin is an Independent Risk Factor for Short-and Long-Term Mortality in Medical Intensive Care Unit Patients. *Crit Care Med* **36**, 759–765.
26. Brekke PH, Omland T, Holmedal SH, Smith P, Soyseth V. (2008) Troponin T Elevation and Long-Term Mortality After Chronic Obstructive Pulmonary Disease Exacerbation. *Eur Respir J* **31**, 563–570.
27. Roe MT, Chen AY, Mehta RH, Li Y, Brindis RG, Smith SC Jr, Rumsfeld JS, Gibler WB, Ohman EM, Peterson ED. (2007) Influence of Inpatient Service Specialty on Care Processes and Outcomes for Patients with Non ST-Segment Elevation Acute Coronary Syndromes. *Circulation* **116**, 1153–1161.
28. Chan MY, Becker RC, Harrington RA, Peterson ED, Armstrong PW, White H, Fox KA, Ohman EM, Roe MT. (2008) Noninvasive, Medical Management for Non-ST-Elevation Acute Coronary Syndromes. *Am Heart J* **155**, 397–407.
29. Zia MI, Goodman SG, Peterson ED, Mulgund J, Chen AY, Langer A, Tan M, Ohman EM, Gibler WB, Pollack CV Jr, Roe MT. (2007) Paradoxical Use of Invasive Cardiac Procedures for Patients with Non-ST Segment Elevation Myocardial Infarction: An International Perspective from the CRUSADE Initiative and the Canadian ACS Registries I and II. *Can J Cardiol* **23**, 1073–1079.
30. Cannon CP, McCabe CH, Stone PH, Rogers WJ, Schactman M, Thompson BW, Pearce DJ, Diver DJ, Kells C, Feldman T, Williams M, Gibson RS, Kronenberg MW, Ganz LI, Anderson HV, Braunwald E. (1997) The Electrocardiogram Predicts One-Year Outcome of Patients with Unstable Angina and Non-Q Wave Myocardial Infarction: Results of the TIMI Registry ECG Ancillary Study. *J Am Coll Cardiol* **30**, 133–140.
31. Goodacre S, Nicholl J, Dixon S, Cross E, Angelini K, Arnold J, Revill S, Locker T, Capewell S, Quinney D, Campbess S, Morris F. (2004) Randomized Controlled Trial and Economic Evaluation of a Chest Pain Observation Unit Compared with Routine Care. *BMJ* **328**, *254.*

32. Roberts RR, Zalenski RJ, Mensah EK, Rydman RJ, Ciavarella G, Gussow L, Das K, Kampe LM, Dickover B, McDermott MF, Hart A, Straus HE, Murphy DG, Rao R. (1997) Costs of an Emergency Department-Based Accelerated Diagnostic Protocol vs Hospitalization in Patients with Chest Pain: A randomized Controlled Trial. *JAMA* **278**, 1701–1702.

33. Farkouh ME, Smars PA, Reeder GS, Zinsmeister AR, Evans RW, Meloy TD, Kopecky SL, Allen M, Allison TG, Gibbons RJ, Gabriel SE, for the Chest Pain Evaluation in the Emergency Room (CHEER) Investigators. (1998) A Clinical Trial of A Chest-Pain Observation Unit for patients with Unstable Angina. *N Engl J Med* **339**, 1882–1888.

34. Aroney CN, Dunlevie HL, Bett JHN. (2003) Use of an Accelerated Chest Pain Assessment Protocol in Patients at Intermediate Risk of Adverse Cardiac Events. *MJA* **178**, 370–374.

35. Steele R, McNaughton T, McConahy M, Lam J. (2006) Chest Pain in Emergency Department Patients: If the Pain is Relieved by Nitroglycerin, is it More Likely to be Cardiac Chest Pain? *CJEM* **8**, 164–169.

36. Swap CJ, Nagurney JT. (2005) Value and Limitations of Chest Pain History in the Evaluation of Patients with Suspected Acute Coronary Syndromes. *JAMA* **294**, 2623–2629.

37. Chan GW, Sites FD, Shofer FS, Hollander JE. (2003) Impact of Stress Testing on 30-Day Cardiovascular Outcomes for Low-Risk Patients with Chest Pain Admitted to Floor Telemetry Beds. *Am J Emerg Med* **21**, 282–287.

38. Meyer MC, Mooney RP, Sekera AK. (2006) A Critical Pathway for Patients with Acute Chest Pain and Low Risk for Short-Term Adverse Cardiac Events: Role of Outpatient Stress Testing. *Ann Emerg Med* **47**, 435.e1–e3.

39. Amsterdam EA, Kirk JD, Diercks DB, Turnipseed SD, Lewis WR. (2004) Early Exercise Testing for Risk Stratification of Low-Risk Patients in Chest Pain Centers. *Crit Pathw Cardiol* **3**, 114–120.

40. Richards D, Meshkat N, Chu J, Eva K, Worster A. (2007) Emergency Department Compliance with Follow-Up for Outpatient Exercise Stress Testing: A Randomized Controlled Trial. *CJEM* **9**, 435–440.

41. Davis C, VanRiper S, Longstreet J, Moscucci M. (1997) Vascular Complications of Coronary Interventions. *Heart Lung* **26**, 118–127.

42. Hollander JE, Robey JL, Chase MR, Brown AM, Zogby KE, Shofer FS. (2007) Relationship Between a Clear-Cut Alternative Noncardiac diagnosis and 30-Day Outcome in Emergency Department Patients with Chest Pain. *Acad Emerg Med* **14**, 210–215.

43. Miller CD, Lindsell CJ, Khandelwal S, Chandra A, Pollack CV, Tiffany BR, Hollander JE, Gibler WB, Hoekstra JW. (2004) Is the Initial Diagnostic Impression of "Noncardiac Chest Pain" Adequate to Exclude Cardiac Disease? *Ann Emerg Med* **44**, 565–574.

44. Hess EP, Wells GA, Jaffe A, Stiell IG. (2008) A Study to Derive a Clinical Decision Rule for Triage of Emergency Department Patients with Chest Pain: Design and Methodology. *BMC* **8**.

45. Giannoglou GD, Antoniadis AP, Chatzizisis YS, Damvopoulou E, Parcharidis GE, Louridas GE. (2008) Sex-Related Differences in the Angiographic Results of 14,500 Cases Referred for Suspected Coronary Artery Disease. *Coron Artery Dis* **19**, 9–14.

46. Patel H, Rosengren A, Ekman I. (2004) Symptoms in Acute Coronary Syndromes: Does Sex Make a Difference? *Am Heart J.* **148**, 27–33.

47. DeVon HA, Ryan CJ, Ochs AL, Shapiro M. (2008) Symptoms Across the Continuum of Acute Coronary Syndromes: Differences Between Women and Men. *Am J Crit Care* **17**, 14–24.

48. Kaul P, Chang WC, Westerhout CM, Graham MM, Armstrong PW. (2007) Differences in Admission Rates and Outcomes Between Men and Women Presenting to Emergency Departments with Coronary Syndromes. *CMAJ* **177**, 1193–1199.

49. Amsterdam EA, Kirk JD, Diercks DB, Lewis WR, Turnipseed SI, Immediate exercise testing to evaluate low-risk patients presenting to the emergency department with chest pain. *J Am Coll Cardiolol* 2002 Jul 17; 40(2): 251–256.

50. Fava S, Azzopardi J, Agius-Muscat H. (1997) Outcome of Unstable Angina in Patients with Diabetes Mellitus. *Diabet Med* **14**, 209–213.
51. Pitsavos C, Kourlaba G, Panagiotakos DB, Stefanadis C. (2007) Characteristics and In-Hospital Mortality of Diabetics and Nondiabetics with Acute Coronary Syndrome; the GREECS Study. *Clin Cardiol* **30**, 239–244.
52. Alexander KP, Newby LK, Cannon CP, Armstrong PW, Gibler WB, Rich MW, Vand de Werf F, White HD, Weaver WD, Naylor MD, Gore JM, Krumholz HM, Ohman M. (2007) Acute Coronary Care in the Elderly, Part I: Non-ST-Segment-Elevation Acute Coronary Syndromes: A Scientific Statement for Healthcare Professionals From the American Heart Association Council on Clinical Cardiology: In Collaboration With the Society of Geriatric Cardiology. *Circulation* **115**, 2549–2569.
53. Avezum A, Makdisse M, Spencer F, Gore JM, Fox KA, Montalescot G, Eagle KA, White K, Mehta RH, Knobel E, Collet JP; GRACE Investigators. (2005) Impact of Age on Management and Outcome of Acute Coronary Syndrome: Observations from the Global Registry of Acute Coronary Events (GRACE). *Am Heart J* **149**, 67–73.
54. Devlin G, Gore JM, Elliott J, Wijesinghe N, Eagle KA, Avezum A, Huang W, Brieger D; for the GRACE Investigators. (2008) Management and 6-Month Outcomes in Elderly and Very Elderly Patients with High-Risk Non-ST-Elevation Acute Coronary Syndromes: The Global Registry of Acute Coronary Events. *Eur Heart J*. April 2 (Epub-accessed April 8, 2008).
55. Weber JE, Shofer FS, Larkin GL, Kalaria AS, Hollander JE. (2003) Validation of a Brief Observation Period for Patients with Cocaine-Associated Chest Pain. *N Engl J Med* **348**, 510–517.
56. Turnipseed SD, Richards JR, Kirk JD, Diercks DB, Amsterdam EA. (2003) Frequency of Acute Coronary Syndrome in Patients Presenting to the Emergency Department with Chest Pain After Methamphetamine Use. *J Emerg Med* **24**, 369–373.
57. Diercks DB, Kirk JD, Turnipseed SD, Amsterdam EA. (2007) Evaluation of Patients with Methamphetamine-and Cocaine-Related Chest Pain in a Chest Pain Observation Unit. *Crit Pathw Cardiol* **6**, 161–164.

Chapter 10
Short-Stay Unit Requirements

Louis Graff IV

Abstract Chest pain units (CPU) are specialized units in the acute care hospital that are designed and staffed to provide the highest quality, most cost efficient services to patients with chest pain. Patients are identified for evaluation and management in a CPU by cardiac risk stratification by the physician upon their presentation to the hospital. Those with low risk, negative cardiac biomarkers, and an EKG negative for acute findings are appropriate for the CPU. Monitoring requirements for patients in a CPU bed need to be at the level of those patients in a hospital intensive care unit, telemetry, or emergency department bed. Staffing requirements are similar to an emergency department or a hospital telemetry unit. With a properly structured and staffed CPU, the highest quality patient care and optimal outcome can be provided to the patient who presents to the physician with chest pain or chest pain equivalent and possible cardiac disease.

Keywords Chest pain unit · Observation · Risk stratification · Chest pain

Chest pain units (CPU) are specialized units in the acute care hospital that are designed and staffed to provide the highest quality, most cost efficient services to patients with chest pain. Their value has been recognized by the relevant professional societies [1, 2]. Studies with historical and randomized controls have shown that they are an important tool for the care of the chest pain patient [3, 4]. Many aspects of the requirements for a CPU bed are identical to those for any acute care hospital bed. But the CPU has certain unique requirements in monitoring and unit staffing.

Patients are identified for evaluation and management in a CPU by cardiac risk stratification by the physician upon their presentation to the hospital [5]. Those with moderate to high risk of active ACS are admitted to the hospital.

L. Graff (✉)
University of Connecticut School of Medicine, Farmington, CT, USA
e-mail: louisgraff4@aol.com

W.F. Peacock, C.P. Cannon (eds.), *Short Stay Management of Chest Pain*,
DOI 10.1007/978-1-60327-948-2_10,
© Humana Press, a part of Springer Science+Business Media, LLC 2009

Those with very low risk are discharged home for outpatient management. Those with low risk, negative cardiac biomarkers, and an EKG negative for acute findings are appropriate for the CPU. Approximately one half of patients who will be identified during hospital evaluation to have acute myocardial infarction are not identified upon their initial evaluation in the hospital [6]. Upon admission to the CPU or the hospital their initial diagnosis is non-ACS such as heart failure, respiratory disease such as asthma, or noncardiac, non-respiratory disease such as peptic ulcer [6]. This proportion is increasing over time as the population ages, which results in more patients presenting with atypical symptoms such as shortness of breath, syncope, weakness rather than classic chest pain [6, 7]. Thus the CPU is needed to clarify which patients actually have acute ACS once they are identified by the physician during the initial contact as possible ACS.

Monitoring requirements for patients in a CPU bed need to be at the level of those patients in a hospital intensive care unit, telemetry, or emergency department bed. Electrocardiographic monitors are needed to constantly record the patient's EKG, heart rate, blood pressure, oximetry, respiratory rate, and ST segments. The monitors need to be configured by CPU staff to alarm at significant abnormalities of these parameters. There needs to be ready availability of resuscitation equipment and medicines. While the physical location of the CPU bed may vary in a hospital from adjacent to the emergency department or upstairs throughout the hospital, the requirements for vigilant electrocardiographic monitoring do not. This monitoring continues throughout the finite time of the patient being evaluated in the CPU.

The monitoring of the patient during their CPU stay is integral to the evaluation process [3, 4]. Those patients with a negative evaluation in the CPU, including electrocardiographic monitoring, are safe to be discharged home for outpatient management. Those who develop findings of acute myocardial ischemia or injury are admitted to the acute care hospital. A portion of these patients are identified by the development of positive cardiac biomarkers. Another portion of these patients are identified by EKG findings of active cardiac disease either on the serial EKG or by the electrocardiographic alarms of abnormal vital signs, changes in continuous ST segments, or development of significant arrhythmias. The patient can be kept on static electrocardiographic monitors or on mobile telemetry monitors depending upon the CPU's capabilities and the judgment of the clinician as to what is most appropriate for the patient.

Staffing requirements are similar to an emergency department or a hospital telemetry unit [5]. Nurses need to have adequate training on the institution's protocols for ruling out ACS. They need to be kept updated in their skills in evaluating electrocardiographic monitors and in advanced cardiac life support protocols for managing complications of cardiac disease. The nurse-to-patient ratio should be appropriate with a lower ratio possible with additional staffing of nurse extenders such as techs and aids. Physicians need to have the training to manage patients with acute, dangerous conditions that are identified in CPUs such as acute myocardial infarction, pulmonary edema, cardiac arrhythmias, and shock. They need to be immediately available for intervention if the CPU patient develops an acute condition as well as available for prompt disposition when the patient has finished their CPU evaluation. The physician-to-patient ratio should be appropriate with a lower ratio possible with additional staffing of physician extenders such as physician assistants, nurse practitioners, and residents [8]. Active physician and nursing CPU leadership is required for the success of the program since the protocols to evaluate and manage patients in the CPU can be complex and labor intensive [2, 9]. Regulatory requirements from the Joint Commission, State Department of Health, and other regulatory bodies must be met for the CPU to remain in business and consequently the physician and nursing leadership is responsible to maintain a program for the continuous monitoring of outcomes of care provided to patients in the CPU.

With a properly structured and staffed CPU, the highest quality patient care and optimal outcome can be provided to the patient who presents to the physician with chest pain or chest pain equivalent and possible cardiac disease [10].

References

1. D. Adams, Jeffrey L. Anderson, Elliott M. Antman, et al. ACC/AHA 2007 Guidelines for the management of patients with unstable Angina/Non_ST-elevation myocardial infarction. *J. Am. Coll. Cardiol.* 2007; 50:1–157.
2. Graff L, Joseph A, Andelmann R, et al. American College of Emergency Physicians: Chest pain units in emergency departments, a report from the Short Term Observation Services Section. *Am J Cardiol* 1995; 76:1036–1039.
3. Graff LG, Dallara J, Ross MA, et al. Impact on the care of the emergency department chest pain patient from the Chest Pain Evaluation Registry (CHEPER) study. *Am J Cardiol* 1997; 80:563–568.
4. Gomez MA, Anderson JL, Karagounis LA, Muhlestein JB, Mooers FB. An emergency department-based protocol for rapidly ruling out myocardial ischemia reduces hospital time and expense: Results of a randomized study (ROMIO). *J Am Coll Cardiol* 1996; 28:25–33.
5. Ross M, Graff L. Principles of observation medicine. *Emerg Med Clin North Am* 2001; 19:1–17.
6. Graff LG, Wang Y, Borkowski B, Tuozzo K, Foody J, Krumholz H, Radford MJ. Delay in the diagnosis of acute myocardial infarction: Effect on quality of care and its assessment. *Acad Emerg Med* 2006; 13(9):931–938.
7. Graff L, Palmer AC, LaMonica P, Wolf S. Triage of patients for a rapid (5-minute) electrocardiogram: A rule based on presenting chief complaints. *Ann Emerg Med* 2000; 36:554–560.
8. Graff L, Radford M. Formula for emergency physician staffing. *Amer J Emerg Med* 1990; 8:194–199.
9. Brillman J, Dunbar L, Graff L, et al. American College of Emergency Physicians Section of Observation Services: Management of observation units. *Ann Emerg Med* 1995; 25:823–830.
10. Graff L, Prete M, Werdmann M, Monico E, Smothers K, Krivenko C, Maag R, Joseph A. Improved outcomes with implementation of emergency department observation units within a multihospital network. *J Qual Improv* 2000; 26:421–427.

Chapter 11
Medical Therapy in Patients Managed in a Chest Pain Observation Unit

James McCord

Abstract There are no randomized controlled trials that demonstrate that any medical therapy reduces adverse events in patients with undifferentiated chest pain evaluated in chest pain units (CPUs). Many of the millions of patients that present to the emergency departments (EDs) in the United States with chest pain are managed in CPUs, but the vast majority of these patients do not suffer an acute coronary syndrome (ACS). Studies have shown that only ~2% of patients evaluated in CPUs are diagnosed with myocardial infarction (MI) (Newby et al. Am J Cardiol 85(7):801–5, 2000; Farkouh et al. N Eng J Med 339(26):1882–8, 1998). This chapter will address the role of aspirin (ASA), nitrates, heparin, and beta blockers in the patients with undifferentiated chest pain in the CPU.

Keywords Pharmacotherapy · Chest pain unit · Observation unit · Aspirin

Aspirin Therapy

The administration of ASA in the setting of STEMI led to a dramatic 25% decrease in mortality equaling that of fibrinolytic therapy [1]. In addition, ASA therapy has been shown to decrease adverse cardiac events in the setting of unstable angina (UA) and non-ST elevation MI (NSTEMI) [2–5]. ASA is inexpensive and has been shown to be safe and well tolerated in multiple randomized controlled trials [2, 6–11]. American Heart Association/American College of Cardiology and European Society of Cardiology guidelines recommend the administration of ASA when the diagnosis of ACS is definite or suspected [12, 13]. One post hoc study demonstrated decreased mortality

J. McCord (✉)
Heart and Vascular Institute, Henry Ford Hospital, 2799 W. Grand Blvd., Detroit, MI 48202, USA
e-mail: Jmccord1@hfhs.org

W.F. Peacock, C.P. Cannon (eds.), *Short Stay Management of Chest Pain*,
DOI 10.1007/978-1-60327-948-2_11,
© Humana Press, a part of Springer Science+Business Media, LLC 2009

rates with out of hospital administration of ASA in patients with suspected ACS [14]. The International Consensus Conference on Cardiopulmonary Resuscitation Writing Group stated that it is reasonable for ASA to be administered in the pre-hospital setting [15].

ASA is inexpensive, safe, and highly efficacious in patients with ACS. Patients with undifferentiated chest managed in a CPU should have received ASA prior to transfer to the CPU. For patients that did not receive ASA prior to transfer to the CPU, ASA should be given to the patient in the CPU. For patients that cannot receive ASA due to an allergy other anti-platelet agents such as clopidogrel should probably not be administered until a diagnosis of ACS is made.

Anticoagulation

There are no randomized placebo-controlled trials that show an improvement in mortality for anticoagulants in the setting of UA/NSTEMI. Unfractionated heparin (UFH) or low molecular weight heparin (LMWH) have been studied in six small randomized placebo-controlled studies that showed a 54% decrease in the combined endpoint of either death or myocardial infarction (MI) in UA/NSTEMI [16–21]. There have been nine trials that have compared UFH to LMWH in UA/NSTEMI [9, 21–28]. In four of these trials the LMWH enoxaparin had lower rates of death or MI when compared with UFH. LMWH can easily be administered in the emergency department as a subcutaneous injection. In addition, the other anticoagulants such as bivalirudin [29] and fondaparinux [30] have been shown to decrease adverse cardiac events in the setting of UA/NSTEMI.

The most significant complication of UFH/LMWH use is bleeding. An analysis of four major trials with UFH and LMWH demonstrated a rate of major bleeding of 1–6.7%, and a transfusion rate of 0.6–12.2% [31]. In the international GRACE registry of over 24,000 ACS patients, the overall rate of major bleeding was 3.9%, but in the United States the major bleeding rate was significantly higher at 6.9%. In the ACTION registry in the United States (formerly known as CRUSADE) in over 30,000 ACS patients the major bleeding rate was 11.5%. The bleeding complications were in part attributed to excessive dosing of 13.8% with LMWH and 32.8% with UFH [32]. Major bleeding in ACS is associated with higher mortality rates. In a combined analysis of the CURE and OASIS-2 trials in patients who suffered a major bleed, the 30-day mortality rate was 12.8% as compared to only 2.5% without. The administration of either UFH or LMWH should be in patients with definite ACS or in patients with high clinical suspicion for ACS [12]. These therapies can lead to significant bleeding complications and should not be used in patients with undifferentiated chest pain in a CPU.

Nitrates

Although an overview of several small studies of nitroglycerin (NTG) in MI in the pre-fibrinolytic era suggests a 35% reduction in mortality [33], two large randomized placebo-controlled studies (ISIS-4,GISSI-3) did not show any improvement for NTG in AMI [34, 35]. Most studies of NTG in UA/NSTEMI have been small and uncontrolled. There are no randomized placebo-controlled studies that suggest symptom relief or reduction in cardiac events in UA/NSTEMI. Patients with known coronary artery disease are advised to use SL NTG at home in the setting of chest pain in the hope of symptom relief, and in patients with ST segment elevation on the electrocardiogram NTG should be administered to evaluate for possible coronary vasospasm [12].

The use of SL NTG in the ED in patients with undifferentiated chest pain is commonly employed. However, the relief or non-relief of chest pain does not assist in the identification of the patient with ACS and should have no impact on the triage decision of these patients [36, 37]. NTG is known to improve esophageal spasm and likely has a significant placebo effect in this setting. The constant administration of NTG, either in the form of nitropaste or intravenous infusion, should not be employed in the CPU.

Beta Blockers

The benefit of routine intravenous beta blocker in the setting of STEMI in the fibrinolytic era has been challenged by two large randomized trials [38, 39]. A meta-analysis of early beta blocker therapy in STEMI found no significant decrease in mortality [40]. More recently the large ACS COMMIT trial (93% STEMI, 7% NSTEMI) studied early intravenous therapy of beta blocker followed by oral administration demonstrated no improvement in mortality or adverse events at 8 days [43]. An overview of double-blind randomized trials of patients with UA or evolving MI suggested a 13% reduction in the risk of progression to MI [42]. However, these trials were conducted prior to the routine use of ASA, clopidogrel, GP IIb/IIIa inhibitors, and revascularization. Also these trial lacked sufficient power to assess mortality in UA. Pooled results from five trials in patients with ACS undergoing percutaneous intervention demonstrated a 6-month mortality rate of 1.7% in patients receiving beta blockers and 3.7% in patients that did not [43]. These findings, however, were post hoc and not randomized.

There should be selective use of beta blockers in the CPU. Patients with atrial fibrillation may need beta blocker therapy for rate control, especially if they are taking it chronically. Patients that are taking a beta blocker at home may need this to be continued. However, patients that will be undergoing some form of stress testing may need to have the beta blocker withheld or the dose decreased to ensure an adequate heart rate response during testing. For the average patient in the CPU who has not already been on a beta blocker it should not be administered either intravenously or orally in the CPU.

Conclusion

The overwhelming majority of low-risk patients with undifferentiated chest pain that are evaluated in a CPU are not diagnosed with an ACS. The only medical therapy that should be routinely administered to this patient population is ASA, as it is inexpensive, safe, well-tolerated, and highly effective across the spectrum of ACS. UFH and LMWH should not be administered routinely but should only be considered in the small fraction of patients that ultimately are diagnosed with ACS. NTG, which has never been shown to improve mortality or adverse cardiac events in ACS, should not be given in a continuous fashion either intravenously or transdermal, but could be considered in patients with definite ACS for control of symptoms. Sublingual NTG may be given as an attempt in symptom relief but does not assist in identifying patients with symptoms that are truly from ACS. Finally beta blockers are not generally recommended but may be given to patients who were already taking them or when they have another indication such as atrial fibrillation.

References

1. Randomised trial of intravenous streptokinase, oral aspirin, both, or neither among 17,187 cases of suspected acute myocardial infarction: ISIS-2. ISIS-2 (Second International Study of Infarct Survival) Collaborative Group. Lancet. 1988 Aug 13;2(8607):349–60.
2. Lewis HD, Jr., Davis JW, Archibald DG, Steinke WE, Smitherman TC, Doherty JE, 3rd, et al. Protective effects of aspirin against acute myocardial infarction and death in men with unstable angina. Results of a Veterans Administration Cooperative Study. The New England Journal of Medicine. 1983 Aug 18;309(7):396–403.
3. Cairns JA, Gent M, Singer J, Finnie KJ, Froggatt GM, Holder DA, et al. Aspirin, sulfinpyrazone, or both in unstable angina. Results of a Canadian multicenter trial. The New England Journal of Medicine. 1985 Nov 28;313(22):1369–75.
4. Theroux P, Ouimet H, McCans J, Latour JG, Joly P, Levy G, et al. Aspirin, heparin, or both to treat acute unstable angina. The New England Journal of Medicine. 1988 Oct 27;319(17):1105–11.
5. The RISC Group. Risk of myocardial infarction and death during treatment with low dose aspirin and intravenous heparin in men with unstable coronary artery disease. Lancet. 1990 Oct 6;336(8719):827–30.
6. Steering Committee of the Physicians' Health Study Research Group. Final report on the aspirin component of the ongoing Physicians' Health Study. The New England Journal of Medicine. 1989 Jul 20;321(3):129–35.
7. Collaborative meta-analysis of randomised trials of antiplatelet therapy for prevention of death, myocardial infarction, and stroke in high risk patients. BMJ (Clinical Research) ed. 2002 Jan 12;324(7329):71–86.
8. ISIS-2 (Second International Study of Infarct Survival) Collaborative Group. Randomized trial of intravenous streptokinase, oral aspirin, both, or neither among 17,187 cases of suspected acute myocardial infarction: ISIS-2. Journal of the American College of Cardiology. 1988 Dec;12(6 Suppl A):3A–13A.
9. Low-molecular-weight heparin during instability in coronary artery disease, Fragmin during Instability in Coronary Artery Disease (FRISC) study group. Lancet. 1996 Mar 2; 347(9001):561–8.

10. Hansson L, Zanchetti A, Carruthers SG, Dahlof B, Elmfeldt D, Julius S, et al. Effects of intensive blood-pressure lowering and low-dose aspirin in patients with hypertension: principal results of the Hypertension Optimal Treatment (HOT) randomised trial. HOT Study Group. Lancet. 1998 Jun 13;351(9118):1755–62.

11. Gurfinkel EP, Manos EJ, Mejail RI, Cerda MA, Duronto EA, Garcia CN, et al. Low molecular weight heparin versus regular heparin or aspirin in the treatment of unstable angina and silent ischemia. Journal of the American College of Cardiology. 1995 Aug;26(2):313–8.

12. Anderson JL, Adams CD, Antman EM, Bridges CR, Califf RM, Casey DE, Jr., et al. ACC/AHA 2007 guidelines for the management of patients with unstable angina/non-ST-Elevation myocardial infarction: A report of the American College of Cardiology/American Heart Association Task Force on Practice Guidelines (Writing Committee to Revise the 2002 Guidelines for the Management of Patients With Unstable Angina/Non-ST-Elevation Myocardial Infarction) developed in collaboration with the American College of Emergency Physicians, the Society for Cardiovascular Angiography and Interventions, and the Society of Thoracic Surgeons endorsed by the American Association of Cardiovascular and Pulmonary Rehabilitation and the Society for Academic Emergency Medicine. Journal of the American College of Cardiology. 2007 Aug 14;50(7):e1–e157.

13. Erhardt L, Herlitz J, Bossaert L, Halinen M, Keltai M, Koster R, et al. Task force on the management of chest pain. European Heart Journal. 2002 Aug;23(15):1153–76.

14. Barbash IM, Freimark D, Gottlieb S, Hod H, Hasin Y, Battler A, et al. Outcome of myocardial infarction in patients treated with aspirin is enhanced by pre-hospital administration. Cardiology. 2002;98(3):141–7.

15. 2005 American Heart Association Guidelines for Cardiopulmonary Resuscitation and Emergency Cardiovascular Care. Circulation. 2005 Dec 13;112(24 Suppl):IV1–203.

16. Telford AM, Wilson C. Trial of heparin versus atenolol in prevention of myocardial infarction in intermediate coronary syndrome. Lancet. 1981 Jun 6;1(8232):1225–8.

17. Williams DO, Kirby MG, McPherson K, Phear DN. Anticoagulant treatment of unstable angina. The British Journal of Clinical Practice. 1986 Mar;40(3):114–6.

18. Theroux P, Waters D, Qiu S, McCans J, de Guise P, Juneau M. Aspirin versus heparin to prevent myocardial infarction during the acute phase of unstable angina. Circulation. 1993 Nov;88(5 Pt 1):2045–8.

19. Neri Serneri GG, Gensini GF, Poggesi L, Trotta F, Modesti PA, Boddi M, et al. Effect of heparin, aspirin, or alteplase in reduction of myocardial ischaemia in refractory unstable angina. Lancet. 1990 Mar 17;335(8690):615–8.

20. Holdright D, Patel D, Cunningham D, Thomas R, Hubbard W, Hendry G, et al. Comparison of the effect of heparin and aspirin versus aspirin alone on transient myocardial ischemia and in-hospital prognosis in patients with unstable angina. Journal of the American College of Cardiology. 1994 Jul;24(1):39–45.

21. Cohen M, Theroux P, Borzak S, Frey MJ, White HD, Van Mieghem W, et al. Randomized double-blind safety study of enoxaparin versus unfractionated heparin in patients with non-ST-segment elevation acute coronary syndromes treated with tirofiban and aspirin: the ACUTE II study. The Antithrombotic Combination Using Tirofiban and Enoxaparin. American Heart Journal. 2002 Sep;144,(3):470–7.

22. Cohen M, Demers C, Gurfinkel EP, Turpie AG, Fromell GJ, Goodman S, et al. A comparison of low-molecular-weight heparin with unfractionated heparin for unstable coronary artery disease. Efficacy and Safety of Subcutaneous Enoxaparin in Non-Q-Wave Coronary Events Study Group. The New England Journal of Medicine. 1997 Aug 14;337(7):447–52.

23. Klein W, Buchwald A, Hillis SE, Monrad S, Sanz G, Turpie AG, et al. Comparison of low-molecular-weight heparin with unfractionated heparin acutely and with placebo for 6 weeks in the management of unstable coronary artery disease. Fragmin in unstable coronary artery disease study (FRIC). Circulation. 1997 Jul 1;96(1):61–8.

24. Comparison of two treatment durations (6 days and 14 days) of a low molecular weight heparin with a 6-day treatment of unfractionated heparin in the initial management of unstable angina or non-Q wave myocardial infarction: FRAX.I.S. (FRAxiparine in Ischaemic Syndrome). European Heart Journal. 1999 Nov;20(21):1553–62.

25. Goodman SG, Fitchett D, Armstrong PW, Tan M, Langer A. Randomized evaluation of the safety and efficacy of enoxaparin versus unfractionated heparin in high-risk patients with non-ST-segment elevation acute coronary syndromes receiving the glycoprotein IIb/ IIIa inhibitor eptifibatide. Circulation. 2003 Jan 21;107(2):238–44.

26. Blazing MA, de Lemos JA, White HD, Fox KA, Verheugt FW, Ardissino D, et al. Safety and efficacy of enoxaparin vs unfractionated heparin in patients with non-ST-segment elevation acute coronary syndromes who receive tirofiban and aspirin: a randomized controlled trial. JAMA. 2004 Jul 7;292(1):55–64.

27. Antman EM, McCabe CH, Gurfinkel EP, Turpie AG, Bernink PJ, Salein D, et al. Enoxaparin prevents death and cardiac ischemic events in unstable angina/non-Q-wave myocardial infarction. Results of the thrombolysis in myocardial infarction (TIMI) 11B trial. Circulation. 1999 Oct 12;100(15):1593–601.

28. Ferguson JJ, Califf RM, Antman EM, Cohen M, Grines CL, Goodman S, et al. Enoxaparin vs unfractionated heparin in high-risk patients with non-ST-segment elevation acute coronary syndromes managed with an intended early invasive strategy: primary results of the SYNERGY randomized trial. JAMA. 2004 Jul 7;292(1):45–54.

29. Stone GW, McLaurin BT, Cox DA, Bertrand ME, Lincoff AM, Moses JW, et al. Bivalirudin for patients with acute coronary syndromes. N Engl J Med. 2006 Nov 23; 355(21):2203–16.

30. Yusuf S, Mehta SR, Chrolavicius S, Afzal R, Pogue J, Granger CB, et al. Comparison of Fondaparinux and enoxaparin in acute coronary syndromes. N Engl J Med. 2006 Apr 6; 354(14):1464–76.

31. Petersen JL, Mahaffey KW, Hasselblad V, Antman EM, Cohen M, Goodman SG, et al. Efficacy and bleeding complications among patients randomized to enoxaparin or unfractionated heparin for antithrombin therapy in non-ST-Segment elevation acute coronary syndromes: a systematic overview. JAMA. 2004 Jul 7;292(1):89–96.

32. Alexander KP, Chen AY, Roe MT, Newby LK, Gibson CM, Allen-LaPointe NM, et al. Excess dosing of antiplatelet and antithrombin agents in the treatment of non-ST-segment elevation acute coronary syndromes. JAMA. 2005 Dec 28;294(24):3108–16.

33. Yusuf S, Collins R, MacMahon S, Peto R. Effect of intravenous nitrates on mortality in acute myocardial infarction: an overview of the randomised trials. Lancet. 1988 May 14;1(8594):1088–92.

34. ISIS-4: a randomised factorial trial assessing early oral captopril, oral mononitrate, and intravenous magnesium sulphate in 58,050 patients with suspected acute myocardial infarction. ISIS-4 (Fourth International Study of Infarct Survival) Collaborative Group. Lancet. 1995 Mar 18;345(8951):669–85.

35. GISSI-3: effects of lisinopril and transdermal glyceryl trinitrate singly and together on 6-week mortality and ventricular function after acute myocardial infarction. Gruppo Italiano per lo Studio della Sopravvivenza nell'infarto Miocardico. Lancet. 1994 May 7;343(8906):1115–22.

36. Henrikson CA, Howell EE, Bush DE, Miles JS, Meininger GR, Friedlander T, et al. Chest pain relief by nitroglycerin does not predict active coronary artery disease. Annals of internal medicine. 2003 Dec 16;139(12):979–86.

37. Diercks DB, Boghos E, Guzman H, Amsterdam EA, Kirk JD. Changes in the numeric descriptive scale for pain after sublingual nitroglycerin do not predict cardiac etiology of chest pain. Annals of emergency medicine. 2005 Jun;45(6):581–5.

38. Roberts R, Rogers WJ, Mueller HS, Lambrew CT, Diver DJ, Smith HC, et al. Immediate versus deferred beta-blockade following thrombolytic therapy in patients with acute myocardial infarction. Results of the Thrombolysis in Myocardial Infarction (TIMI) II-B Study. Circulation. 1991 Feb;83(2):422–37.

39. Van de Werf F, Janssens L, Brzostek T, Mortelmans L, Wackers FJ, Willems GM, et al. Short-term effects of early intravenous treatment with a beta-adrenergic blocking agent or a specific bradycardiac agent in patients with acute myocardial infarction receiving thrombolytic therapy. Journal of the American College of Cardiology. 1993 Aug;22(2):407–16.

40. Freemantle N, Cleland J, Young P, Mason J, Harrison J. beta Blockade after myocardial infarction: systematic review and meta regression analysis. BMJ (Clinical Research) ed. 1999 Jun 26;318(7200):1730–7.

41. Chen ZM, Pan HC, Chen YP, Peto R, Collins R, Jiang LX, et al. Early intravenous then oral metoprolol in 45,852 patients with acute myocardial infarction: randomised placebo-controlled trial. Lancet. 2005 Nov 5;366(9497):1622–32.

42. Yusuf S, Wittes J, Friedman L. Overview of results of randomized clinical trials in heart disease. II. Unstable angina, heart failure, primary prevention with aspirin, and risk factor modification. JAMA. 1988 Oct 21;260(15):2259–63.

43. Ellis K, Tcheng JE, Sapp S, Topol EJ, Lincoff AM. Mortality benefit of beta blockade in patients with acute coronary syndromes undergoing coronary intervention: Pooled results from the Epic, Epilog, Epistent, Capture and Rapport Trials. Journal of Interventional Cardiology. 2003 Aug;16(4):299–305.

Chapter 12
Provocative Testing

J. Douglas Kirk, Michael C. Kontos, and Ezra A. Amsterdam

Abstract Most patients presenting to the emergency department with symptoms suggestive of acute coronary syndrome (ACS) have a benign condition. However, management of this population remains a major challenge. An important contemporary approach to this problem has been the development of chest pain units (CPU) in which low-risk patients are managed by accelerated diagnostic protocols. If the initial evaluation is nondiagnostic, patients receive provocative testing and the safety of stress testing in this context has been well established. Negative provocative testing allows direct discharge with outpatient follow-up, while a positive test results in admission for further evaluation. The most frequently applied test is treadmill electrocardiography but stress (exercise or pharmacologic) myocardial perfusion imaging or stress echocardiography is also utilized in many institutions. Test selection depends on physician and institutional preference, the patient's ability to exercise, and interpretability of the electrocardiogram. Each method of provocative testing has advantages and limitations in terms of logistics, complexity, cost, ease of interpretation, and accuracy. However, each has clearly demonstrated its utility in contributing to safe, accurate, and efficient assessment of low-risk patients with possible ACS.

Keywords Acute coronary syndrome · Stress testing · Myocardial imaging · Myocardial perfusion

Introduction

Safe, cost-effective management of patients presenting with chest pain remains an important challenge [1, 2]. The principle goal in the evaluation of these patients is recognition of those with acute coronary syndrome (ACS) or other

J.D. Kirk (✉)
Department of Emergency Medicine, University of California, Davis, Medical Center,
4150 V Street, PSSB Suite 2100, Sacramento, CA 95817, USA
e-mail: jdkirk@ucdavis.edu

W.F. Peacock, C.P. Cannon (eds.), *Short Stay Management of Chest Pain*,
DOI 10.1007/978-1-60327-948-2_12,
© Humana Press, a part of Springer Science+Business Media, LLC 2009

potentially life-threatening causes of chest pain [3–5]. Although ACS is the primary focus of the initial evaluation in patients presenting to the emergency department (ED) with chest pain, the etiology in the majority of these patients is relatively benign, such as musculoskeletal, gastroesophageal, and anxiety disorders [2]. The clinical challenge is efficient identification of the latter groups to reduce unnecessary hospitalization of patients who do not have ACS without compromising the care of patients at risk. The development of chest pain units (CPU), which are described in earlier chapters, is a response to this need. The focus of these units is management of the lower risk population that comprises chest pain patients presenting without initial, objective evidence of myocardial infarction (MI) or ischemia in whom an abbreviated evaluation can determine the need for admission or the safety of discharge [6–10]. It is further emphasized that the primary goal of evaluation in this setting is to identify or exclude ACS rather than to detect coronary artery disease (CAD). Therefore, the utility of the methods of evaluation in these patients should be viewed from this perspective.

This approach is often referred to as an accelerated diagnostic protocol (ADP). This process usually entails a brief period (3–9 h) of clinical observation, serial 12-lead electrocardiograms (ECG), continuous telemetry monitoring, and measurement of serial cardiac injury markers [6–10]. Positive findings indicate ACS and mandate admission for further management. Negative findings are consistent with absence of MI and no evidence of ischemia at rest. Although ADPs utilizing newer technology have enhanced identification of patients with ACS, this strategy alone is insufficient to exclude patients who have ischemia alone, without MI, who remain at significant risk. In most institutions ADPs have incorporated additional "provocative" diagnostic testing to detect underlying CAD as a surrogate marker for patients who have unstable angina after myocardial necrosis has been excluded. This cautious approach has been supported by reports of failure to recognize ACS and inadvertent discharge of as many as 5% of apparently low-risk patients who demonstrate a nearly twofold increase in 30-day mortality compared to patients who were appropriately recognized [11]. In addition, failure to recognize MI or ischemia is one of the leading causes of malpractice awards against emergency physicians, thereby reinforcing this conservative approach [12]. The utility of ADPs has been well demonstrated with this method, as indicated by its safety and the very low clinical risk in patients designated as appropriate for early discharge.

The choice of diagnostic test typically includes exercise treadmill testing (ETT), stress myocardial perfusion imaging (MPI), or stress echocardiography. Rest MPI or echocardiography has also been applied in some institutions. Patients with a positive provocative test are admitted for further evaluation, most often coronary angiography, and those with a negative result are discharged to outpatient follow-up. This chapter will focus on the "secondary risk stratification" afforded by this additional diagnostic testing and will address appropriate test selection with patient type.

Patient Selection

Critical to the success of an ADP that utilizes early provocative testing in patients with undifferentiated chest pain is the identification of those with low clinical risk on presentation to the ED. For both efficient resource utilization and superior diagnostic accuracy, it is fundamental to match the risk of disease with the complexity of diagnostic testing.

There is substantial evidence that among ED patients with chest pain, a low-risk group can be identified. These patients have a low occurrence of adverse cardiac events and neither require nor benefit from intensive care. Of patients admitted for "rule out MI," those with a <5–10% probability of MI can generally be identified by the type of chest pain, cardiac history, and resting ECG [13]. Goldman et al. extended this approach in over 10,000 patients, demonstrating that the initial clinical assessment could distinguish those with <1% risk of adverse events [14] (Fig. 12.1). The initial ECG alone provides

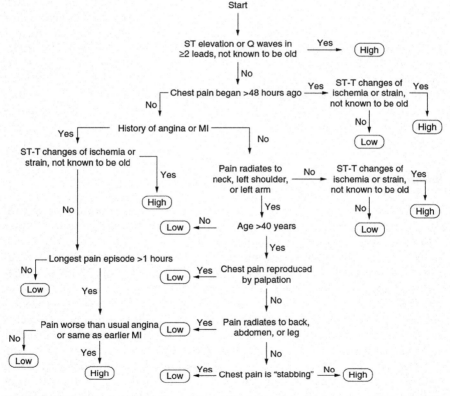

Fig. 12.1 Algorithm for evaluating patients with chest pain in the emergency room. The Goldman algorithm divides patients into groups at high risk (≥7%) and low risk (<7%) for an acute episode of myocardial ischemia. Adapted with permission from Zalenski et al. [82]

important prognostic data. Although not optimally sensitive for the diagnosis of MI, a normal ECG in patients with chest pain portends a favorable prognosis, with a high likelihood of a benign clinical course and fewer adverse events than in patients with abnormal ECGs [15]. An important concept to emerge from these studies is that although the cause of chest pain is frequently elusive, basic clinical tools provide powerful estimates of cardiac risk. This reliable identification of low-risk groups is fundamental to the safety and feasibility of an ADP.

Test Selection

The selection of a specific diagnostic test, and whether or not imaging is incorporated, is most commonly dependent upon the patient's ability to exercise and the ability to interpret the stress ECG. However, institutional expertise in differing modalities and test availability, particularly after hours, are also important determinants of test selection. In many institutions, these factors drive the choice of diagnostic test strategy regardless of the actual indication for more complex testing. ETT is the most frequently used strategy in current ADPs and remains as the cornerstone of diagnostic testing for inducible ischemia, and by inference, CAD, in CPUs. It is against this standard that ETT is recommended as a first-line test unless the clinical circumstances described below preclude its use. Advantages and disadvantages of diagnostic tests that utilize a cardiac imaging modality should be weighed before choosing a particular test in a given patient.

Inability to Exercise

In patients who cannot exercise because of physical limitations, peripheral arterial disease, or pulmonary disease, pharmacologic stress testing with either MPI or echocardiography is usually indicated. Pharmacologic stress MPI can be performed with either a vasodilator (dipyridamole or adenosine) or dobutamine, with vasodilators considered as the preferred agents. Both dipyridamole and adenosine have been well studied and are highly effective in diagnosis and risk stratification. Sensitivities and specificities for diagnosing CAD are similar to that of exercise stress MPI [16]. However, when compared to patients undergoing exercise stress MPI, the incidence of cardiac death in patients after pharmacologic stress MPI is higher, even in those patients with normal imaging [17]. This higher risk is related to the underlying comorbidities precluding exercise, rather than reduced prognostic accuracy of the test in this group of patients. In patients with contraindications to vasodilators such as bronchospastic disease, dobutamine can be used as an alternative stress agent. Because dobutamine has not been studied as extensively as the two vasodilators, tends to have more side effects, and does not produce the degree of coronary flow heterogeneity as the other agents, it should be used only in patients who have contraindications to vasodilator stress agents [18].

Rest MPI, in which a technetium (Tc-99m)-based isotope is injected during or shortly after symptoms in the ED, is a related technique that can provide similar risk stratification (discussed in detail below). This strategy relies on the patients rest symptoms to serve as the "stress" portion of the study. A perfusion defect indicates acute ischemia, acute infarction, or old infarction. Normal perfusion is associated with very low clinical risk, allowing patients to be discharged home with further outpatient routine rest/stress MPI if indicated to detect underlying CAD.

Baseline ECG Changes

The other common indication for using imaging in conjunction with stress testing is baseline ECG abnormalities that preclude accurate interpretation of the stress ECG. Imaging in conjunction with stress testing should be used if the baseline ECG shows widespread ST depression such as accompanies left bundle branch block (LBBB), left ventricular hypertrophy (LVH) with significant ST segment changes, ventricular paced rhythm, or preexcitation [19]. Although exercise capacity can be assessed, exercise-induced ischemia cannot be reliably determined with the stress ECG. In patients with LVH, with or without resting ST segment abnormalities, ST depression during exercise often occurs in the absence of significant CAD. In these patients, stress MPI has been shown to have similar diagnostic sensitivity and specificity to those observed in patients without LVH [20].

Patients who have underlying LBBB represent a special subset in whom pharmacologic stress MPI is preferable to exercise for both diagnosis and risk stratification. There appears to be an increased prevalence of myocardial perfusion defects primarily involving the interventricular septum during exercise imaging, in the absence of significant CAD [21]. These defects may be reversible or fixed, and are often absent during vasodilator stress, indicating that ischemia is an unlikely etiology. Therefore, MPI with pharmacologic vasodilation appears to be more accurate for identifying CAD in these patients [22].

Stress echocardiography also provides additional risk stratification and plays an important role in these patients. In the patient with baseline ECG abnormalities who can exercise, stress echocardiography is an equally appropriate test, so that the ultimate test selected is often dependent upon institutional or operator expertise. Stress echocardiography can be performed with standard echocardiography equipment and the results are available immediately after testing. Unlike all other imaging techniques, it is noninvasive and poses no risk from radiation exposure. Echocardiography can also provide structural and functional data, as well as findings that suggest other nonischemic etiologies for the patients' symptoms, including pulmonary embolism, valvular heart disease, cardiomyopathies, and pericardial disease [23].

Rather than proceeding immediately to stress echocardiography, some have advocated using rest echocardiography in selected patients with ongoing symptoms upon presentation. This strategy, similar to rest MPI's ability to detect perfusion defects, is based on the premise that the echocardiogram will detect wall motion abnormalities if symptoms are related to ischemia or infarction. Study results using this strategy have been mixed and few clinicians rely primarily on this approach alone as part of an ADP.

Added Value of Cardiac Imaging

In contrast to the patients with abnormal rest ECGs, those with normal ECGs constitute a large, important subgroup of patients undergoing evaluation for chest pain. The presence of a normal rest ECG identifies a low-risk group with an excellent prognosis after MI is excluded [24]. The exercise ECG also has a higher specificity in these patients than in those who have rest ST-T changes or LVH.

Several studies have examined the incremental value of stress MPI compared with ETT in patients with a normal rest ECG not taking digoxin [25, 26]. In a study of 1,659 low-risk patients without known CAD, Ladenheim et al. found that in the subgroup of 1,451 patients who had a normal rest ECG, the MPI results did not add additional information over pretest data [25]. Another report analyzed outcomes of 3,058 consecutive patients with a normal rest ECG who underwent exercise dual isotope MPI [26]. There were 70 adverse events (2.3%) during a mean follow-up of 1.6 ± 0.5 years. After adjusting for pretest indicators of risk, stress MPI yielded incremental value to predict adverse events, but not in low-risk patients. Patients with a low pretest probability of CAD had an adverse event rate of only 0.4%, suggesting that stress MPI would be unlikely to be cost-effective. However, for patients who had an intermediate to high likelihood of CAD prior to stress testing, the cost per adverse event identified was $25,134.

Recommendations for Choice of Diagnostic Test

The current American College of Cardiology/American Heart Association (ACC/AHA) guidelines for stress testing as well as for management of non-ST elevation myocardial infarction/unstable angina (NSTEMI/UA) recommend that ETT without imaging should be performed as the initial test in low- to intermediate-risk patients who have ischemic symptoms, who can exercise, do not have significant baseline ECG changes that preclude interpretation, and are not taking digoxin [19, 27]. Patients with abnormal ECGs will need the addition of cardiac imaging with either MPI or echocardiography. Patients unable to walk will require pharmacological stress testing with imaging. Of note, because of the additional diagnostic and prognostic information obtained, stress MPI or echocardiography is often employed as a sole strategy to evaluate all patients presenting with chest pain, despite the absence of an indication for complex testing in lower risk patients. Although the aforementioned subsets of patients benefit from imaging, in others, the additional information obtained is likely not cost-effective and routine ETT would be the appropriate first choice for testing. The clinical application of ETT, MPI, and stress echocardiography are described in the following sections.

Exercise Treadmill Testing

ETT is an important component of the diagnostic evaluation of patients with suspected CAD, regardless of the setting. It is most often performed with ECG monitoring alone and is still the procedure of choice in majority of ADPs. Exceptions to its use include inability to exercise or resting ECG abnormalities that preclude accurate interpretation of stress-induced alterations. In these situations, stress testing in conjunction with imaging, either MPI or echocardiography is appropriate.

The exercise ECG detects myocardial ischemia due to underlying CAD as a result of mismatch of oxygen supply and demand. Although the diagnostic reliability of a negative ETT has been validated in low-risk populations based on comparisons with coronary angiography, it is even more useful in providing critical prognostic information and is frequently used to predict future adverse cardiac events [28]. Depending on the results of the information obtained from the ETT, patients with positive tests are typically referred for further evaluation. In those in whom the suspicion is low, repeat testing with imaging can be used. For patients who have high-risk findings, the next step is frequently coronary angiography and revascularization if appropriate. In most cases, those with negative exercise tests benefit little from further evaluation. Thus, a negative test in a low-risk population provides objective, reliable evidence of low clinical risk.

Test Performance and Interpretation

Most stress test protocols incorporate a series of stages with gradually increasing speed and/or incline that produce a predictable increase in cardiac workload. The most commonly used are the Bruce protocol and a variant that uses two "warm-up" stages referred to as a modified Bruce protocol (Table 12.1). Both a clinician and a technician are in attendance, constantly observing the patient's clinical status. A 12-lead ECG is monitored continuously and blood pressures are taken with each 3-min stage. It has been demonstrated that both

Table 12.1 Minutes exercised, percent grade, speed, and estimate of work for each stage of the modified Bruce protocol

Stage	Minutes	Grade (%)	Speed (mph)	METS
0	3	0	1.7	2.3
½	6	5	1.7	3.5
1	9	10	1.7	4.7
2	12	12	2.5	7.0
3	15	14	3.4	10.1
4	18	16	4.2	12.9
5	21	18	5.0	15.0

Stages 0 and ½ precede the typical Bruce protocol (stages 1–5); METS, metabolic equivalents.

clinical and ECG responses to exercise can be useful in determining patients' risk. The usual ECG criteria for a positive test for myocardial ischemia are ≥1.0 mm horizontal or downsloping ST segment deviation 60–80 ms after the J point. Additional alterations of exercise test variables that indicate an abnormal test and are associated with an increased risk of future adverse events are described in Table 12.2 [29, 30]. The occurrence of one or more of these variables identifies a high-risk group that may benefit from coronary angiography and revascularization. A negative test is usually defined as the one in which the patient achieves ≥85% of age-predicted maximal heart rate without the aforementioned ST segment deviation. A nondiagnostic test is defined as no significant ST deviation but failure to reach the 85% age-predicted target heart rate. The majority of the latter are treated as a negative test unless exercise capacity is poor (<2 stages of the standard Bruce protocol), in which case a more definitive test not dependent upon exercise is advised.

Table 12.2 Stress testing variables associated with high risk

- ≥1 mm of downsloping or flat ST segment depression
- ST selgment depression at a low cardiac workload or of prolonged duration
- Multiple leads with ST segment depression
- Exercise-induced angina
- Fall in systolic blood pressure below baseline during exercise
- bPoor exercise capacity
- ST segment elevation
- Ventricular arrhythmias
- Chronotropic incompetence

In low-risk patients undergoing ETT as part of a CPU evaluation, only a minority will have positive tests, and nearly half are found to be false positives on more definitive testing. While this lack of specificity may initially be a cause for concern, many of these false positives can be recognized during the initial exercise test. The degree of ST segment deviation and the point at which it occurs during the test are helpful in determining whether a test is a true or false positive result. The less the ST segment deviation and the higher the cardiac workload (measured in exercise time, metabolic equivalents [METS], or rate-pressure product [systolic blood pressure × heart rate]) at which it occurs, the higher the likelihood that the test result is a false positive. ST segment deviation in patients with excellent functional capacity and no angina also suggest a false positive test. In addition, the relationship between the ST segment response and heart rate during recovery is an important discriminating feature between true and false positive stress tests [31]. If resolution of ST segment deviation begins as or before the heart rate begins to fall, it suggests a false positive test. Thus while the general rule is to follow-up a positive stress test with a more definitive study, a false positive test can frequently be predicted with reasonable reliability based upon the characteristics of the initial stress test.

While most ADPs historically incorporate a "cooling off" period prior to ETT, others have advocated a more direct approach with earlier ETT in stable patients with normal initial cardiac injury markers and a normal or nondiagnostic ECG [32, 33]. This approach is now more widely applicable since most ADPs have markedly shortened the observation period as cardiac injury markers measured in shorter intervals have improved the early identification of patients with ACS. The protocol described in Table 12.3 provides practical

Table 12.3 Exercise treadmill test protocol

Eligible patients:

All patients with chest pain suspicious of myocardial ischemia
No other serious etiology for chest pain is considered or found (e.g., pulmonary embolism, aortic dissection, esophageal rupture)
Clinically stable and without evidence of left ventricular dysfunction
ECG normal or only minor nonspecific repolarization abnormalities
Exclusion criteria:
Inability to exercise adequately
ECG abnormalities precluding accurate interpretation (e.g., bundle branch block, left ventricular hypertrophy with strain, or digitalis effect)
ED evaluation:
Physical examination not suggestive of left ventricular dysfunction or significant valvular disease
Equal arm blood pressures
Chest radiograph not suggestive of aortic dissection or congestive heart failure
Negative troponin I and myoglobin upon arrival
ETT procedure (Modified Bruce Protocol):
Test endpoints
Symptom limited
Fall in systolic blood pressure ≥ 10 mmHg
Coupling of ventricular ectopics
Sustained supraventricular tachycardia
1 mm ST segment depression (horizontal or downsloping) or elevation 80 ms after the J point*

ECG, electrocardiogram; ETT, exercise treadmill testing. * Criteria for a positive test. Adapted with permission from Kirk et al. [1].

recommendations for performing an ETT and can be used as a guideline to implement stress testing in any ED or CPU, allowing for varying degrees of pretest observation and sampling of ECGs and cardiac injury markers.

Prognostic Scores

The use of ETT scores as an additional management tool can add prognostic information to the individual patient's clinical data, allowing comparison of patients or groups of patients. This method of risk stratification is useful in the assessment of undifferentiated chest pain patients typically seen in the ED and can easily be incorporated into the pathway of an ADP. The most commonly used and the best validated is the Duke Treadmill Score, which is calculated by measuring the exercise time in minutes on a Bruce protocol, minus five times the ST segment deviation in millimeters, minus four times the exercise-induced angina (0 = none, 1 = nonlimiting, and 2 = exercise limiting) [34]. Based on the score, patients are classified as low ($\geq +5$), moderate (–10 to +4), and high (≤ -11) risk. One easily remembered reference value is that a patient must exercise >5 min, without chest pain or ECG changes to be considered low risk. In a large study of patients undergoing exercise testing for risk assessment, prognosis was related to the risk category as determined by the Duke score, even after adjustment for other clinical predictors of risk. Five-year survival was 65% in high-risk patients, 90% in moderate-risk patients, and over 97% in low-risk patients [35].

Others have demonstrated that patients with excellent exercise tolerance (≥ 10 METS) or a heart rate >160 beats per minute infrequently have three vessel (15%) or left main (1%) disease and have an excellent prognosis (1% mortality/year), irrespective of the ECG findings [36]. Peak exercise capacity has been shown to be the strongest predictor of mortality, regardless of the presence or absence of CAD [30]. Similar to poor peak exercise capacity, a delay in heart rate recovery (less than 12–18 beats per minute decrease at 1 min post-exercise) is also associated with a worse prognosis. A study of 2,428 patients undergoing exercise testing with 6-year follow-up demonstrated a nearly two-fold increase in adjusted mortality in patients with abnormal heart rate recovery [37]. A limitation of these two variables is that they better predict mortality, both cardiac and noncardiac, rather than of CAD, and therefore may have less application in patients undergoing an ETT from a CPU.

Supervision and Post-Discharge Testing

Other important considerations include supervision and interpretation of the test and timing (predischarge or outpatient) of the ETT. In many cases these tests have been performed by cardiologists who provide consultation to selected patients with negative findings during an ADP. This may be unfortunately associated with an inherent delay due to lack of availability of cardiologists. With increased frequency, ETT is performed by other personnel such as physician extenders or nurses with subsequent interpretation by a cardiologist [38]. While it is not practical to train general emergency physicians to perform ETT, other unique groups have successfully performed these tests. At the University of California (Davis) Medical Center CPU, we employ staff physicians with special training in the assessment of patients with chest pain and performance of ETT to provide testing. The interreader reliability between these physicians and cardiologists in 645 patients who underwent stress testing in the CPU was very high with discrepancies found in only 11 patients (1.7%, kappa = 0.96), the majority of which were clinically insignificant [39]. These data suggest that noncardiologists with special training in ETT can reliably perform and interpret these studies. This is critically important to the applicability of this procedure as a risk stratification tool.

Recommendations for the timing (index visit or outpatient) of stress testing is not thoroughly evidence based. Most ADPs advocate early testing but this would require institutions to have 24/7 availability, and most do not. This limitation frequently leads to holding patients in EDs or observation units until the test is available, usually during the daytime. Weekends may offer additional challenges. Alternatively, an ETT can be performed shortly (within 72 h) after discharge. This approach is based on the general recommendation from the 2007 ACC/AHA guidelines for NSTEMI/UA [27] and refers to low-risk patients without further ischemic discomfort, normal or nondiagnostic ECGs, and normal cardiac injury markers. This recommendation is principally based on expert opinion (a consensus level of evidence). While there are no randomized clinical trials addressing this situation, several observational studies have examined the clinical course of patients who were referred for outpatient ETT [40–42]. Patient selection was typically at the physician's discretion and follow-up was not rigorously adhered to. Despite these limitations, adverse events were rare. Nonetheless, predischarge stress testing should be encouraged if possible and if not, testing within 72 h is a reasonable alternative.

Utility of Exercise Stress Testing in an ADP

Stress testing is now a "routine" in most EDs or CPUs and is considered a part of standard of care. Current practice is predicated on nearly two decades of experience from a variety of institutions that have incorporated some form of provocative testing into their ADPs. One of the first described was a relatively conservative approach compared to today's standards [6]. It consisted of a 9-h observation period in the ED's chest pain center, during which ~1000 patients underwent continuous ST segment monitoring, serial measurement of CK-MB and ECGs, and a resting echocardiogram. Patients without evidence of cardiovascular disease on this stepwise approach underwent ETT, which had a negative predictive value of 98.7% and enabled 82% of the patients to be discharged from the ED. A follow-up study to this initial report demonstrated that patients with positive, nondiagnostic, and negative ETT had cardiac event rates of 26, 3, and 0.9%, respectively, during 1-year follow-up [43]. This approach led to compelling data from a number of subsequent studies that suggested performing ETT as part of an ADP was safe and cost-effective [7, 8, 44].

This observational data has been confirmed in two randomized controlled trials that compared ADPs with ETT to usual care with hospital admission. Of the 50 patients randomized to ADP care in the first trial, 49 had MI excluded and 41/44 (93%) had a negative ETT; the other 3 were false positives. At 1 month, there were no adverse cardiac events in either the ADP or inpatient groups. Although this was a very low-risk population, the length of stay and associated costs in the ADP group were nearly half the control group, demonstrating the utility of this approach [9]. In the second study, investigators randomized patients to a 6-h ADP ($n = 212$) or standard inpatient care ($n = 212$) [10]. Those with negative ECGs and cardiac injury markers underwent ETT, which was positive in 55 patients who were admitted for further work-up and negative in 97 who were discharged home. Adverse cardiac event rates were 3.8% in the ADP group and 8% in the inpatient group. In addition to a shorter length of stay, half the patients in the ADP group avoided hospital admission.

At the majority of centers that have incorporated ETT as a risk stratification tool, it has been employed after a negative ADP evaluation, which by today's standards typically included a relatively long period of observation (6–12 h in most, but up to 48 h in some cases). Clinical outcomes were comparable to those of traditional inpatient evaluation; however, the timing of ETT is variable. Our use of ETT at the University of California, Davis, differs in that it is frequently performed shortly after identification of low risk by history, a resting ECG, and an initial negative cardiac troponin and myoglobin. We have employed an "immediate" ETT protocol (Table 12.3) in more than 4000 appropriately selected, low-risk patients with chest pain over the past decade. Our preliminary report in 93 patients suggested this approach was safe and had the potential for major cost savings [45]. The majority of patients had negative tests and there were no complications from exercising patients who presented with acute chest pain. A follow-up study of 212 patients modified this approach in several significant respects. Patients with a prior history of CAD were not excluded and ETT was performed by staff physicians (internists) in our CPU. Serial cardiac injury markers were not measured (although a majority had negative initial cardiac injury makers) [32]. There were no adverse effects of ETT. Of the 28 (13%) patients who had positive tests, 10 were diagnosed with UA and 3 with MI on further testing. Negative ETTs were found in 125 (59%) and 59 (28%) were nondiagnostic (negative for ischemia but failed to achieve target heart rate). All patients with negative ETTs and 93% of those with nondiagnostic tests were discharged home from the ED. Follow-up at 30 days revealed no adverse cardiac events in patients discharged from the ED. This data suggest that nearly 90% of these low-risk patients could be safely discharged home based on the results of ETT. More importantly, it demonstrated the safety of shortening the ADP in selected patients on the basis of the initial presentation.

A larger study was needed to confirm the feasibility of this strategy before advocating its general use. Using the same protocol, 1000 heterogeneous patients, including 7.5% with a prior history of CAD were included (33). Nearly identical to our prior experience, the ETT was negative in 64%, positive in 13%, and nondiagnostic in 23%. There were no complications of testing and 80% of patients were safely discharged home from the ED. During the 30-day follow-up there were no mortality and cardiac events in the three groups as described in Table 12.4. Compared to a negative exercise test, the relative risk of a cardiac event or the diagnosis of CAD was 38-fold for a nondiagnostic test and 114-fold for a positive test.

Table 12.4 Exercise treadmill test results of low-risk patients with chest pain

Test result	N	Adverse events	Diagnosis of CAD
Negative	640	1 MI	1
Positive	125	4 MI	33
		12 revascularizations	
Nondiagnostic	235	7 revascularizations	25

CAD, coronary artery disease; MI, myocardial infarction.

Emerging from these studies is recognition of the common occurrence and excellent predictive value of negative ETT in patients identified as low risk [6–10, 32, 33, 43, 44]. Further, although the positive predictive value is modest, positive tests are infrequent and result in the need for further evaluation in only small numbers of patients. Therefore, the utility of a strategy incorporating ETT into an ADP was confirmed by its ability to safely and efficiently reduce unnecessary admissions in low-risk patients while avoiding inappropriate discharge of patients with ACS not identified by routine measurement of cardiac injury markers and ECGs. Estimates of cost-effectiveness indicate the potential for substantial savings for similar reasons.

Myocardial Perfusion Imaging

A number of studies have demonstrated that stress testing with MPI or echocardiography provides more information than ETT alone in patients presenting to the ED with chest pain [16, 46]. The additional information that is obtained, including the amount of infarcted or jeopardized myocardium and the extent of ischemia, have significant prognostic value, and the addition of gating provides quantitative information on systolic function [47]. Studies of large patient samples have demonstrated that estimation of the severity of systolic dysfunction is an excellent predictor of cardiac mortality. In contrast, markers of induced ischemia (exertional symptoms, ECG changes, and extent of reversible perfusion defects) are better predictors of the subsequent development of acute ischemic syndromes [47]. Similar to ETT, results should not be considered simply as positive or negative; rather, accurate diagnosis and risk stratification should include the extent and severity of ischemia, either quantitatively [48, 49] or semiquantitatively [50], as well as exercise duration, symptoms, and stress ECG results.

Practical Applications of Stress Imaging

At peak stress (exercise or pharmacologic), the radiopharmaceutical is injected intravenously. The patient is then imaged by a gamma camera to quantitate myocardial perfusion with stress. These images are subsequently compared with those obtained at rest. Areas that show similarly decreased perfusion at stress and rest are consistent with prior MI, whereas areas with normal perfusion at rest but perfusion defects during on stress images are consistent with myocardial ischemia. The specific area of perfusion abnormality reflects the involved coronary artery, and the size of the perfusion abnormality correlates with the severity of CAD.

The choice of radiopharmaceutical used with stress MPI is made by the individual laboratory performing the test. Thallium-201 (Tl-201) was one of the first isotopes used for stress MPI. It is injected at peak stress and the patient is imaged within 5–10 min. Over the next 3–4 h, there is equilibration of blood and myocardial Tl-201 concentration (redistribution). Repeat images at rest are obtained 3–4 h later.

The limitations of Tl-201 (including soft tissue attenuation of the low-energy emissions and poor count statistics) prompted the development of the Tc-99m agents, which have largely replaced Tl-201. The technetium agents have improved imaging characteristics compared to Tl-201 due to higher photon energy and shorter half-life, allowing larger doses. These advantages are somewhat offset by increased uptake in abdominal organs and lack of redistribution. Tc-99m based agents that are currently available for clinical use include sestamibi (Cardiolite) and tetrofosmin (Myoview).

As a result of the higher photon energy available from Tc-99m agents, MPI can be gated with the ECG and provides good-quality images. Images of the heart (8–16 frames) are captured at multiple points in the cardiac cycle. The reconstructed images allow display of myocardial wall thickness, motion, and perfusion simultaneously by connecting the individual frames into cine loop format (similar to animation and motion pictures). Gated imaging also provides assessment of ventricular volume and ejection fraction. The accuracy of wall motion assessment and ejection fraction calculation by gated imaging has compared favorably to other imaging techniques.

In general most patients should be without food for 2–4 h prior to stress testing. This is particularly true for those who are undergoing pharmacologic stress testing with either dipyridamole or dobutamine, as these medications can provoke nausea and vomiting. Similar to ETT patients, in those who undergo stress MPI but do not achieve an adequate heart rate response, ischemia may be missed or underestimated. Iskandrian et al. reported that in patients who underwent stress MPI, the degree of coronary stenosis was underestimated in those who did not achieve adequate heart rate, defined as either 85% of age-predicted maximal heart rate or a positive stress ECG [51]. An important advantage of imaging in conjunction with stress testing is the ability to also assess systolic function, one of the most important prognostic indicators in patients with CAD. This can be done quantitatively with programs that allow direct measurement of left ventricular volumes and calculation of ejection fraction in conjunction with stress MPI. For patients who have ischemia on stress testing, the greater the degree of systolic dysfunction, the higher the likelihood of worse outcomes.

Stress MPI using Tc-99m isotopes is typically performed in either a 1- or 2-day protocol depending on the patient's size. For the 1-day protocol, patients are given a low dose of isotope for the rest images and a higher dose for the stress imaging. However, for obese patients, a higher dose of isotope is required to provide adequate cardiac imaging and a 2-day protocol is required. Typically, the patient undergoes stress testing first, and if the images are abnormal, rest images are performed the following day to determine if the defect is reversible, indicating ischemia, or is fixed, reflecting infarction. If the stress images are normal, no further imaging is usually required. Some institutions use a dual isotope protocol to improve patient throughput. In appropriate patients, injection of Tl-201 is performed at rest, with imaging a few minutes later. Stress MPI using a Tc-99m isotope can then be immediately performed.

Nonimaging Variables

A number of variables that are associated with increased prognostic risk with ETT do not confer similar risk in patients undergoing pharmacologic stress testing. Chest pain, which has important prognostic implications in patients undergoing ETT, is found to some degree in majority of the patients undergoing vasodilator stress testing. Patients undergoing dobutamine stress testing may have chest pain from ischemia, but this symptom is as likely to be related to rapid heart rate and sensation of increased force of cardiac contraction. The diagnostic accuracy of the stress ECG for a similar heart rate achieved in patients undergoing dobutamine stress testing is probably the same as for ETT. In contrast, the ECG is highly specific in patients undergoing vasodilator stress testing, and a positive ECG, even in the setting of normal perfusion, is usually associated with an increased risk of cardiovascular events. Hypotension, which is a predictor of worse outcomes in patients undergoing ETT, is fairly common during vasodilator testing and confers no additional risk. Hypotension with dobutamine stress testing is usually not associated with worse long-term outcomes.

Image Interpretation

Perfusion defects are graded in a variety of ways that usually provide a quantitative/semiquantitative assessment of the extent of perfusion abnormality as well as its severity. Defect grade is usually quantified as either not present, low, moderate, or high grade (little to no visible perfusion). Size is quantified by the percent of left ventricular involvement: a small defect, <5%; moderate, 5–15%; and large, >15% of the left ventricle. A limitation of MPI is the presence of attenuation defects. In women there can be variable attenuation by breast tissue that shifts across the anterior wall. This degree of variability can result in the false positive appearance of a defect consistent with ischemia when none is present. Attenuation defects can also occur in men with obese abdomens in which the diaphragm is displaced upward resulting in an apparent defect in the inferior wall. The presence of normal wall motion in those areas makes ischemia less likely.

Patients who have normal perfusion imaging have a very low risk of subsequent coronary events. In a summary of 16 studies involving 27,855 patients, the average cardiac event rate ranged from 0 to 1.6% with an average 1-year event rate of 0.6% [52]. This event rate varies based on the gender and the type of stress (pharmacologic vs. exercise). Patients undergoing pharmacologic stress imaging and those with diabetes have a higher likelihood of subsequent death or MI over the next 1 year [53].

Regardless of how the degree of abnormality is calculated, a greater degree of abnormality predicts an increased risk of subsequent events. This is important because subsequent observational data have confirmed that patients who have small defects have a low event rate and therefore, a low likelihood of benefiting from invasive treatment. In most cases, unless symptoms persist, this group should undergo medical treatment alone. Of concern is the potential for a patient with a single defect who has multivessel CAD. This may occur because MPI as well as stress echocardiography may underestimate the degree of abnormality for a variety of reasons. These include "balanced ischemia" in which relative perfusion is decreased in all parts of the heart, so that the presence of three vessel disease or left main disease would be missed. However, it is likely these patients would have poor exercise tolerance and stress-induced deterioration of systolic function. Another reason for missing multiple areas of ischemia is the presence of severe stenosis in an artery resulting in ischemia early in exercise prior to the appearance of ischemia in other areas supplied by significant but less severe CAD. Therefore, patients who have ischemia at low workloads are at higher risk than those in whom ischemia develops at higher workloads.

A number of schemes have been developed to try to identify those patients at risk for worse outcomes. These include combining the results of the stress ECG results and MPI with a clinical risk factor score. One scale gave one point for male gender, history of MI, diabetes and insulin use, and one point for each year in age greater than 40 [54]. In patients with a cardiac risk score >5, MPI could further stratify risk. However, in those patients who had low scores, MPI afforded no additional value. In patients with normal MPI but positive stress ECG, the latter is most likely a false positive result. A number of studies have evaluated outcomes with this discrepancy in stress ECG and MPI and found an annual cardiac death and MI rate similar to that of patients with normal scans, with the risk about 1% [55]. However, this discrepancy needs to be considered with the patient's symptoms and degree of exercise tolerance.

Pharmacological Stress Imaging

In patients who are unable to exercise, pharmacological stress using one of several agents is an alternative. Dipyridamole and adenosine are vasodilators that result in perfusion defects as the result of induced flow heterogeneity, in which increase in flow in normal arteries is greater than in arteries with significant stenoses. In minority of cases this may result in a coronary steal phenomenon with true ischemia. Patients are given a short continuous infusion, with the isotope administered at the time of peak drug effect (3 min after dipyridamole or during the adenosine infusion). Patients who are undergoing vasodilator stress should be without caffeine for a minimum of 12 h (and preferably 24 h) prior to injection, as this substance can interfere with vasodilatory actions of dipyridamole and adenosine. In contrast, dobutamine acts by stimulating beta I and II and alpha I receptors, resulting in increased contractility at low doses and increased heart rate and blood pressure at higher doses. The increased hemodynamic burden can induce left ventricular wall motion abnormalities and perfusion defects due to regional myocardial dysfunction in segments supplied by obstructive CAD. A variety of different infusion protocols have been used but in general, most use 3 min infusion stages in which dobutamine dose is sequentially increased from 10, 20, 30, and 40 mg/kg/min. In many cases if the target heart rate is not reached, atropine is added in 0.25 mg increments to a total of 2 mg.

Acute Rest Imaging

An alternative mechanism for early identification of high-risk patients who are initially considered low risk is rest MPI in the acute setting. One of the two Tc-99m isotopes are used, which are taken up by the myocardium in relation to coronary flow. Patients can be injected in the ED while experiencing symptoms and imaged after clinical stabilization. The images obtained subsequently provide a "snap shot" of coronary blood flow at the time of injection. In addition, simultaneous assessment of wall motion and thickening are obtained, allowing differentiation of perfusion defects resulting from artifacts or soft tissue attenuation from those occurring as a result of ischemia [56]. Ejection fraction is also obtained, providing a quantitative determination of systolic function.

Numerous studies have demonstrated that rest MPI can accurately identify high-risk patients [57–61, 63, 64, 66] (Table 12.5). In addition, rest MPI offers a statistically significant increase in both diagnostic and prognostic information to the ECG and clinical variables. These findings were confirmed in a prospective, randomized, multicenter trial of 2,475 patients who presented to the ED with chest pain and nonischemic ECGs [60]. Patients were randomized to receive usual care with or without the addition of rest MPI. Sensitivity of the two strategies was similar, as both treatment strategies missed one patient with MI, resulting in sensitivities of 96 and 97%, respectively. Patients in the rest MPI arm had a significantly lower hospitalization rate, which translated into an estimated cost savings of $70 per patient.

Table 12.5 Diagnostic accuracy of rest myocardial perfusion imaging in patients with acute chest pain and a nonischemic electrocardiogram

Reference	Year	N	Isotope	Sensitivity (%)	Specificity (%)	NPV (%)	Outcome
Varetto et al. [57]	1993	64	Tc-mibi	100	92	100	CAD
Hilton et al. [61]	1994	102	Tc-mibi	94	83	99	CAD/AMI
Tatum et al. [66]	1997	438	Tc-mibi	100	78	100	AMI
Kontos et al. [58]	1997	532	Tc-mibi	93	71	99	AMI
Heller et al. [63]	1998	357	Tc-tet	90	60	99	AMI
Kontos et al. [59]	1999	620	Tc-mibi	92	67	99	AMI
Udelson et al. [60]	2002	1215	Tc-mibi	96	NR	99	AMI
Schaeffer et al. [64]	2007	479	Tc-mibi	77	92	99	ACS

ACS, acute coronary syndrome; AMI, acute myocardial infarction; CAD, angiographic coronary artery disease; NPV, negative predictive value; NR, not reported; Tc-mibi, Tc-99m-Sestamibi; Tc-tet, Tc-99m-Tetrofosmin. Adapted with permission from Kontos and Tatum [83].

Rest MPI has certain limitations for evaluating chest pain patients. A perfusion defect can indicate acute ischemia, acute infarction, or remote infarction. Differentiating MI is readily accomplished by the presence of elevated cardiac injury markers. To differentiate prior infarction from acute ischemia, repeat imaging during a pain-free state can be performed. Resolution of a perfusion defect indicates that the initial defect was secondary to acute ischemia; if the defect remained unchanged, prior MI would be the more likely etiology. Sensitivity of imaging is dependent on the total ischemic area; patients with small areas of myocardium at risk (3–5% of the left ventricle) may not be detected. Therefore, optimal use is typically in conjunction with at least one set of cardiac injury markers, which offer complementary information to the MPI. By definition, cardiac injury markers are abnormal only in patients with myocardial necrosis and are negative in patients who have ischemia alone. However, in both settings perfusion will be abnormal. Further, rest MPI can quantify the ischemic area, which may be a better way to assess overall ischemic risk than cardiac injury markers alone.

Despite the application of this relatively complex and expensive technology, rest MPI can be cost-effective, as the number of patients requiring admission is reduced [61–63]. These observational studies suggest cost reductions occur when rest MPI is used as an integral part of patient management and are the result of a number of factors. Low-risk patients can be discharged directly from the ED, rather than admitted or undergo a more prolonged observation. Early identification of patients with atypical symptoms and a nonischemic ECG who are actually having MI can avoid inappropriate discharge. By more appropriate selection of diagnostic procedures, the rate of coronary angiography in low-risk patients can be reduced [61, 63]. In recognition of the high diagnostic utility of this approach, current guidelines indicate that rest MPI has a class 1 indication for evaluating patients with a nonischemic ECG [52].

Incorporating Rest Imaging into an ADP

Ideal candidates for rest MPI are patients who have a nondiagnostic ECG and negative initial cardiac injury markers. Its optimal use is in patients who will be discharged home and have stress testing as an outpatient if imaging is negative. Implementation of this technique in the ED requires coordination among radiologists, cardiologists, emergency physicians, and other support personnel for optimal utility. In low-risk patients injected during anginal symptoms, normal rest images markedly reduce the likelihood of ACS, and in younger patients, subsequent stress testing may not be necessary. If the likelihood of CAD on the basis of clinical variables is relatively low and the rest ECG is normal, rest MPI can be followed by ETT. However, in the presence of an abnormal rest ECG, or if the patient is unable to adequately exercise, stress testing with imaging, either echocardiography or more commonly MPI, with exercise or pharmacological stress, would be appropriate.

One limitation of rest MPI is in the patient whose symptoms have resolved prior to or shortly after arrival to the ED. In patients injected while pain free, suggesting resolution of ischemia, risk in the subsequent 2–3 days is low but ACS has not absolutely been excluded. Some centers perform rest MPI only in patients with ongoing symptoms, resulting in a higher prevalence of abnormal images. Symptom-free patients, rather than undergoing imaging, are admitted for observation, have serial cardiac injury markers obtained and undergo stress testing if negative. An alternative method is to perform the aforementioned dual isotope protocol, using rest Tl-201 imaging, and if negative, stress imaging with a Tc-99m based isotope.

The ability to have imaging available during all hours is a potential logistical issue. In a study by Schaeffer et al., patients presenting from 12 am to 6 am were injected with Tc-99m-sestamibi and imaging was delayed until morning [64]. There was no difference in diagnostic accuracy in patients receiving delayed imaging compared to those who presented when imaging was immediately available. As an alterative, patients can be injected early after arrival by either an ED physician or radiology technologist, with images obtained after the arrival of an on-call nuclear medicine technologist.

Although not normally considered candidates for rest MPI because of their higher pretest likelihood of ischemia or old infarction, rest MPI can provide useful additional diagnostic information in selected subgroups of patients with known CAD. This should be limited to patients with a nonischemic ECG who have atypical symptoms, particularly if the symptoms differ from their typical angina. However, patients with prior MI, especially those with Q waves on the ECG, are likely to have perfusion defects, and if MI is excluded, subsequent repeat rest imaging after a pain-free period is required to differentiate new ischemia from old infarction. Another group of patients in whom rest MPI can be used as an alternative to admission are those presenting with cocaine-associated chest pain. In a study of 216 consecutive patients with chest pain after recent cocaine use who underwent rest MPI, only five (2.3%) patients had abnormal studies, including two with acute MI [65].

Clinicians from the Virginia Commonwealth University Medical Center have developed and implemented a systematic chest pain protocol designed for all chest pain patients, with MPI used for the evaluation of lower risk patients [66]. All patients presenting to the ED with suspected myocardial ischemia are assigned to a triage risk level based on the probability of having ACS derived from clinical and ECG variables. After the initial evaluation, patients with ST segment elevation (level 1), ST segment depression or ischemic T-wave inversion (level 2) or those with known CAD experiencing typical symptoms (level 2) are admitted directly to the coronary care unit. Patients considered low to moderate risk (levels 3 and 4) for ACS (e.g., absence of ischemic ECG changes or history of CAD) undergo further risk stratification using rest MPI [66]. Level 3 patients are admitted as observation patients and undergo a rapid rule-in protocol. Level 4 patients remain in the ED. If images are either negative or unchanged from previous studies, patients are discharged home and scheduled for outpatient ETT. If MPI is positive, they are admitted and advanced to the level 2 treatment protocol.

The role of rest MPI is different between level 3 patients and level 4 patients. In level 3 patients, a positive MPI identifies a high-risk patient in whom early initiation of aggressive treatment is indicated, with the potential for early intervention. The combination of negative MPI and negative cardiac injury markers, on the other hand, identifies patients who can safely undergo early ETT and discharge. In contrast, the role of MPI in level 4 patients is to diagnose unsuspected ACS and prevent their inadvertent discharge from the ED. Outpatient follow-up ETT is used to exclude significant CAD in appropriately selected patients.

This simple risk stratification scheme accurately separates patients into high- , intermediate-, and low-risk groups. The ability of MPI to further risk stratify lower risk patients was confirmed as outcomes in patients with positive MPI were similar to those of high-risk level 2 patients [66]. This strategy also allows patients without prior MI who have large perfusion defects to be referred directly to coronary angiography and revascularization (Fig. 12.2).

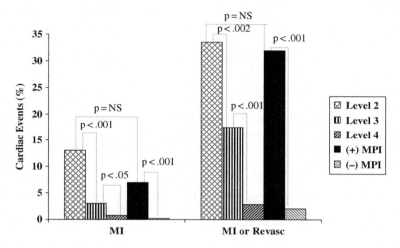

Fig. 12.2 Cardiac outcomes compared to the initial triage level assignment and the myocardial perfusion imaging results. The incidence of MI or revascularization was significantly different among level 2 (*hatched bars*), level 3 (*vertical bars*), and level 4 (*diagonal bars*) patients. Patients who had positive imaging (*dark bars*) had an incidence of MI or revascularization similar to the level 2 patients. Adapted with permission from Tatum et al. [66]

Echocardiography

Echocardiography is a valuable technique that provides tomographic imaging of the heart. It is noninvasive, portable, and presents no risk to the patient. Echocardiography can provide structural and functional data, as well as findings that suggest nonischemic etiologies for the patients' symptoms [23].

Abnormalities in diastolic function occur within seconds after the onset of myocardial ischemia. Shortly thereafter wall thickening is impaired and the amount of endocardial excursion is reduced [67, 68]. These developments typically precede ECG abnormalities and chest pain onset [69]. Unfortunately, similar to MPI, there is a minimum threshold of myocardium that has to be ischemic before abnormalities can be detected, which may limit this strategy's applicability. Animal studies have shown that wall motion may remain normal or near normal if <20% of the thickness of the myocardium is involved or if the circumferential extent of infarction is <12% [70]. However, an advantage of echocardiography in detecting ACS in the pain-free patient is that wall motion can remain abnormal for hours to days after an ischemic event, even in the absence of necrosis ("myocardial stunning") [71].

Stress Echocardiography

Protocols for stress echocardiography are similar to that for stress MPI, although dobutamine is the only agent used for pharmaocologic testing. Accurate determination of the severity of ischemia usually requires completion of imaging within 30–45 s of exercise cessation. The degree of abnormality is typically calculated by dividing the left ventricle into 16 segments, with each scored as 0 (normal), 1 (hypokinesis), 2 (akinesis), and 3 (dyskinesis). The total score is determined, and then divided by the number of segments visualized to derive a wall motion score index (normal = 1.0). Systolic function can be semiquantitatively determined based on ejection fraction or degree of wall motion abnormality. Similar to MPI, the degree of stress abnormality correlates with risk.

Stress echocardiography has been evaluated in several studies in the ED. It not only assists in the diagnosis of CAD, but identifies patients' risk for future adverse cardiac events after MI has been excluded. In the largest study of this type, Bholasingh studied 404 patients in the ED with dobutamine stress echocardiography [72]. After exclusion of 23 patients with poor echocardiographic windows and 4 patients who had significant baseline echocardiographic abnormalities, the remaining 377 patients demonstrated 26 positive and 351 negative tests. The negative predictive value for adverse cardiac events (death, MI, UA, revascularization) was 96%. In a multivariate analysis a positive study had independent prognostic value (OR 7.1; 95% CI 2.5–20.2).

One randomized multicenter trial compared dobutamine stress echocardiography (107 patients) to ETT (89 patients) in the ED [73]. Patients with a negative evaluation in the dobutamine stress echocardiography group had no adverse events at 2 months compared to 9 patients (11%) evaluated with ETT ($p = 0.004$). In a multivariate analysis, positive dobutamine stress echocardiography was the only independent predictor of an adverse event (OR 7.0; 95% CI 1.4–35.8), with a negative predictive value of 91% at 6 months [74]. This finding in a small number of patients requires corroboration by additional studies.

An important advantage of echocardiography is that in low-risk patients who have normal wall motion on rest echocardiography, stress testing can be performed immediately. Trippi et al. reported a unique strategy in which low-risk patients were identified by the ED physician and an on-call sonographer performed rest images. Subsequently, dobutamine stress echocardiography was performed, with digitized images transmitted telephonically for remote interpretation by the on-call cardiologist [75]. This protocol was found to be safe and substantially decreased the time to exclude ACS.

Rest Echocardiography

Several studies using rest echocardiography in the ED to risk stratify patients have found a high diagnostic accuracy [76, 77]. In one study, rest echocardiography was performed in 262 patients within 4 h of ED arrival. Forty-five patients (17%) had adverse events, which included MI in 23 and revascularization in an additional 22. Sensitivity for identifying patients with these events was significantly higher for rest echocardiography (91%) than the ECG (40%). Its negative predictive value was also high, as only 4 of the 166 patients (2%) who had a negative echocardiogram had an adverse event. In a multivariate model, the only independent predictors of adverse events were male gender (OR 2.4, 95% CI 1.1–5.3) and positive echocardiography (OR 24, 95% CI 9–65). Importantly, addition of the echocardiography results to the clinical, historical, and ECG data provided significant incremental diagnostic information. In contrast, Gibler et al. found that echocardiography had limited sensitivity but excellent specificity when used as part of a diagnostic chest pain pathway [6]. Differences between this study and the former ones include a low incidence of cardiac events (only 4% had ACS) and imaging performed late in the ADP.

Limitations of echocardiography in the chest pain patient include the presence of wall motion abnormalities (at times segmental), in patients with myocarditis, prior MI and left bundle branch block. Confirming acute ischemia in a patient with significant systolic dysfunction can also be difficult. However, most of these cases identify a higher risk patient in whom early discharge may not be appropriate. Although theoretically echocardiography can provide alternative diagnoses (such as aortic stenosis or pericardial effusion) or discover other significant findings (such as ventricular thrombus), studies have shown this is uncommon (<2%) [78]. Because of these logistic difficulties, optimal use of rest echocardiography appears to be in patients in whom other diagnoses, such as pericarditis or pulmonary embolism, are also being strongly considered. Results can then be used to further determine if and what additional diagnostic tests are needed.

Comparison of Stress Echocardiography and Stress MPI

In patients who require imaging, both echocardiography and MPI can be used. Both techniques have advantages and disadvantages (Table 12.6). A summary of studies indicates that the overall diagnostic performance of stress echocardiography and stress MPI appears to be similar (16,46) (Table 12.7). Comparison of the accuracy of the two techniques is limited, as few studies performed both tests in the same patients. In the head-to-head studies, stress echocardiography appeared to be more specific, while stress MPI was more sensitive. In addition, there are few studies that included only ED patients undergoing chest pain evaluation, and they are further limited by small numbers and few adverse

Table 12.6 Advantages and disadvantages of stress echocardiography and stress myocardial perfusion imaging

Stress echocardiography	Stress myocardial perfusion imaging
Less expensive	More expensive
No radiation	Radiation
Results available shortly after testing	Processing required
Measures function	Measures perfusion
Qualitative	Quantitative
Variable windows	Tissue attenuation
Good prognostic information	Excellent prognostic information
Shorter testing time	Longer testing time

Table 12.7 Sensitivity and specificity of exercise and pharmacologic stress echocardiography and myocardial perfusion imaging

	N	Sensitivity	Specificity
Exercise echo	3420	86	81
Exercise MPI	4480	87	73
Dobutamine echo	3280	82	84
Pharmacologic MPI	2492	87	73

Echo, echocardiography; MPI, myocardial perfusion imaging.
Pharmacologic is with either dipyridamole or adenosine.

outcomes. In one of the few studies performed in ED chest pain patients, Conti et al. reported on 503 patients with a nonischemic ECG who after ED evaluation, underwent ETT, stress echocardiography, and stress MPI [79]. Patients with a positive test underwent coronary angiography to establish a diagnosis of CAD. Sensitivity (85 vs. 86%) and specificity (95 vs. 90%) were similar in stress echocardiography and stress MPI, respectively. Although specificity of ETT (95%) was similar to the other two tests, sensitivity was significantly lower at 43%.

Although both stress MPI and stress echocardiography have higher diagnostic accuracy than ETT alone, they are more expensive. Therefore, an important consideration is whether the additional information is worth the additional cost. Unfortunately, there are few direct comparisons of cost-effectiveness for evaluating low to intermediate chest pain patients with respect to the choice of imaging. Two analyses of cost-effectiveness using observational data on outcomes to evaluate various diagnostic strategies for patients with chest pain have been reported [80, 81]. The former concluded that for patients with typical angina, the use of exercise echocardiography instead of ETT improved survival at a cost of $32,000 per quality-adjusted life-year; for patients with atypical angina, the cost per quality-adjusted life-year increased to $41,900. Exercise MPI also improved outcomes, but was more expensive per improved quality-adjusted life-year with costs of $38,000 and $54,900, respectively. These cost-effectiveness ratios are similar to those of other medically accepted interventions. A second analysis that assumed a higher specificity for stress echocardiography than the prior study (88 vs. 77%) concluded that stress echocardiography was a more cost-effective strategy than MPI, with total costs equal to or lower than those of exercise ETT [81]. These cost-effectiveness analyses suffer from a number of limitations. These include the assumption that the relative sensitivity and specificity of the test is fixed, when it likely varies by relative experience and expertise of the interpreter, even at the same institution. Additionally, most cost-effectiveness analyses employ decision-analytic or simulation models that often rely on assumptions rather than on actual practice patterns.

Other important considerations are that stress MPI is more sensitive for detection of single-vessel disease, more easily quantifies extent of ischemia, and appears to be more reproducible. Finally, given the importance of physician's interpretation for assessing the results of either diagnostic test or the overall similarity in costs, when imaging is required, an important consideration should include the logistics and local expertise of the center, rather than perceived differences in the diagnostic accuracy of the two methods.

Summary

The focus of chest pain units has evolved primarily for the management of the lower risk population. The initial goal in low-risk patients presenting with chest pain is to exclude ACS rather than to discover the presence of CAD. ADPs are critical for the early identification of patients with ACS but should also gateway patients with negative evaluations to further diagnostic testing to identify occult CAD. The secondary risk stratification afforded by this approach is predicated upon proper identification of low-risk patients and appropriate test selection. The utility of this strategy has been well demonstrated, as indicated by its safety and the very low clinical risk in patients discharged home.

The selection of a specific diagnostic test, and whether or not imaging is incorporated, is most commonly dependent upon the patient's ability to exercise and the interpretability of the ECG. However, institutional expertise and test availability, particularly after hours, are critical considerations. ETT without imaging should be performed in low- to intermediate-risk patients who can exercise and do not have significant baseline ECG changes that preclude stress ECG interpretation. Patients with abnormal ECGs usually require the addition of cardiac imaging; both stress echocardiography and MPI can be utilized as their diagnostic performance appears to be similar. However, given the importance of logistics and local expertise, these factors should drive the choice between these studies. Pharmacological stress imaging is required in patients with the inability to exercise sufficiently. Importantly, all patients discharged home after a negative assessment should receive appropriate outpatient follow-up to determine the need for additional evaluation.

References

1. Kirk JD, Diercks DB, Turnipseed SD, et al. Evaluation of chest pain suspicious for ACS: Use of an ADP in a chest pain evaluation unit. Am J Cardiol 2000; 85(5A):40B–48B.
2. Amsterdam EA, Lewis WR, Kirk JD, Diercks DB, Turnipseed S. Acute ischemic syndromes: Chest pain center concept. Card Clinics 2001; 20(1):117–136.
3. Braunwald E, Antman E, Beasley JW, et al. ACC/AHA guidelines for the management of patients with unstable angina and on-ST segment elevation myocardial infarction. J Am Coll Cardiol 2000;36:970–1062.
4. Hutter AM, Amsterdam EA, Jaffe AS. Task force 2: ACSs: Section 2B-Chest discomfort evaluation in the hospital, 31st Bethesda Conference. J Am Coll Cardiol 2000;35:853–62.
5. Lee TH, Goldman L. Evaluation of the patient with acute chest pain. N Engl J Med 2000; 342:1187–1195.
6. Gibler WB, Runyon JP, Levy RC, et al. A rapid diagnostic and treatment center for patients with chest pain the ED. Ann Emerg Med1995; 25:1–8.
7. Zalenski RJ, Rydman RJ, McCarren M, et al. Feasibility of a rapid diagnostic protocol for an ED chest pain unit. Ann Emerg Med 1997; 29:99–108.
8. Mikhail MG, Smith FA, Gray M, et al. Cost-effectiveness of mandatory stress testing in chest pain center patients. Ann Emerg Med1997; 29:88–98.
9. Gomez MA, Anderson JL, Karagounis LA, et al. An ED-based protocol for rapidly ruling out myocardial ischemia reduces hospital time and expense: results of a randomized study (ROMIO). J Am Coll Cardiol 1996; 28:25–33.
10. Farkouh ME, Smars PA, Reeder GS, et al. A clinical trial of a chest-pain observation unit for patients with unstable angina: Chest pain evaluation in the emergency room (CHEER) investigators. N Engl J Med 1998;39:1882–8.
11. Pope JH, Aufderheide TP, Ruthazer R, et al. Missed diagnoses of acute cardiac ischemia in the ED. N Engl J Med 2000;342:1163–70.
12. Karcz A, Holbrook J, Burke MC, Doyle MJ, Erdos MS, Friedman M, Green ED. Massachusetts emergency medicine closed malpractice claims: 1988–1990. Ann Emerg Med1993; 22:553–559.
13. Lee TH, Cook EF, Weisberg M, et al. Acute chest pain in the emergency room: Identification and examination of low-risk patients. Archives of Int Med 1985; 145:65.
14. Goldman L, Cook EF, Johnson PA, et al. Prediction of the need for intensive care in patients who come to EDs with acute chest pain. N Engl J Med 1996;334:1498.
15. Brush JE, Jr, Brand DA, Acampora D, et al. Use of the initial electrocardiogram to predict in-hospital complications of acute myocardial infarction. N Engl J Med 1980;312:1137–41.
16. Ritchie JL, Bateman TM, Bonow RO, et al. Guidelines for clinical use of cardiac radionuclide imaging: Report of the American College of Cardiology/American Heart Association Task Force on Assessment of Diagnostic and Therapeutic Cardiovascular Procedures (Committee on Radionuclide Imaging), developed in collaboration with the American Society of Nuclear Cardiology. J Am Coll Cardiol 1995;25:521–547
17. Hachamovitch R, Berman DS, Shaw LJ, et al. Incremental prognostic value of myocardial perfusion single photon emission computed tomography for the prediction of cardiac death: Differential stratification for risk of cardiac death and myocardial infarction. Circulation 1998;97:535–43.
18. Gibbons RJ, Chatterjee K, Daley J, et al. ACC/AHA/ACP-ASIM guidelines for the management of patients with chronic stable angina: A report of the American College of Cardiology/American Heart Association Task Force on Practice Guidelines. J Am Coll Cardiol 1999;33:2092–2197.
19. Gibbons RJ, Balady GJ, Bricker JT, et al. ACC/AHA 2002 guideline update for exercise testing: summary article: A report of the American College of Cardiology/American Heart Association Task Force on practice guidelines (committee to update the 1997 exercise testing guidelines). Circulation2002; 106:1883.

20. Elhendy A, van Domburg RT, Sozzi FB, et al. Impact of hypertension on the accuracy of exercise stress myocardial perfusion imaging for the diagnosis of coronary artery disease. Heart 2001;85:655–61.
21. DePuey EG, Guertler-Krawczynska E, Robbins WL. Thallium-201 SPECTainocornary artery disease patients with left bundle branch block. J Nucl Med 1988;29:1479–85.
22. O'Keefe JH Jr, Bateman TM, Silvestri R, et al. Safety and diagnostic accuracy of adenosine thallium-201 scintigraphy in patients unable to exercise and those with left bundle-branch block. Am Heart J 1992;124:614–21.
23. Ribeiro A, Lindmarker P, Juhlin Dannfelt A, Johnsson H, Jorfeldt L. Echocardiography Doppler in pulmonary embolism: Right ventricular dysfunction as a predictor of mortality rate. Am Heart J 1997; 134:479–487.
24. Elveback LR, Connolly DC, Leton LJ III. Coronary heart disease in residents of Rochester, Minnesota. VII: Incidence, 1950 through 1982. Mayo Clin Proc 1986;61:896–900
25. Ladenheim ML, Kotler TS, Pollock BH, et al. Incremental prognostic power of clinical history, exercise electrocardiography and myocardial perfusion scintigraphy in suspected coronary artery disease. Am J Cardiol 1987;59:270–7
26. Hachamovitch R, Berman DS, Kiat H, et al. Value of stress myocardial perfusion single photon emission computer tomography in patients with normal resting electrocardiograms: An evaluation of incremental prognostic value and cost-effectiveness. Circulation 2002;105:823–9.
27. Anderson JL, Adams, CD, Antman EM, et al. ACC/AHA 2007 guidelines for the management of patients with unstable angina/non-ST elevation myocardial infarction. J Am Coll Cardiol. 2007;50:e1–157.
28. Hung J, Chaitman BR, Lam J, Lesperance J, Dupras G, Fines P, Cherkaoui O, Robert P, Bourassa MG. A logistic regression analysis of multiple noninvasive tests for the prediction of the presence and extent of coronary artery disease in men. Am Heart J 1985 Aug;110(2):460–9.
29. Weiner DA, Ryan TJ, McCabe CH, et al. Prognostic importance of a clinical profile and exercise test in medically treated patients with coronary artery disease. J Am Coll Cardiol 1984; 3:772.
30. Myers J, Prakash M, Froelicher V, et al. Exercise capacity and mortality among men referred for exercise testing. N Engl J Med 2002; 346:793.
31. Okin PM, Kligfield P. Heart rate adjustment of ST segment depression and performance of the exercise electrocardiogram: A critical evaluation. J Am Coll Cardiol 1995; 25:1726–35.
32. Kirk JD, Turnipseed SD, Lewis WR, et al. Evaluation of chest pain in low risk patients presenting to the ED: The role of immediate exercise testing. Ann Emerg Med 1998; 32:1–7.
33. Amsterdam EA, Kirk JD, Diercks DB, et al. Immediate exercise testing for assessment of clinical risk in patients presenting to the ED with chest pain: Results in 1,000 patients. J Am Coll Cardiol 2002; 40:251–6.
34. Mark DB, Hlatky MA, Harrell FE Jr, et al. Exercise treadmill score for predicting prognosis in coronary artery disease. Ann Int Med 1987;106:793.
35. Shaw LJ, Peterson ED, Shaw LK, et al. Use of a prognostic treadmill score in identifying diagnostic CAD subgroups. Circulation 1998;98:1622.
36. McNeer JF, Margolis JR, Lee KL, et al. The role of the exercise test in the evaluation of patients for ischemic heart disease. Circulation 1978; 57:64.
37. Cole CR, Blackstone EH, Pashkow FJ, et al. Heart-rate recovery immediately after exercise as a predictor of mortality. N Engl J Med 1999; 341:1351.
38. Squires RW, Allison TG, Johnson BD, Gau GT. Non-physician supervision of cardiopulmonary exercise testing in chronic heart failure: Safety and results of a preliminary investigation. J Cardiopulm Rehabil 1999 Jul–Aug;19 (4):249–53
39. Kirk JD, Turnipseed SD, Diercks DB, et al. Interpretation of immediate exercise treadmill test: Inter-reader reliability between cardiologist and noncardiologist in a chest pain evaluation unit. Ann Emerg Med 2000; 36:10–14.

40. Meyer MC, Mooney RP, Sekera AK. A critical pathway for patients with acute chest pain and low risk for short-term adverse cardiac events: Role of outpatient stress testing. Ann Emerg Med 2006; 47:427–35.
41. Lai C, Noeller TP, Schmidt K, et al. Short-term risk after initial observation for chest pain. J Emerg Med 2003; 25: 357–62.
42. Manini AF, Gisondi MA, van der Vlugt, TH, Schreiber DH. Adverse cardiac events in ED patients with chest pain six months after a negative inpatient evaluation for acute coronary syndrome. Acad Emerg Med 2002; 9: 896–902
43. Diercks DB, Gibler WB, Liu T, et al. Identification of patients at risk by graded exercise testing in an ED chest pain center. Am J Cardiol 2000; 86(3): 289–92.
44. Polanczyk CA, Johnson PA, Hartley LH, et al. Clinical correlates and prognostic significance of early negative exercise tolerance test in patients with acute chest pain seen in the hospital ED. Am J Cardiol 1998; 81:288.
45. Lewis WR, Amsterdam EA. Utilities and safety of immediate exercise treadmill test of low-risk patients admitted to the hospital for suspected AMI. Am J Cardiol 1994;74:987–90.
46. Cheitlin MD, Alpert JS, Armstrong WF, et al. ACC/AHA guidelines for the clinical application of echocardiography: A report of the American College of Cardiology/American Heart Association Task Force on Practice Guidelines (Committee on Clinical Application of Echocardiography): Developed in collaboration with the American Society of Echocardiography. Circulation 1997;95:1686–1744.
47. Sharir T germano G, Kang X, et al. prediction of myocardial infarction versus cardiac death by gated myocardial perfusion SPECT: Risk stratification by the amount of stress-induced ischemia and the poststress ejection fraction. J Nucl Med 2001;42:831–7
48. Germano G, Kavanagh PB, Waechter P, et al. A new algorithm for the quantitation of myocardial perfusion SPECT. I: Technical principles and reproducibility. J Nuc Med. 2000;41:712–9.
49. Sharir Y, Germano G, Waechter PB, et al. A new algorithm for the quantitation of myocardial perfusion SPECT, II: Validation and diagnostic yield. J Nucl Med. 2000;41:720–7.
50. Berman DS, Kiat H, Friedman JD, et al. Separate acquisition rest thallium-201/stress technetium-99m sestamibi dual-isotope myocardial perfusion single-photon emission computed tomography: A clinical validation study. J Am Coll Cardiol. 1993;22:1455–64.
51. Iskandrian AS, Heo J, Kong B, Lyons E. Effect of exercise level on the ability of thallium-201 tomographic imaging in detecting coronary artery disease: Analysis of 461 patients. J Am Coll Cardiol. 1989 Nov 15;14 (6):1477–86.
52. Klocke FJ, Baird MG, Lorell BH, et al. American College of Cardiology; American Heart Association; American Society for Nuclear Cardiology. ACC/AHA/ASNC guidelines for the clinical use of cardiac radionuclide imaging – executive summary: A report of the American College of Cardiology/American Heart Association Task Force on Practice Guidelines (ACC/AHA/ASNC Committee to Revise the 1995 Guidelines for the Clinical Use of Cardiac Radionuclide Imaging). J Am Coll Cardiol. 2003 Oct 1;42 (7):1318–33
53. Hachamovitch R, Hayes S, Friedman JD, Cohen I, Shaw LJ, Germano G, Berman DS. Determinants of risk and its temporal variation in patients with normal stress myocardial perfusion scans: What is the warranty period of a normal scan? J Am Coll Cardiol. 2003 Apr 16;41 (8):1329–40.
54. Poornima IG, Miller TD, Christian TF, et al. Utility of myocardial perfusion imaging in patient with low-risk treadmill scores. J Am Coll Cardiol. 2004;43:194–9.
55. Fagan LF, Shaw L, Kong, BA. Prognostic value of exercise thallium scintigraphy in patients with good exercise tolerance and a normal or abnormal exercise electrocardiogram and suspected or confirmed coronary artery disease. Am J Cardiol. 1992 Mar 1;69 (6):607–11.
56. Kontos MC, Haney A, Jesse RL, Ornato JP, Tatum J. Perfusion Defects in the Absence of Abnormal Wall Motion and Thickening Are Not Clinically Significant in Chest Pain Patients Undergoing Acute Rest Myocardial Perfusion Imaging. J Am Coll Cardiol 2006;47:108A.

57. Varetto T, Cantalupi D, Altieri A, Orlandi C. Emergency room technetium-99m sesta-mibi imaging to rule out acute myocardial ischemic events in patients with nondiagnostic electrocardiograms. J Am Coll Cardiol 1993; 22:1804–1808.
58. Kontos MC, Jesse RL, Schmidt KL, Ornato JP, Tatum JL. Value of acute rest sestamibi perfusion imaging for evaluation of patients admitted to the emergency department with chest pain. J Am Coll Cardiol 1997 Oct;30 (4):976–82
59. Kontos MC, Jesse RL, Anderson FP, Schmidt KL, Ornato JP, Tatum JL. Comparison of myocardial perfusion imaging and cardiac troponin I in patients admitted to the emer-gency department with chest pain. Circulation. 1999 Apr 27;99 (16):2073–8.
60. Udelson JE, Beshansky JR, Ballin DS, Feldman JA, Griffith JL, Handler J et al. Myo-cardial perfusion imaging for evaluation and triage of patients with suspected acute cardiac ischemia: A randomized controlled trial. JAMA 2002;288:2693–700.
61. Hilton TC, Thompson RC, Williams HJ, Saylors R, Fulmer H, Stowers SA. Technetium-99m sestamibi myocardial perfusion imaging in the emergency room evaluation of chest pain. J. Am. Coll. Cardiol. 1994;23:1016–22
62. Hilton TC, Fulmer H, Abuan T, Thompson RC, Stowers SA, Fulmer H et al. Ninety-day follow-up of patients in the ED with chest pain who undergo initial single-photon emission computed tomography perfusion scintigraphy with technetium 99m-labeled sestamibi. J Nucl Cardiol 1996;3:308–11.
63. Heller GV, Stowers SA, Hendel RC, Herman SD, Daher E, Ahlberg AW et al. Clinical value of acute rest technetium-99m tetrofosmin tomographic myocardial perfusion ima-ging in patients with acute chest pain and nondiagnostic electrocardiograms. J Am Coll Cardiol 1998;31:1011–17.
64. Schaeffer MW, Brennan TD, Hughes JA, Gibler WB, Gerson MC. Resting radionuclide myocardial perfusion imaging in a chest pain center including an overnight delayed image acquisition protocol. J Nucl Med Technol. 2007 Dec;35 (4):242–5.
65. Kontos MC, Schmidt KL, Nicholson CS, Ornato JP, Jesse RL, Tatum JL. Myocardial perfusion imaging with technetium-99m sestamibi in patients with cocaine-associated chest pain. Ann Emerg Med 1999 Jun;33 (6):639–45.
66. Tatum JL, Jesse RL, Kontos MC, Nicholson CS, Schmidt KL, Roberts CS, Ornato JP. Comprehensive strategy for the evaluation and triage of the chest pain patient. Ann Emerg Med 1997 Jan;29 (1):116–25.
67. Theroux P, Ross J, Jr., Franklin D, Kemper WS, Sasyama S. Regional Myocardial function in the conscious dog during acute coronary occlusion and responses to mor-phine, propranolol, nitroglycerin, and lidocaine. Circulation 1976; 53:302–314.
68. Weyman AE, Franklin TD, Egenes KM, Green D. Correlation between extent of abnor-mal regional wall motion and myocardial infarct size in chronically infarcted dogs. Circulation 1997; 56:72–78.
69. Hauser AM, Gangadharan V, Ramos RG, Gordon S, Timmis GC. Sequence of mechan-ical, electrocardiographic and clinical effects of repeated coronary artery occlusion in human beings: Echocardiographic observations during coronary angioplasty. J Am Coll Cardiol 1985; 45:193–197.
70. Lieberman AN, Weiss JL, Jugdutt BI et al. Two-dimensional echocardiography and infarct size: Relationship of regional wall motion and thickening to the extent of myo-cardial infarction in the dog. Circulation 1981;63:739–46.
71. Kloner RA, Jennings RB. Consequences of Brief Ischemia: Stunning, Preconditioning, and Their Clinical Implications. Part 1. Circulation 2001; 104:2981–2989.
72. Bholasingh R, Cornel JH, Kamp O, et al. Prognostic value of predischarge dobutamine stress echocardiography in chest pain patients with a negative cardiac troponin T. J Am Coll Cardiol. 2003;41 (4):596–602.
73. Nucifora G, Badano LP, Sarraf-Zadegan N, et al. Comparison of early dobutamine stress echocardiography and exercise electrocardiographic testing for management of patients presenting to the ED with chest pain. Am J Cardiol 2007;100 (7):1068–73.

74. Geleijnse ML, Elhendy A, Kasprzak JD, et al. Safety and prognostic value of early dobutamine-atropine stress echocardiography in patients with spontaneous chest pain and a non-diagnostic electrocardiogram. Eur Heart J 2000;21 (5):397–406.
75. Trippi JA, Lee KS, Kopp G, Nelson DR, Yee KG, Cordell WH. Dobutamine stress tele-echocardiography for evaluation of ED patients with chest pain. J Am Coll Cardiol 1997; 30:627–632.
76. Sabia P, Afrookteh A, Touchstone DA, Keller MW, Esquivel L, Kaul S. Value of regional wall motion abnormality in the emergency room diagnosis of acute myocardial infarction. A prospective study using two-dimensional echocardiography. Circulation 1991; 84:I85–92.
77. Kontos MC, Arrowood JA, Paulsen WH, Nixon JV, Paulsen WH. Early echocardiography can predict cardiac events in ED patients with chest pain. Ann Emerg Med 1998; 31:550–557.
78. Lim SH, Sayre MR, Gibler WB. 2-D echocardiography prediction of adverse events in ED patients with chest pain. Am J Emerg Med 2003;21 (2):106–10.
79. Conti A, Sammicheli L, Gallini C, et al. Assessment of patients with low-risk chest pain in the ED: Head-to-head comparison of exercise myocardial SPECT. Am Heart J 2005;5:894–901.
80. Kuntz KM, Fleischmann KE, Hunink MG, Douglas PS. (1999) Cost-effectiveness of diagnostic strategies for patients with chest pain. Ann Inter Med 1999;130:709–718
81. Garber AM and Solomon NA. Cost-effectiveness of alternative test strategies for the diagnosis of coronary artery disease. Ann Int Med 1999; 130:719–728
82. Zalenski RJ, McCarren M, Roberts R, et al. An evaluation of a chest pain diagnostic protocol to exclude acute cardiac ischemia in the ED. Arch Int Med 1997;157:1085
83. Kontos MC, Tatum JL. Imaging in the Evaluation of the Patient with Suspected Acute Coronary Syndrome. Cardiology Clinics 2005; 23 (4):517–530

Chapter 13
Use of Multislice CT and MRI for the Evaluation of Patients with Chest Pain

Brian O'Neil, Michael J. Gallagher, and Gilbert L. Raff

Abstract Approximately 6 million patients are evaluated annually in United States emergency departments for acute chest pain (McCaig and Burt, National Hospital Ambulatory Medical Care Survey 2003. National Center for Health Statistics: Hyattsville, MD, 2005). Delineation of the presence or absence of an acute coronary syndrome must be accurate and efficient. The latest estimate is that 2% of patients with an acute coronary syndrome are inappropriately sent home from the emergency department (Pope et al. N Engl J Med 2000;342:1163–1170; Lee and Goldman, N Engl J Med 2000;342:1163–1170). These patients suffer higher morbidity than admitted patients. Missed ACS was the number one payout per case and that accounts for 41% of claims paid. So not surprisingly physicians do not want to miss ACS, resulting in an annual cost of US$10 to $13 billion to rule out ACS (McCaig and Burt, The National Hospital Ambulatory Medical Care Survey. Centers for Disease Control and Prevention's National Center for Health Statistics, 2005).

Coronary CT angiography (CCTA) has great promise as a tool to expedite the triage of acute chest pain patients. The direct visualization of the coronary anatomy, the ability to simultaneously image the rest of the thorax to exclude aortic dissection and pulmonary embolism and the ability to provide alternate causes of chest pain, such as pneumonia, pericardial fluid, and esophageal inflammation. This chapter will examine the use of coronary CT angiography and MRI for the evaluation of acute chest pain.

Keywords CT angiography · Cardiac MRI · Low-risk chest pain patients · CTA triage of ED chest pain patients · CTA vs. MPI in ED chest pain patients

B. O'Neil (✉)
Department of Emergency Medicine, William Beaumont Hospital,
Royal Oak, MI, USA
e-mail: boneil@med.wayne.edu

W.F. Peacock, C.P. Cannon (eds.), *Short Stay Management of Chest Pain*,
DOI 10.1007/978-1-60327-948-2_13,
© Humana Press, a part of Springer Science+Business Media, LLC 2009

Overview of CT Technology

The advent of helical/spiral CT imaging technology and the dramatic advances in the temporal and spatial resolutions of CT [6] have made it possible to visualize the coronary arteries with systems able to synchronize the image reconstruction with the cardiac phase [7, 8]. Gantry rotation times have decreased to 330 ms and providing a temporal resolution of a completed image in 165 ms with dual X-ray sources improving the temporal resolution (i.e., 83 ms). Improved detector and collimator hardware now provide submillimeter image resolution (0.4–0.5 mm). The high-resolution 64-slice scanners have become standard for CCTA (Fig. 13.1). Such scanners decrease breath-hold time and reduce cardiac motion artifacts which have increased the overall percentage of "interpretable" scans, and allowed imaging without the need for beta blockade in many patients. Challenges remain in imaging patients with heavily calcified coronary arteries, coronary artery stents, and markedly obese patients.

The Accuracy of Coronary CT Angiography

The ability of CCTA to quantitate coronary artery lesion severity correlates well with invasive coronary angiography (Pearson correlation, $r = 0.72$) [9–11]. The considerable standard deviation in these early studies, however, limits its quantitative accuracy (see Fig. 13.2).

Diagnostic Accuracy of CT in Emergency Department Patients with Acute Chest Pain – Initial Experience

At least six recent studies have evaluated the safety and diagnostic accuracy of 64-slice CCTA for triage of emergency department patients with acute chest pain [12–17]. In aggregate, 376 emergency department patients (predominantly low to intermediate pretest coronary risk) with acute chest pain were prospectively followed over a 30-day to 15-month follow-up period after diagnosis by CCTA. All six studies excluded patients with abnormal cardiac biomarkers or ischemic electrocardiographic changes, and two of the six studies excluded patients with preexisting CAD [15, 17]. Overall, an adjudicated diagnosis of acute coronary syndrome occurred in 72 (19.1%) of the 376 study patients. The absence of significant coronary artery stenosis by CCTA accurately excluded the presence of ACS in 373 of the 376 patients, resulting in a combined study mean negative predictive value of 99%. This suggests that CCTA can identify a subset of ED chest pain patients who can be safely discharged home on the basis of CT findings.

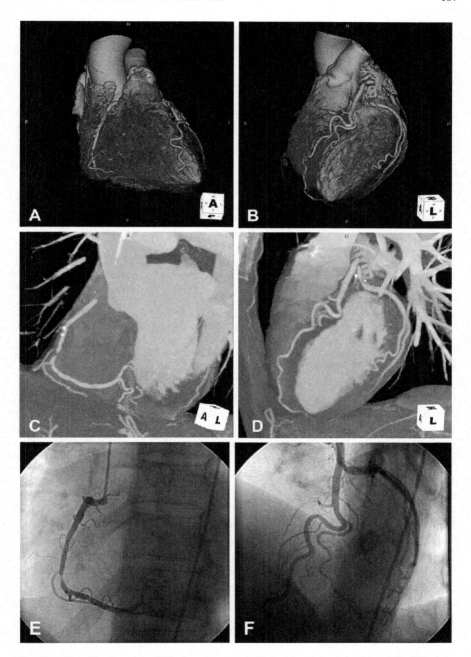

Fig. 13.1 Visualization of calcified and non-calcified coronary atherosclerotic plaques by 64-slice coronary CT angiography. (**A**, **B**) Volume rendering technique demonstrates stenosis of the right coronary artery below the acute marginal branch (**A**), as well as nodular coronary calcifications largely extrinsic to the right coronary lumen and (**B**) normal left coronary artery.

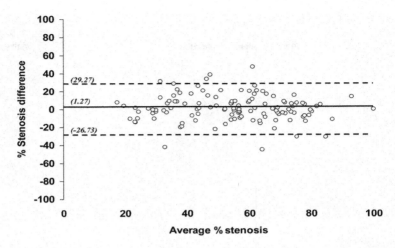

Fig. 13.2 Figure taken from a diagnostic accuracy study of 64-slice coronary computed tomography angiography (CCTA) in 70 consecutive patients who underwent elective invasive coronary angiography for suspected coronary artery disease [9]. Bland–Altman analysis of the differences of percent diameter stenosis measured by CCTA vs. quantitative coronary angiography (QCA) during invasive catheterization, compared to the average percent diameter stenosis by the two methods. The mean difference was 1.3 ± 14.0% (*central line*). A total of 94% of the values lie within 1.96 standard deviations of the mean (*outer lines*). There was no significant correlation between stenosis difference and stenosis severity (Spearman correlation = –0.07, $p = 0.59$)

In one of these studies, we reported the results of a randomized trial in 197 low-risk acute chest pain patients evaluated by either early CCTA or by a standard diagnostic protocol [17]. Patients randomized to immediate CCTA were eligible for discharge with normal or minimally abnormal results (<25% stenosis), patients with severe stenosis (>70%) were referred for immediate invasive angiography, whereas patients with intermediate-grade stenosis underwent additional stress testing. The two groups were compared for safety, diagnostic accuracy, and efficiency. Among patients randomized to CCTA, 75% had decisive triage by CCTA alone (67% were immediately discharged and 8% were referred for immediate catheterization, which revealed significant disease in seven of eight referred cases). Importantly, CCTA alone was not considered adequate for diagnosis in 24 of 99 cases, owing either to lesions of unclear hemodynamic significance (stenosis = 26–70%) in 13 patients or to non-diagnostic quality scans in 11 patients (all 24 underwent non-invasive stress testing). Among the

◀━━━

Fig 13.1 (continued) (**C, D**) Maximum intensity projection images of the same arteries demonstrate severe non-calcified stenosis of the right coronary artery and superficial calcified plaque. (**E, F**) Invasive coronary angiography of the same arteries

patients discharged immediately, none had a major cardiac event or subsequent diagnosis of CAD over a 6-month follow-up period. The overall diagnostic accuracy of CCTA was 94% and the negative predictive value was 100%. Diagnostic efficiency, defined as time from randomization to definitive diagnosis, showed that the CCTA approach was more rapid (3.4 vs. 15.0 h) and reduced costs by 15% Table 13.1.

Additional centers have published their data on the 30-day cardiovascular event rates of the first 54 patients evaluated by a similar strategy. Hollander et al. evaluated low-risk chest pain patients with a TIMI score < 3, no acute ischemia on ECG and negative initial enzymes with CT coronary angiography in the ED. Of the 54 patients evaluated, 46 patients (85%) were immediately

Table 13.1 Early and 6-month clinical outcomes

	MSCT $n = 90$	Standard of Care $n = 98$	p Value
Index visit outcomes			
Test complications	0(0%)	0(0%)	NA
Direct ED discharges	88(88.1%)	95(96.9%)	0.03
Acute myocardial Infraction	0(0%)	0(0%)	NA
Death	0(0%)	0(0%)	NA
In-hospital diagnostic cath	11(11.1%)	3(3.1%)	0.03
Positive caths	9(9.1%)	1(1%)	0.02
In-hospital PCI	3(3.0%)	1(1.0%)	0.62
In-hospital CABC	2(2.0%)	0(0%)	0.60
6-month outcomes			
Test complications	0(0%)	0(0%)	NA
Unstable angina	0(0%)	0(0%)	NA
Myocardial infraction	0(0%)	0(0%)	NA
Death	0(0%)	0(0%)	NA
Late ED R/O ischemia	6(6.1%)	6(6.1%)	1.00
Late office R/O ischemia	2(2.0%)	2(2.0%)	1.00
Late diagnostic cath	1(1.0%)	4(4.1%)	0.21
Late stress/MSCT test	1(1.0%)	3(2.0%)	0.37
Cath cumulative	12(12%)	7(7.1%)	0.24
True-positive cumulative	8/12(67.7%)	1/7(14.3%)	0.08
True-negative cumulative	1/12(8.3%)	4/7(57.1%)	0.04
False-positive cumulative	3(25%)	2(28.5%)	1.00
False-negative cumulative	0(0%)	0(0%)	NA
Cath-accuracy cumulative	9(75%)	5(71.4%)	1.00
Clinically correct diagnosis	96/99(97.0%)	96/98(98.0%)	1.00
Late tests cumulative	2(2.0%)	7(7.1%)	0.10
Diagnostic efficecy	94/99(94.9%)	89/98(90.8%)	0.26
PCI cumulative	4(4.0%)	1(1.0%)	0.37
CABC cumulative	2(2.0%)	0(0%)	0.50

CABC - corenary artery bypass grafting; Cath - carolac cathetorization/invasive coronary angiography; ED - emergency department; MSCT - multi-slice computed tomography; PCI - percutaneous coronary intervention; R/O - rule out.

released from ED and none had cardiovascular complications within 30 days. Of note discharged patients were not required to receive a second set of enzymes as in other studies. The other eight were admitted after CT coronary angiography: one with >70% stenosis, five with 50–69% stenosis, and two had 0–49% stenosis. Of these patients, three patients had non-invasive testing; one had reversible ischemia and the catheterization confirmed the CTA results. They concluded in the evaluation of ED patients with low-risk chest pain that CT coronary angiography may safely allow rapid discharge of patients with negative studies.[1]

Calcium Scoring in Addition to the CCTA

The inclusion of the calcium score into the chest pain protocol is controversial. Studies have evaluated the extent of coronary artery disease (CAD) on 64-slice contrast-enhanced multidetector-computed tomography in patients who underwent investigation of a chest pain syndrome, who had a zero or low coronary calcium score (CS). In 668 consecutive patients, 39% acute and 61% with long-term presentation, obstructive (>50% lesion) CAD was present in 27 of 231 patients (7%) with a zero calcium score and in 17% with a low calcium score (1–100). Of the 27 patients with obstructive CAD on multidetector-computed tomography, invasive coronary angiography confirmed these findings in 21 of 23 patients (positive predictive value 91%). To further examine this very issue we performed a retrospective analysis of two prospective previously published studies on the use of MDCT coronary angiography in the diagnosis of ED patients with acute chest pain. This study was designed to determine the incidence of catheterization-proven non-calcified plaque and lesions >50% luminal stenosis in patients with absent or minimal coronary calcification. Among the 300 ED patients enrolled into these two prospective trials, 198 underwent both coronary artery calcium scoring and MDCT coronary angiography. The primary end points of this study were (1) the incidence of catheterization-proven lesions >50% luminal stenosis in patients with absent or minimal coronary calcification (CAC <20 Agatston units) and (2) the overall incidence of non-calcified plaque (MDCT stenosis >25%) in patients with a CAC <20 Agatston units. Surrogate outcomes for those not receiving cardiac catheterization were the diagnosis of an acute coronary syndrome which includes myocardial infarction documented by cardiac enzymatic criteria, unstable angina defined as chest pain, and invasive angiographic evidence of at least one coronary stenosis >70% (or stenosis >50% with a positive stress test), or death of a presumed cardiac etiology. Of the 175 patients with interpretable MDCT images, 118 had no coronary calcification (CAC = 0), 23 had minimal coronary calcification (CAC = 1–20), 17 had mild calcifications (CAC = 20–100), and 17 had at least moderate calcification

(CAC>100) (Fig. 13.1). Among the 141 patients with calcium scores under 21, 4/141 (2.8%) had coronary stenoses over 50% on invasive angiography (three with maximum QCA stenosis >90%, one with 65% stenosis). These patients represented 4/16 (25%) of all the study patients with lesions over 50% proven by invasive coronary catheterization. An additional 5/141 (7.1%) patients with minimal coronary calcification had catheterization-proven moderate coronary artery disease (maximum stenosis 26–50%). Among the 17 patients with calcium scores between 20 and 100, 4/17 (23.5%) had coronary stenoses over 50% on invasive angiography (all with maximum QCA stenosis >70%). These patients represented 4/16 (25%) of all the study patients with lesions over 50% proven by invasive coronary catheterization. An additional $X/17$ (Y%) patients with minimal coronary calcification had catheterization-proven moderate coronary artery disease (maximum stenosis between 26 and 50%). In total, 22 (15.6%) patients with CAC < 20 had significant (i.e., >25% stenosis) non-calcified coronary artery atherosclerotic plaque. Nine of the 22 patients with MDCT-proven non-calcified plaque underwent invasive cardiac catheterization; four had severe CAD; and five had moderate CAD upon invasive catheterization. Therefore, the efficacy of calcium scoring as a risk stratification tool is poor in this patient population. We have subsequently dropped this measure from our routine protocol and in doing so have further reduced the radiation exposure.

Coronary CTA and Identification of Unstable Plaques

Our institution has recently published data from a sampling of patients that show CCTA has the ability to recognize vulnerable plaques and provide additional relevant information beyond angiography alone.[2] Complex plaque morphology is the angiographic hallmark of unstable coronary lesions. Invasively, complex lesions are characterized by haziness, irregularity, frank ulceration, intraplaque contrast persistence, and luminal filling defect. Computed tomographic coronary angiography (CTA) features of plaques in patients with acute coronary syndromes (ACS) are just being identified. However, the CTA correlates of angiographically diagnosed, complex unstable coronary lesions have not been fully delineated. The CTA-documented lesion morphology was strikingly similar to invasive angiographic features indicative of plaque disruption, including lesion haziness (55%), irregularity (55%), ulceration (67%), and intraplaque contrast penetration (62%). On CTA images, complex lesions typically appeared bulky, hypodense, eccentric (index = 0.33 ± 0.29), and positively remodeled (index = 1.5 ± 0.77), with features similar to complex ruptured plaque seen by intravascular ultrasound. Given the increasing use of CTA to evaluate acute chest pain, characterization of plaque instability has considerable clinical implications. Further studies will be necessary to establish the sensitivity, specificity, and predictive accuracy of CTA for characterization of complex plaque.

The "Triple Rule-Out" CT Protocol

Given the robust clinical performance of CCTA for exclusion of acute coronary syndrome in emergency department patients, as well as the widespread use and proven clinical accuracy of CT angiography for diagnosis of acute aortic dissection [18–22] and pulmonary embolism [23–27], a "triple rule-out" scan protocol to simultaneously exclude all three potentially fatal causes of acute chest pain with a single scan is an attractive option. Once 64-slice CT scanners became widely available, the technical limitations of combined simultaneous evaluation of all three vascular areas have been largely overcome. A conventional cardiac CTA "field of view" already includes the anatomy between the carina and the diaphragm. The technical challenge of a "triple rule-out" scan protocol is to obtain high and consistent contrast intensity in all three vascular beds. Combined simultaneous evaluation for the pulmonary, coronary, and thoracic aortas requires a carefully tailored imaging and injection protocol (see Fig. 13.3 example). In evaluating one such protocol, we prospectively imaged 50 ED chest pain patients who underwent

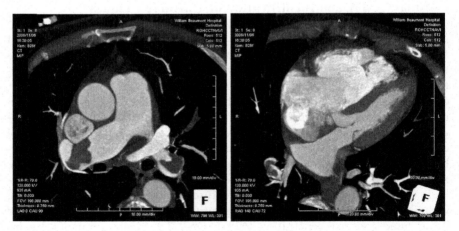

Fig. 13.3 "Triple rule-out" scan acquisition in a 79-year-old female with acute chest pain, non-specific electrocardiogram changes, and negative cardiac biomarkers. (**A**) Axial 5 mm maximum intensity projection images show uniform enhancement of the ascending aorta and main pulmonary artery bifurcation. Bilateral large pulmonary emboli are seen, as well as (**B**) marked right heart enlargement. The patient was also noted to have >50% mixed calcified and non-calcified plaque in the proximal left anterior descending coronary artery

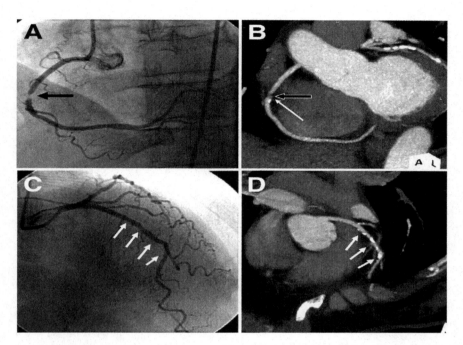

Fig. 13.4 Putative CT differences between unstable and stable plaque in the same patient. Panels A–D show comparative images in a patient with unstable, ruptured right coronary artery (RCA) lesion, but stable plaque in the LAD and circumflex arteries. Invasive angiography (**A**) documents the complex plaque severely narrowing the mid-RCA (*black arrow*). The CTA **Fig 13.4** (continued) images (**B**) are concordant, revealing a bulky, eccentric, and hypodense RCA lesion (*black arrow*) with intraplaque contrast penetration indicative of ulceration and rupture (*white arrow*). Panel C shows stable plaque in the left coronary artery from same patient. Invasive angiogram (**C**) demonstrates non-complex mild plaque in the mid-LAD (*white arrows*). The CTA image (**D**) similarly reveals mild non-complex plaque with punctate calcific elements and moderate luminal narrowing (*white arrows*) but lacking the bulky, hypodense-disrupted features characteristic of complex plaques

single-acquisition 64-slice CT angiography to evaluate the enhancement of the coronary, pulmonary, and thoracic vasculature [28]. We used a "tri-phasic" injection protocol that delivers the standard 100 mL of iodinated contrast at 5 mL/s typical for CCTA examinations, followed by an additional 30 mL at 3 mL/s to maintain pulmonary artery opacification, followed by a standard saline flush injection. This protocol is easy to achieve with commercially available radiographic injectors. Importantly, a caudal–cranial scan acquisition was used (as opposed to the standard CCTA cranial–caudal technique) to scan the distal pulmonary arteries at the base of the lung earlier, as these are most subject to problems with low-contrast intensity. Mean coronary artery, pulmonary artery, and aortic enhancement values were consistently higher than 250 Hounsfield units, and right atrial

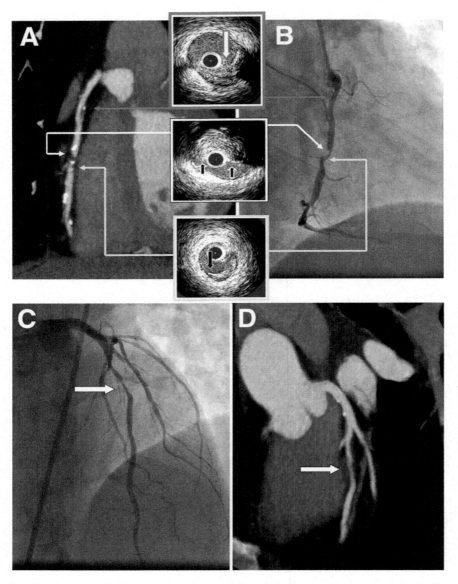

Fig. 13.5 Putative CT differences between unstable and stable plaque in the same patient. The CTA image (**A**) documents an ulcerated, bulky, eccentric, hypodense mid-RCA lesion; IVUS confirms complex morphology with bulky, eccentric, disrupted plaque in the proximal (*middle box, white arrows*) and distal (*lower box, yellow arrows*) aspects of this lesion. Invasive angiography (**B**) reveals a concordant bulky, eccentric, scalloped complex RCA lesion (*white* and *yellow arrows*). Proximally to the culprit lesion, CTA documents a bulky, eccentric, hypodense lesion (*red arrows*) confirmed by IVUS (*upper red box*), which is less apparent by invasive imaging. An invasive angiogram (**C**) demonstrates non-complex stenotic plaque in the mid-LAD (*white arrow*). The CTA image (**D**) similarly reveals non-complex plaque lacking the bulky, hypodense-disrupted CTA features characteristic of complex plaques

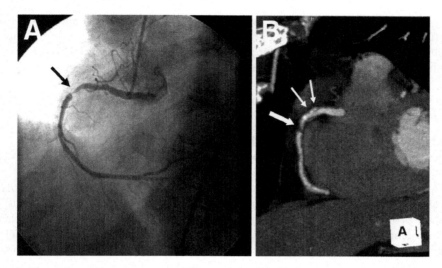

Fig. 13.6 CTA can identify more than one complex plaque. The CTA can identify more than one complex plaque apart from the angiogram-identified culprit vessel. The comparative angiographic images document ruptured plaque by both techniques, but significant plaque extension is underappreciated by invasive angiography. Invasive image (**A**) reveals a complex ruptured plaque in the right coronary artery (*black arrow*). The CTA image (**B**) similarly demonstrates the same complex ruptured plaque characterized by a hazy, hypodense-ulcerated plaque (*large white arrow*); however, more proximally, there is also a bulky lucent lesion with intraplaque contrast penetration (*small white arrows*) or spotty calcification, which are both signs of a complex vulnerable plaque that was not apparent by invasive imaging. A fair amount of data shows that patients with ACS may have multiple ruptured plaques. This may be detectable by CTA

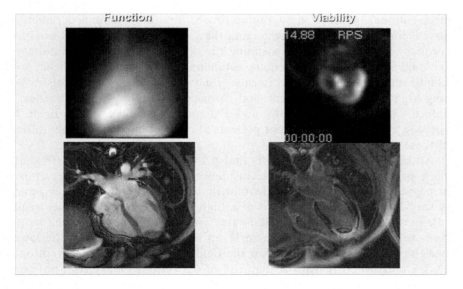

Fig. 13.7 Spect MPI vs. MRI

enhancement did not interfere with interpretation of the coronary arteries. Although feasibility studies of this and similar protocols are promising, large-scale clinical trials assessing the clinical accuracy of such "triple rule-out" protocols are not yet available.

Dedicated Coronary vs. "Triple Rule-Out" Scan Protocol – Radiation Dose Considerations

In spite of these technical advances, important radiation safety concerns remain that should limit indiscriminate application of a "triple rule-out" scan protocol. The effective radiation dose of a scan is calculated as the dose–length product (measured and displayed by the scanner on each patient) multiplied by the European Commission thoracic conversion factor (0.017) to yield the effective dose in milliSieverts (mSv). Thus, the radiation dose is directly proportional to the scan length in centimeters. Compared to the usual radiation dose of a standard CCTA (generally ranging from 8 to 22 mSv, depending on body habitus, gender, and scan protocol), the effective radiation dose of a "triple rule-out" scan is often increased by 50%, simply due to the increased field of view. By comparison, rest-stress radionuclide scans typically involve exposures in the range of 8–16 mSv, while diagnostic invasive angiography doses range from 5 to 13 mSv. Further, among patients who undergo CCTA as a primary triage test in the ED, there is a subset who also require a non-invasive stress test (often a radionuclide test), followed in some cases by diagnostic and interventional invasive angiographic procedures. This combined radiation dose is a cause for concern, changing the 0.6 mm high resolution used for coronary CTA to 2 mm for scanning the upper lung fields (since pulmonary angiography does not require submillimeter resolution) in theory can significantly reduce radiation dosage. Innovative imaging protocols involving tight heart rate control and "prospective gating" can drastically reduce radiation exposure (to under 5 mSv) but these are difficult to apply in emergency department patients and is not currently being utilized in these patients.

An additional consideration is that prior studies of patients with acute chest pain have shown that the incidence of "occult" pulmonary embolism or aortic dissection in patients without suggestive signs or symptoms is very low. Thus, unless there is a high index of suspicion, the "triple rule-out" should be avoided. It is also worthy of note that if the suspicion is high the entire thoracic aorta up to the aortic arch and the lower two-thirds of the lung are within the field of view during a conventional CCTA and would reveal the majority of dissections and central pulmonary emboli without additional radiation.

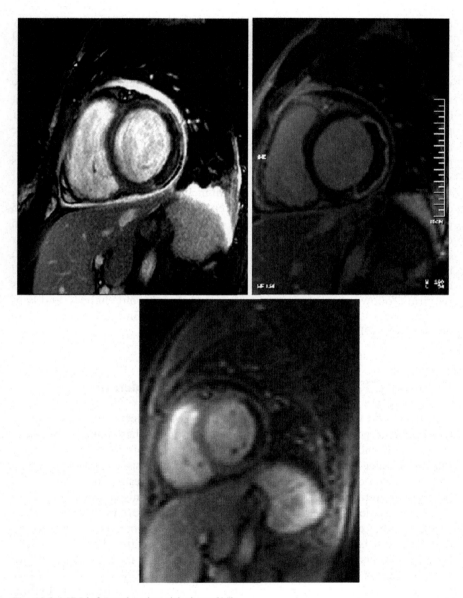

Fig. 13.8 MRI infarcted and at risk tissue [35]

Assessment for Non-Cardiac, Extravascular Pathology: Value Added

Well over 50% of acute chest pain cases represent non-cardiac conditions [15]. In patients who undergo a dedicated CCTA, images of non-cardiac thoracic structures are contained in the field of view and therefore available to the expert reader. Diseases that can be detected (in addition to aortic and pulmonary arterial pathology) include pericardial thickening and/or effusions, esophageal pathology, pneumonia, pulmonary nodules, pneumothoraces, mediastinal masses, pleural effusions and masses, as well as chest wall abnormalities. Previous studies have demonstrated that up to one in six patients without coronary abnormalities detected on CT was diagnosed with non-cardiac findings that could explain their presenting symptoms [29]. These findings suggest that for patients with acute chest pain, a comprehensive review of the thoracic cardiac and non-cardiac structures should be undertaken. We evaluated patients undergoing CT for additional findings beyond CAD that either provided physicians with a plausible etiology for CP or findings requiring further work-up. Chest findings considered not clinically significant included lymphadenopathy < 1 cm, calcified lesions, atelectasis, fatty liver or renal or hepatic cysts. We evaluated 145 patients, 11 or 8% had >50% stenosis on CTA, 8/11 had ≥70% stenosis on cardiac catheterization, and no PEs or aortic dissections were found. Eleven or eight percent had non-cardiac findings aiding in the physician's diagnosis, which included eight Hiatal hernias, two pulmonary infiltrates not seen on CXR, and one pericardial effusion. An additional 34 or 23% had significant findings requiring follow-up, primarily pulmonary nodules, thyroid changes, and lymphadenopathy >1 cm. Total percent of significant findings were 39% in patients with CTA/chest CT.

Coronary CTA Limitations and Protocol Considerations

Coronary CTA has several important limitations that affect its usefulness in the triage of emergency department patients with acute chest pain. It has been convincingly shown that the heart rate and regularity of the rhythm is closely related to image quality and accuracy of coronary stenosis estimation [9]. It is a common practice to premedicate patients who have resting heart rates >65 beats per minute with beta blocking drugs, and to administer sublingual nitroglycerin to patients to enhance image quality. We surveyed our research logs and noted that about 15% of screened patients had some contraindication to beta antagonists. If available, dual-source CCTA obviates the need for beta blocker administration in most patients. At this time, most facilities do not perform CCTA in patients with irregular rhythms; however, recent hardware and software improvements allow imaging of patients with irregular rhythms including atrial fibrillation. It is essential to screen patients in the ED for a history of iodine allergy and to avoid administration of contrast in patients with diminished creatinine clearance.

Importantly, a major limitation is that CCTA presently provides data regarding anatomical lesions only, not their physiologic impact on coronary blood flow. For this reason, in our series 15% of ED patients with acute chest pain required additional non-invasive stress imaging owing to intermediate severity lesions detected on CCTA [17]. Finally, the importance of a team approach to implementation of a CCTA emergency department triage protocol cannot be overstated. Emergency department physicians and cardiologists must be well educated regarding the application and inherent limitations of CCTA, and a complete review of cardiac and adjacent structures available from the CT data should be performed by physicians with appropriate background and level of experience.

There are now over 30 published studies comparing CCTA to quantitative invasive coronary angiography, encompassing over 2,000 patients [30, 9, 10, 31–33]. Among the 18 studies in which per-patient analyses are available (involving 1,329 patients, using either 16 or 64-slice CT), the mean subject-weighted sensitivity and specificity for the detection of significant CAD (i.e., $\geq 50\%$ luminal stenosis) were 97 and 84%, respectively [34]. Analysis of just the 64-slice studies revealed a sensitivity and specificity of 98 and 93%, respectively. Importantly, the combined results from all 18 studies demonstrated a mean per-patient negative predictive value of 97%. These data support the hypothesis that a normal CCTA may obviate the need for invasive angiography in properly selected clinical circumstances. These studies validate that patients at the opposite ends of the disease spectrum (i.e., those with <25 vs. >70% maximal luminal stenoses) can be accurately triaged by CCTA alone, while patients with lesions of intermediate severity (25–70% stenosis) may require functional testing.

The Use of Magnetic Resonance Imaging in the Emergency Department

The number of clinical studies of MRI use in ED patients is low. Therefore broad conclusions and recommendations are difficult. A review of the evidence to date shows that MRI has some promise both as an anatomical and a functional assay. Kwong et al. demonstrated in 161 consecutive patients presenting with 30 min of CP and non-STEMI ECGs that rest MRI with perfusion, LV function, and Gadolinium enhancement for MI, showed equivalent sensitivity and improved specificity as compared to ECG criteria and worse sensitivity and equivalent specificity to TIMI risk scoring at at 6.8whs for ACS outcomes. Of note the incidence of ACS was 16% with 10 NSTEMI and 15 unstable angina with significant stenosis. The test took on an average 58 ± 10 min to complete. The use of adenosine Stress MRI was studied by Ingkanisorn et al. in 135 ED patients with 30 min chest discomfort, negative troponin >6 h after last episode of discomfort, and a non-diagnostic ECG.[3] Outcome was the 1 year incidence of death, AMI, stenosis >50%, or abnormal correlative stress test. Twenty (14.8%) patients experienced an outcome, 15 had >50% stenosis, 2 abnormal stress, 1 AMI, and 1 death. None of the patients with a normal adenosine CMR had an adverse outcome at 1 year. Cardiac risk factors and CMR were both significant predictors of the defined outcome by Kaplan–Meier analysis. Multiple studies have been performed comparing multidetector CTA and MRI for stenotic accuracy. Kefer et al. found in 52 patients scheduled for catheterization received both MRI and 16-slice MDCT.[4] CTA had better sensitivity and equivalent specificity and diagnostic accuracy as MRI with correlation of 0.6 for MRI and 0.75 CTA for the prediction of degree of coronary artery stenosis. Gerber et al. evaluated 27 patients undergoing catheterization; CTA and MRI had high negative predictive values for segmental stenosis: 93% (168 of 180 segments) for CT and 90% (198 of 220 segments) for MRI.[5] However, the overall diagnostic accuracy favored MR imaging 80% (234/294 segments) vs. CTA 73% (214/294 segments, $p < 0.05$). The use of MRA for the detection of CAD has been studied a few of small observational trials. Muller et al. produced the best results to date and showed in 35 patients with significant stenosis >50% MRA had a positive predictive value of 87% and a negative predictive value of 93%.[6] Kim in 109 patients undergoing cardiac catheterizations, in whom 636 out of 759 proximal and middle distal segments were interpretable there was low specificity of 42% and a diagnostic accuracy of 72%. Testing took on an average 70 min to complete.[7] Further, Kessler et al. found that in 73 patients the sensitivity was 65% and specificity 88%.[8] Nikolaou et al. in 20 patients evaluatal for significant stenosis >50%, MDCT as compared to MRA had better sensitivity (85 vs. 79%) and specificity (77 vs. 70%).[9] Liu et al. compared 64-slice MDCT and MRA in patients with elevated calcium scores. In 18 patients who received both MDCT and MRA compared techniques on lesions with Ca + + score >100. Coronary MRA had higher image quality for coronary segments with nodal calcification than for coronary segments with diffuse calcification. Coronary MRA had better specificity than coronary MDCTA for the detection of significant stenosis in patients with high calcium scores in MRI imaging.[10] In summary, the pros of MRI are as follows: they provide excellent details of cardiac ischemia and viability, provide excellent evaluation of myocardial function, and can also visualize aorta and lungs with a sensitivity and specificity comparable to nuclear imaging without radiation exposure. The cons of MRI are as follows: it does not visualize the coronary anatomy, there is limited experience and availability; to date there is no proven advantage over nuclear/echo, it is more expensive, and exposure to gadolinium can lead to nephrogenic systemic fibrosis. The use of MRA for the detection of CAD displayed only fair sensitivity and specificity when compared to cardiac catheterization. In the small studies comparing MDCT to MRA, MDCT appeared superior; however, MRA may be useful in patients with nodal calcification and potentially coronary stents. In particular, only adenosine stress testing has been studied in ED chest pain patients.

Conclusions

Computed tomography has evolved over the past two decades into a powerful imaging tool that is now capable of imaging the coronary arteries. In addition to the proven clinical accuracy of CT angiography for the diagnosis of aortic dissection and pulmonary embolism, coronary CTA has been recently validated as a highly sensitive and reliable technique to confirm or exclude significant coronary stenosis in patients with suspected coronary artery disease. Initial experiences suggest that CCTA is an accurate and efficient test for the triage of appropriately selected acute chest pain patients to early discharge or further inpatient diagnosis and treatment. Emergency department patients with a low to intermediate pretest likelihood of coronary disease and negative cardiac biomarkers and electrocardiograms are best suited for CCTA-based triage. Technical advances now permit acquisition of well-opacified images of the coronary arteries, thoracic aorta, and pulmonary arteries from a single CT scan protocol. While this "triple rule-out" technique can potentially exclude fatal causes of chest pain in all three vascular beds, the attendant higher radiation dose of this method precludes its routine use except when there is sufficient support for the diagnosis of either aortic dissection or pulmonary embolism. The use of MRI and MRA in the evaluation of Chest pain patients is less clear due to the paucity of studies; however, stress MRI and the use of MRA in patients with elevated calcium scores may prove useful.

Notes

1. CTA for rapid disposition of low-risk ED patients with chest pain syndromes, Hollander JE, Acad Emerg Med. 2007 Feb;14(2):112–6.
2. Computed tomographic angiographic morphology of invasively proven complex coronary plaques. Goldstein JA, Dixon S, Safian RD, Hanzel G, Grines CL, Raff GL. J. Am. Coll. Cardiol. Img. 2008;1;249–251.
3. Adenosine stress magnetic resonance, Ingkanisorn et al., JACC, 2006;47:1427–32.
4. Head to Head: 16 Slice MDCT vs. MRI, Kefer et al., JACC 2005;46:92–100.
5. Direct comparison of four-section multidetector row CT and 3D navigator MR imaging for detection – initial results. Gerber et al., Radiology. 2005 Jan;234(1):98–108.
6. Muller et al., J Mag Res Imag, 1997;7:644.
7. Kim et al., NEJM, 2001;345:1863.
8. Kessler et al., AM J Cardiol, 1997; 80:989.
9. Nikolaou et al., Eur Radiol, 2002;12:1663.
10. Comparison of 3D free-breathing coronary MR angiography and 64-MDCT angiography for detection of coronary stenosis in patients with high calcium scores. Liu et al. AJR Am J Roentgenol. 2007 Dec;189(6):1326–32.

References

1. McCaig LF, Burt CW, National Hospital Ambulatory Medical Care Survey 2003: Emergency Department Summary: Advance Data from Vital and Health Statistics, No. 358. Hyattsville, MD: National Center for Health Statistics; 2005.
2. Pope JH, Aufderhelde TP, Ruthazer R, et al. Missed diagnoses of acute cardiac ischemia in the emergency department. N Engl J Med 2000;342:1163–1170.
3. Lee TH, Goldman L. Evaluation of the patient with acute chest pain. N Engl J Med 2000; 342:1187–1195.

4. Lee TH, Rouan GW, Weisberg MC, et al. Clinical characteristics and natural history of patients with acute myocardial infarction sent home from the emergency room. Am J Cardiol 1987;60:219–224.

5. Karcz A, Korn R, Burke MC, et al. Malpractice claims against emergency physicians in Massachusetts: 1975–1993. Am J Emerg Med. 1996;14:341–345.

6. Kalendar WA, Seissler W, Klotz E, Vock P. Spiral volumetric CT with single breath-hold technique: continuous transport and continuous scanner rotation. Radiology 1990;176:181–183.

7. Ohnesorge B, Flohr T, Becker C, et al. Cardiac imaging by means of electrocardiographically gated multisection spiral CT: initial experience. Radiology 2000;217:564–571.

8. Achenbach S, Ulzheimer S, Baum U, et al. Noninvasive coronary angiography by retrospectively ECG-gated multislice spiral CT. Circulation 2000;102:2823–2828.

9. Raff GL, Gallagher MJ, O'Neill WW, et al. Diagnostic accuracy of noninvasive coronary angiography using 64-slice spiral computed tomography. J Am Coll Cardiol 2005;46:552–557.

10. Mollet NR, Cademartiri F, van Mieghem CA, et al. High-resolution spiral computed tomography coronary angiography in patients referred for diagnostic conventional angiography. Circulation 2005;112:2318–2323.

11. Leber AW, Knez A, von Ziegler F, et al. Quantification of obstructive and nonobstructive coronary lesions by 64-slice computed tomography. J Am Coll Cardiol 2005;46:147–154.

12. Sato Y, Matsumoto N, Ichikawa M, et al. Efficacy of multislice computed tomography for the detection of acute coronary syndrome in the emergency department. Circ J 2005;69:1047–1051.

13. White CS, Kuo D, Kelemen M, et al. Chest pain evaluation in the emergency department: Can MDCT provide a comprehensive evaluation? AJR 2005;185:533–540.

14. Hoffmann U, Nagurney JT, Moselewski F, et al. Coronary multidetector computed tomography in the assessment of patients with acute chest pain. Circulation 2006;114:2251–2260.

15. Gallagher MJ, Ross MA, Raff GL, et al. The diagnostic accuracy of 64-slice computed tomography coronary angiography compared with stress nuclear imaging in emergency department low-risk chest pain patients. Ann Emerg Med 2007;49:125–136.

16. Rubinshtein R, Halon DA, Gaspar T, et al. Usefulness of 64-slice cardiac computed tomographic angiography for diagnosing acute coronary syndromes and predicting clinical outcome in emergency department patients with chest pain of uncertain origin. Circulation 2007;115:1762–1768.

17. Goldstein JA, Gallagher MJ, O'Neill WW, et al. A randomized controlled trial of multislice coronary computed tomography for evaluation of acute chest pain patients. J Am Coll Cardiol 2007;49:863–871.

18. Willoteaux S, Lions C, Gaxotte V, et al. Imaging of aortic dissection by helical computed tomography (CT). Eur Radiol 2004;14:1999–2008.

19. Yoshida S, Akiba H, Tamakawa M, et al. Thoracic involvement of type A aortic dissection and intramural hematoma: diagnostic accuracy – comparison of emergency helical CT and surgical findings. Radiology 2003;228: 430–435.

20. Hamada S, Takamiya M, Kimura K, et al. Type A aortic dissection: evaluation with ultrafast CT. Radiology 1992;183:155–158.

21. Sebastia C, Pallisa E, Quiroga S, et al. Aortic dissection: diagnosis and follow-up with helical CT. RadioGraphics 1999;19:45–60.

22. Shiga T, Wajima Z, Apfel CC, et al. Diagnostic accuracy of transesophageal echocardiography, helical computed tomography, and magnetic resonance imaging for suspected thoracic aortic dissection. Arch Intern Med 2006;166:1350–1356.

23. Ghaye B, Remy J, Remy-Jardin M. Non-traumatic thoracic emergencies: CT diagnosis of acute pulmonary embolism: the first 10 years. Eur Radiol 2002;12:1886–1905.

24. Anderson DR, Kovacs MJ, Dennie C, et al. Use of spiral computed tomography contrast angiography and ultrasonography to exclude the diagnosis of pulmonary embolism in the emergency department. J Emerg Med 2005;29:399–404.
25. Prologo JD, Gilkeson RC, Diaz M, et al. CT pulmonary angiography: a comparative analysis of the utilization patterns in emergency department and hospitalized patients between 1998 and 2003. Am J Roentgenol 2004;183:1093–1096.
26. Ghanima W, Almaas V, Aballi S, et al. Management of suspected pulmonary embolism (PE) by D-dimer and multi-slice computed tomography in outpatients: an outcome study. J Thromb Haemost 2005;3:1926–1932.
27. Quiroz R, Kucher N, Zou KH. Clinical validity of a negative computed tomography scan in patients with suspected pulmonary embolism: a systematic review. JAMA 2005;293:2012–2017.
28. Vrachliotis TG, Bis KG, Haidary A, et al. Atypical chest pain: coronary, aortic, and pulmonary vasculature enhancement at biphasic single-injection 64-section CT angiography. Radiology 2007;243:Number 2:368–376.
29. Onuma K, Tanabe, Nakazawa G, et al. Noncardiac findings in cardiac imaging with multidetector computed tomography. J Am Coll Cardiol 2006;48:402–406.
30. Leschka S, Alkadhi H, Plass A, et al. Accuracy of MSCT coronary angiography with 64-slice technology: first experience. Eur Heart J 2005;26:1482–1487.
31. Pugliese F, Mollet NR, Runza G, et al. Diagnostic accuracy of non-invasive 64-slice CT coronary angiography in patients with s angina pectoris. Eur Radiol 2006;16:575–582.
32. Ropers D, Rixe J, Anders K, et al. Usefulness of multidetector row spiral computed tomography with 64- × 0.6-mm collimation and 330-ms rotation for the noninvasive detection of significant coronary artery stenoses. Am J Cardiol 2006;97:343–348.
33. Hamon M, Biondi-Zoccai GGL, Malagutti P, Agostoni P, Morello R, Valgimigli M, Hamon M. Diagnostic performance of multislice spiral computed tomography of coronary arteries as compared with conventional invasive coronary angiography: A meta analysis. J Am Coll Cardiol 2006;48:1896–1910.
34. Raff GL, Goldstein JA. Coronary angiography by computed tomography: coronary imaging evolves. J Am Coll Cardiol 2007;49:1830–1833.
35. Raff GL, O'Neill WW, Gentry RE, Dulli A, Bis KG, Shetty AN, Goldstein JA. Microvascular Obstruction and Myocardial Function after Acute Myocardial Infarction: assessment by Using Contrast-enhanced Cine MR Imaging. Radiology 2006;240(2): 629–838.

Chapter 14
Disposition from the Short Stay Unit

Chris A. Ghaemmaghami and William J. Brady

Abstract One of the primary goals in the use of the chest pain unit (CPU) is the identification of patients with possible acute coronary syndromes (ACS). Another important goal of the CPU in this group of patients undergoing evaluation is the distinction of patients that should be admitted to hospital for further inpatient care from those that can be safely discharged without an increased risk of adverse cardiac events. This focus on risk assessment and prevention of events through referral for definitive care when needed is at the core of the CPU's value. Risk assessment is primarily short term in nature in the CPU (e.g., "Is this patient having an ACS now?"), but established processes of care that efficiently dovetail the CPU with the broader outpatient and inpatient settings can have a major impact on long-term event prevention as well. The use of straightforward criteria to select appropriate patients for entry into the CPU and a well-designed observation process employing serial patient assessments and diagnostic testing both aid in distinguishing patients who need admission versus those that can be safely discharged. Discharge planning considerations are also important as is the recognition of nonmedical barrier to safe discharge. The following sections will review these items in more detail such that the clinician-administrator is able to develop a safe, effective, and efficient CPU guideline for disposition of patients with potential ACS.

Keywords Chest pain · Outpatient · Discharge criteria · Acute coronary syndromes

C.A. Ghaemmaghami (✉)
Department of Emergency Medicine, University of Virginia Health System, PO Box 800699, Charlottesville, VA 22908-0699, USA
e-mail: cg3n@virginia.edu

W.F. Peacock, C.P. Cannon (eds.), *Short Stay Management of Chest Pain*,
DOI 10.1007/978-1-60327-948-2_14,
© Humana Press, a part of Springer Science+Business Media, LLC 2009

CPU Patient Entry: Appropriate Patient Selection for "Rule Out ACS"

One of the most important determinants of the success of the disposition process from a short stay unit is appropriate initial patient selection. In most cases, patients are placed in a short stay unit by a referring physician after some level of direct evaluation. In the case of the patient with the chief complaint of chest pain, a basic history, physical examination, 12-lead ECG, and initial serum cardiac marker measurement is assumed to be performed prior to entry into a CPU. The basic information obtained through this process should help to identify either (a) patients at such high risk for ACS or adverse events that inpatient admission is indicated without further testing or (b) patients with syndromes that are clearly nonischemic in origin where initiation of a clinical pathway to rule out ACS would not be appropriate. At the same time, prior to entry into the CPU, practical and logistical factors that prevent safe discharge of the patient from the hospital should be assessed. Early identification of this type of patient will enable the CPU to run more efficiently and will prevent conundrums, and thus an obstacle to efficient throughput, in the final patient disposition. This caveat is particularly important in a setting where shift changes between physicians and nurses will lead to the transfer of care of patients. No one staffing an observation unit wants to inherit a patient without a clearly delineated set of disposition possibilities.

Exclusion of Patients at High Risk for ACS or Adverse Cardiac Events If Discharged

Simply put, patients having grossly abnormal vital signs (e.g., hypotension, respiratory instability), unstable cardiac rhythms, diagnostic ischemic changes on ECG, or elevations of serum cardiac markers in a clearly diagnostic range for significant myocardial injury should not be entered into a CPU pathway. They should be admitted to the hospital. These patients are at high risk for ACS based on their initial physician assessment and should not be placed in the CPU – the diagnostic component of the observation process will in most cases only delay hospital admission and more definitive care. Additionally, when incremental testing strategies involving ECG and serial serum cardiac markers are applied to groups of patients with a high prevalence of ACS, the chance of a false-negative diagnostic work-up increases dramatically. Thus, entering high-risk patients into the CPU results in both decreased efficiency and increased risk for both the patient and the caregiver [1, 2].

Exclusion of Patients at Very Low Risk of ACS from Observation Strategies

Although the diagnosis of subtle or even occult ACS can be difficult, it is occasionally possible to make a definitive non-ACS diagnosis in the patient with signs or symptoms suggestive of ACS. The practical advantage of excluding patients with extraordinarily low-risk scenarios lies primarily in the reduction of overutilization of observation resources. Patients with very low pretest probabilities of ACS (<1 % chance) will be more likely to have false-positive ECG and cardiac marker results than actual ACS [3]. Applying the CPU testing strategy to these patients will result in an increased number of false-positive work-ups, unnecessary imaging or invasive testing, and increased cost and risk to patients.

The ED screening process to find the theoretical "No-risk" patient prior to CPU entry should focus on the identification of common cardiopulmonary processes like pneumonia and pulmonary embolism that can be proven through readily available ED testing (e.g., chest X-ray, CT pulmonary angiography). While some patients can have ACS excluded due to the solid diagnosis of an alternative process, many cannot and physicians should not overreach on this strategy. For example, gastroenterological diagnoses, like gastroesophageal reflux disease (GERD), although common in the ED patient with atraumatic chest pain, cannot be definitively proven in the ED. This difficulty creates a common pitfall for physicians who would like to make a clinical diagnosis of a common disease (GERD) while ignoring the possibility of a subtle ACS. In all cases, the evaluating physician must carefully entertain the possibility that ACS can occur concurrently with ACS mimics [4].

Exclusion of Patients with Logistical and Nonmedical Barriers to Safe Discharge

Before a patient is entered into an observation pathway, a realistic assessment – from a logistical perspective – of whether or not a patient can be discharged in the event that all testing is negative. Frequently nonmedical barriers to safe discharge from the hospital are present and easily recognizable. These factors should be determined by the initial physician prior to entry to the CPU, and these barriers must be addressed prior to signing out the care of a patient to another provider. Many patients presenting to the ED had previously been living independently, but may be judged to now need additional care on a full- or part-time basis. Common reasons for this change in status include progressive or previously unrecognized lack of mobility or cognitive impairment that inhibits the patient's ability to carry out activities of daily living. In the event that no immediate outpatient caregivers can be identified for these patients, appropriate steps should be taken to admit the patient to hospital. Entry into the CPU will only delay this inevitable "social" admission.

Indications for Hospitalization from the Short Stay Unit: Admission Triggers

During the observation period of the CPU stay, the primary goal of the clinical pathway for a potential ACS patient is the continual collection of data aimed at risk assessment. This new information – both objective and subjective in nature – can either confirm the low-risk status of a patient in the CPU or change the assessment of the patient's risk from low/intermediate for ACS into a higher range that may require hospital admission and acute intervention. Although the information is in many cases nonspecific for ACS, the fact that the risk level has been elevated for the individual under evaluation usually results in an immediate disposition decision and removal from the CPU pathway.

Any clinical pathway for observation of patients being evaluated for possible ACS should have defined admission triggers – clinical or diagnostic endpoints that, if found, result in hospital admission with or without acute intervention (Table 14.1). While the activities of the patient undergoing observation are passive, those of the health-care providers are active and include frequent reassessments. The core diagnostic elements of an ACS CPU pathway should include frequent measurement of vital signs, assessment of patient symptoms, repeating and interpreting 12-lead ECG's, and serial serum cardiac marker determination. A second role of the CPU pathway is to give the clinician the opportunity to entertain and definitively make alternative diagnoses during the allotted time; thus, the actual time period of observation is another tool of significant value in the CPU process. Consideration of alternate diagnoses adds accuracy and efficiency to the overall diagnostic process.

Table 14.1 Admission triggers

Clinical factors

    Unexplained bradycardia or tachycardia
    Hypotension
    Severe hypertension
    Progressive or persistent dyspnea
    Intractable or recurring ischemic chest pain
    Severe decrement in patient's functional capacity from baseline

Diagnostic factors

    New or dynamic ECG changes
    New elevations of serum cardiac markers
    Abnormalities on immediate provocative testing

Assessment of Clinical Factors

The assessment of clinical factors is of paramount importance during observation.

Clinical factors include simple measurement of vital signs and reassessment of patients' symptoms. Repeated, routine measurement of vital signs will help to detect early signs of clinical decompensation. These should be scheduled by protocol and recorded diligently.

As a general rule, the development of abnormal vital signs in a patient undergoing an observation protocol in the CPU requires explanation. In the absence of a benign explanation, the patients should be admitted to the hospital for further evaluation.

Heart Rate

Unexplained bradycardia or tachycardia should always be addressed as they may represent significant physiologic impairment. Bradycardia may be an early sign of ischemia or infarction of the conduction system, especially if it involves the AV node; worsening degrees of AV nodal block may indicate progression of an infarction. Tachycardia in the CPU patient has many possible implications. Rhythm identification in the newly tachycardic patient is essential. Sinus tachycardia (ST) may be the only clinical sign of underlying clinical decompensation or early shock. If the underlying etiology is cardiac ischemia, sinus tachycardia may indicate left ventricular dysfunction or a new hemodynamic lesion (e.g., acute mitral regurgitation from papillary muscle dysfunction). Increased adrenergic tone related to ischemia and pain is also a common cause of sinus tachycardia in the ACS patient. The evaluator must always have a high index of suspicion for alternate non-ACS diagnosis in the CPU patient that suddenly develops tachycardia. Sepsis, pneumonia, and pulmonary embolism are all common diseases that may initially present with relatively normal vital signs and diagnostic studies. New rhythms other than sinus tachycardia should be identified and treated appropriately.

Iatrogenic causes for abnormal heart rates in the CPU are common and must be considered. The evaluator always must consider the influence of cardioactive medications (e.g., beta blockers, calcium channel blockers, and other AV nodal slowing agents) that are commonly used in the treatment of cardiac patients. Sinus tachycardia may result as a reflex from use of vasodilators such as nitrates and hydralazine and can also be related to volume depletion resultant from diuretics administration. Bradycardia and hypotension due to vasovagal episodes related to phlebotomy, which by their very nature are transient and self-limited, should not be overly concerning.

Of course, the treating clinicians are the most appropriate personnel to determine the significance of alterations in heart rate and other clinical data; further diagnostic and management decisions are best made by these clinicians.

Blood Pressure

Much like heart rate abnormalities, unexplained hypotension is an ominous sign that should alert the clinician to either severe cardiac dysfunction or the presence of a non-ACS diagnosis. With the exception of iatrogenic hypotension from commonly used medications and vasovagal episodes patients experiencing hypotension in the CPU should be considered for admission. Hypertension, on the other hand, is a much less reliable indicator of acute illness or decompensation. Judicious treatment of hypertension should be considered. Rarely, extreme, isolated hypertension requires hospital admission in this low-risk CPU patient population.

Respiratory Distress and Hypoxemia

Unexplained tachypnea or increased work of breathing at rest may indicate recurrent ischemia, the development of pulmonary edema or pulmonary embolus. Elderly patients in particular commonly present with dyspnea as an anginal equivalent [5]. A careful reexamination of the lungs and jugular venous pressure should be performed if respiratory distress develops. The clinician should consider reimaging the chest with the most appropriate imaging modality.

Recurrent Ischemic Pain

The reoccurrence of ischemic pain at rest during observation should ordinarily be an admission trigger. The logical argument for this disposition decision is that if the patient is having ischemic pain at rest in optimal conditions, then they will certainly continue to have these symptoms at home. Constant intractable pain that is not associated with ECG changes or elevated troponin levels after several hours is far less likely to be of cardiac origin than if the pain is episodic and recurrent. A caveat must be made here: brief episodes of ischemic pain, however, may not result in ECG changes or serum cardiac marker elevations.

Abnormal ECG and Serum Cardiac Marker Testing in the Observation Phase

Dynamic ECG Changes

Rhythm monitoring and repeated 12-lead ECGs based on additional clinical changes are essential parts of observation. Admission triggers related to the ECG are based on the assumption that the initial electrocardiogram has been nondiagnostic (normal, nonspecifically abnormal, or unchanged from previous tracings) with a stable rhythm (Table 14.2).

Table 14.2 Diagnostic ECG triggers for admission

Dynamic ST changes
ST depression
ST elevation
New bundle branch block – not rate-related
New arrhythmias
New 2nd or 3rd AV nodal block
Ventricular tachycardia
Excessive ventricular ectopy

Continuous ECG Rhythm Monitoring

Patients may be placed on continuous ECG rhythm monitoring while undergoing the rule out MI procedure. This step is aimed at the detection of new arrhythmias with particular attention to ventricular arrhythmias and high-grade AV nodal blocks. If these are identified they should result in hospital admission. The detection of atrial arrhythmias like atrial fibrillation/flutter and other supraventricular tachycardias occurs with some frequency and may redirect the evaluation and provide a reasonable alternative diagnosis to ACS.

ST Segment Changes

With changes in symptoms, serial or continuous, 12-lead ECG monitoring is performed to detect diagnostic ST changes that cannot be found through standard telemetry systems (i.e., single or multilead rhythm monitoring). Specifically, dynamic ST segment elevation or depression of greater than or equal to 1 mm as compared to the baseline ECG should warrant concern.

T-Wave Changes

T-wave inversions and flattening are less specific changes than ST segment deviation for acute ischemia. In the CPU, dynamic T-wave changes should be looked at with some skepticism before making an admission decision. One potentially helpful aspect of the inverting T-wave is summarized as such: as the depth of the T-wave inversion increases, the rate of ACS also increases [6]. A few common pitfalls that may occur over the course of hours spent in the CPU that can result in T-wave inversions and/or flattening include different ECG techniques between baseline and repeat 12-lead ECGs and the occurrence or correction of electrolyte abnormalities. Changes in body position can have a major influence in T-wave appearance. A patient sitting upright or lying in lateral decubitus position can have major changes in the anatomical position of the heart inside the thorax. Likewise, changes in lead position can have a major impact in ECG appearance [7, 8]. Almost all ECG machines in use are now digital. The CPU staff should be aware that the different ECG manufacturers may use different software filters that aid in the generation of the tracing. These data processing differences can result in slight variations in the appearance of ECG. Ideally, all 12-lead ECGs for each patient should be performed in the same semi-upright position, using the same machine and leads throughout the observation process for consistency.

Another potential confounder of apparent dynamic ECG findings is the presence of a significant electrolyte disturbance – particularly involving potassium, calcium, and magnesium [9]. It is a common practice in the CPU to correct these abnormalities during the observation period, so it would be expected that the ECG appearance may change as well. The CPU clinicians should be careful to not overreact to normalization of the ECG after the electrolyte corrections. Much less commonly, the treatment of hypothermia can have a similar effect. In any case, hospital admission decisions based on T-wave changes alone should meet some scrutiny.

Abnormal Cardiac Markers

The use of serum cardiac markers for the diagnosis of ACS and for prognostication is discussed more extensively elsewhere in this chapter. This discussion is focused on the use of these markers as a basis for hospital admission from the CPU.

Until recently, the technical limits of most cardiac troponin assays were such that detectable levels of circulating troponin were almost always abnormal with a reasonably high specificity for ACS. Newer, more highly sensitivity cardiac troponin assays (cTnI or cTnT) have the ability to detect very small concentrations of circulating troponin [10]. As a result, a significant percentage of patients in an CPU environment will have detectable troponin levels. Unfortunately, in that a large number of low-risk patients are included in this population, these troponin elevations may not be associated with ACS. In fact, these troponin elevations may be related to other cardiac, non-ACS conditions – decompensated heart failure and hypertensive urgencies/emergencies are among the most common. While these alternative conditions may not represent true ACS, all troponin elevations to date have been associated with increased mortality and short-term adverse outcome rates and deserve appropriately aggressive care.

In order to improve the accuracy of admission decisions for ACS based on serum troponin elevations, two strategies can be incorporated into the CPU guidelines [11].

(a) **Determine a diagnostic cutoff that will be respected at your institution.** With assistance from either the local laboratory or the assay manufacturer, the cardiologists and emergency physicians involved in managing the CPU should agree on an established diagnostic cutoff level that, once met on a single sample, should result in admission. This diagnostic level alone should not actually define AMI or ACS, but it does provide a post-test odds assessment such that ACS is highly probable [10]. When using the high sensitivity assays, this diagnostic cutoff level may be five to ten times higher than the lower limit of detection.

(b) **Measure troponin trends to look for peaking patterns versus plateaus.** Troponin concentrations below the predetermined diagnostic cutoff and above the lower level of detection should be addressed through careful reassessment of the patients and serial measurements. Going back to the bedside with the added knowledge of an indeterminate elevation of troponin can sometimes yield new information from the physical examination or patient history that was not previously discerned. Serial measurements are performed to distinguish trends as well as to detect analytic false-positives. Timing between sample collections in the CPU should be in the range of every 2–4 h [11]. Currently, no data exist supporting sampling intervals of less than 90 min. If a clinical answer is not apparent from reevaluation, then repeat testing for a trend analysis is appropriate.

Trend analysis of nondiagnostic troponin levels will yield one of three patterns: peaking, declining, or a plateau. Peaking patterns are highly specific for acute processes and in the appropriately selected CPU population, ACS is the most common of these. Both declining and plateau patterns frequently indicate subacute, non-ACS processes, the detection of a prior recent ACS which is resolving or analytical errors [12]. In summary, patients with peaking or declining troponin patterns should generally be hospitalized, but those with plateauing patterns should have individualized therapy and disposition, taking into consideration their clinical presentation.

Provocative Testing and Advanced Imaging

The integration of advanced imaging and provocative testing into the CPU protocol is largely determined by local factors, especially resource availability, institutional preference, and expertise. An extensive section on specific aspects of various advanced testing modalities appears elsewhere in this chapter. Admission criteria based on positive results of these advanced tests should be focused on the intention to treat ACS and the need for further invasive testing (i.e., coronary angiography). Most patient with positive tests will require hospital admission, but the demonstration of coronary artery disease alone does not dictate admission if the patient is clinically at low risk for ACS. (See section on outpatient strategies for patients with known CAD.)

Reassessment of Functional Status at the End of the CPU Protocol

After the patient has stabilized and serial cardiac marker and ECGs are nondiagnostic, basic functional status can easily be assessed. The CPU "road test" is a powerful maneuver to help determine appropriateness for discharge. The CPU staff can perform low-level exercise by simply having the patient walk with assistance inside the unit and in the hallways for 1 or 2 min. To be fair, efforts to reproduce the patient's home conditions – baseline supplemental oxygen, use of a walker or a cane – should be made. This exercise test occasionally results in recurrent ischemic symptoms, abnormal blood pressure or heart rate responses, and respiratory distress that were not present at rest. A positive finding on this simple evaluation even prior to the arrangement of provocative testing should result in hospital admission.

Situations When Outpatient Medical Management Strategies for Patients with Known Coronary Artery Disease Are Appropriate

Patients with CAD will become symptomatic at times and present for evaluation. It is impractical to exclude all patients with preexisting CAD from observation protocols because of the high prevalence of CAD. A careful assessment of the presenting symptoms including time course and frequency of symptoms can be helpful to identify patients at low versus high risk of an ACS. These low-risk patients with known CAD will have specific diagnostic and therapeutic goals. Since the presence of CAD is already known in this set of patients, the immediate diagnostic goals in these cases are to exclude myocardial infarction and to observe for continued ischemia. This observation strategy can generally be accomplished in 6–12 h in the CPU through a standard protocol using the ECG and serial serum cardiac marker measurements. Therapeutic goals should include stabilization and optimization of medical management of myocardial oxygen delivery, oxygen demand, and platelet inhibition (e.g., aspirin).

A few specific scenarios involving patients with known CAD are commonly seen in the CPU and may result in outpatient care rather than admission. In some cases, patients with known severe, inoperable or nonintervenable CAD will have been previously evaluated by their physicians, and after careful deliberation between doctor and patient, a long-term plan for medical management may have been decided upon. When these patients present for evaluation with limited ischemic symptoms, they may be discharged home after the successful completion of an observation protocol to rule out AMI. As mentioned previously, recurrent ischemia in the CPU is an indication for hospital admission, including this patient population. Medical therapy can be optimized with the help of the patient's primary team of physicians and close follow-up can be established. These patients should be made aware of the long-term risk of coronary events associated with their disease.

Medication noncompliance is one of the most common reasons for the occurrence of ischemic symptoms in the patient with established CAD. Patients who are noncompliant with antianginals and antihypertensives are relatively straightforward. Ischemic symptoms are the result of a reversible supply–demand mismatch and do not represent an acute coronary event (i.e., plaque rupture or thrombosis). After AMI is excluded, a simple resumption of medications and referral back to the patient's cardiologist or primary care physician should be sufficient. In significant contrast, patients that become symptomatic after non-compliance with antiplatelet agents have a higher risk of acute coronary thrombosis, especially if coronary stents are in place. These patients may have a more significant short-term risk for ACS and may need to be admitted for more aggressive anticoagulation and platelet inhibition even if they rule out successfully for AMI [13, 14].

Finally, some patients with known CAD, yet low risk of ACS, will successfully rule out for AMI by ECG and serial serum markers but will need an outpatient assessment for inducible ischemia to further guide invasive therapy. In contrast to the "medical management only" subset, these nonacute patients would potentially be eligible for surgery or percutaneous coronary intervention (PCI) if indicated. The CPU process allows for outpatient testing of these low-risk patients once they have successfully completed the CPU protocol without demonstration of subjective or objective abnormality; this strategy also assumes that the patient is compliant with medical instructions, follow-up appointments, and precautions. In this subgroup of patients, the short-term rate of adverse cardiac events approaches that of the non-CAD population [15].

Establishment of Follow-up

The final step in the process of CPU evaluation is arrangement of outpatient follow-up. An important distinction between low- and intermediate-risk patients must be kept in mind when arranging follow-up. Intermediate-risk patients should leave the CPU with firm plans for contact with a primary care physician or cardiologist in the very near term, i.e., days not weeks. Cardiac risk factor modification and general reassessment will be the focus of the next outpatient visit. Low-risk patients who do not appear to have cardiac risk factors may not require such close follow-up. Many times, routine follow-up with a primary care physician is adequate.

One of the major determinants of compliance with follow-up plans is access to care. It is strongly recommended that the CPU have plans in place for direct lines of referral with participating primary care clinics and cardiologists who will accept CPU-referred patients. An on call or referral list of outpatient clinic options is frequently available for new patients presenting to hospital-based emergency departments. It may be necessary to use these connections to ensure patients are not lost to follow-up.

It is particularly critical to address access to outpatient care issues in settings where outpatient provocative testing is offered or encouraged [16]. Both immediate and delayed provocative testing models are in use today, although data supporting the safety of delayed testing is sparse [17]. Integrating immediate provocative testing or coronary imaging into CPU guidelines for patients that have no access to scheduled outpatient testing due to payer status or other nonmedical barriers may be necessary. If these tests are not available when the patient presents and the patient has no access, default hospital admission is sometimes advisable. Despite the resultant costs in CPU length of stay and increased hospital admission rates, patient safety must come first. The most elegant plan for outpatient care will fail if the patient cannot logistically comply with it.

It should be noted, however, that each center needs to decide on the balance it strikes between medical paternalism and a patient's responsibility for their own care. If patients have access to outpatient care, lack nonmedical barriers to follow-up, and are given specific scheduled instructions for follow-up, some believe that immediate provocative testing of low-risk patients, although convenient, may not be medically necessary.

The patient should be involved in the discharge planning process so that they are comfortable with the treatment plan, have the opportunity to ask questions, and have a basic understanding of the rationale of the process they have just completed. It is important that the patient not be given the impression that their medical care is not completed; rather, it should be stressed that they have successfully completed the first step of a multistep process of evaluation. Predischarge education and discharge documents should clearly explain that while they do not appear to be having a myocardial infarction at this time, they need to comply with follow-up instructions to help prevent future cardiac events.

Summary

Utilization of the short stay unit for the evaluation of patients with possible ACS is only effective if there is a clear understanding of the various disposition outcomes that are possible. Clarifying specific admission triggers and discharge criteria are essential to maintain an efficient process that improves early recognition and treatment of ACS and accuracy of admissions. A clinical pragmatism is currently required when designing the necessary clinical pathways for admission or discharge because in many critical areas related to observation medicine the level of evidence present in the literature is not strong or does not correlate with the real-world undifferentiated patient population that inevitably presents in the acute care setting. Local solutions that emphasize patient safety and realistic resource utilization should always be sought in these centers and the chosen methods should be refined over time through sound process improvement activities.

References

1. Jackson BR. The dangers of false-positive and false-negative test results: False-positive results as a function of pretest probability. *Clin Lab Med* 2008: 28(2): 305–19.
2. Gill CJ, Sabin I, Schmid CH. Why Clinicians are natural Bayesians. *BMJ* 2005; 330:1080–3.
3. Gluud C, Gluud LL. Evidence based diagnostics. *BMJ* 2005; 330:724–6
4. Hollander JE, Robey JL, Chase MR, Brown AM, Zogby KE, Shofer FS. Relationship between a clear-cut alternative noncardiac diagnosis and 30-day outcome in emergency department patients with chest pain. *Acad Emerg Med* 2007; 14(3): 210–5.
5. Bayer AJ, Chadha JS, Farag RR, et al. Changing presentation of myocardial infarction with increasing old age. *J Am Geriatr Soc* 1986; 34:263–266.
6. Lin KB, Shofer FS, McCusker C, Meshberg E, Hollander JE. Predictive value of T-wave abnormalities at the time of emergency department presentation in patients with potential acute coronary syndromes. *Acad Emerg Med* 2008 Jun;15(6): 537–43.
7. Adams MG, Drew BJ. Body position effects on the ECG: Implication for ischemia monitoring. *J Electrocardiol* 1997; 30: 285.
8. Newlan SP, Meij SH, VanDam TB. Correction of ECG variations caused by body positions changes and electrode placement during ST-T monitoring. *J Electrocardiol* 2001; 34: 213–216.
9. Mirvis DM, Goldberger AL. "Electrocardiography" in Braunwald's Heart Disease: A Textbook of Cardiovascular Medicine, 8th ed. Saunders 2007: pp. 160–186.
10. Wu AH. Jaffe AS. The clinical need for high-sensitivity cardiac troponin assays for acute coronary syndromes and the role for serial testing. *Am Heart J* 2008; 155(2): 208–14.
11. Jaffe AS. Use of Biomarkers in the Emergency Department and Chest Pain Unit. *Cardiol Clin* 2005; 23(4): 453–465.
12. Gupta, S. de Lemos JA. Use and Misuse of Cardiac Troponins in Clinical Practice. *Prog Cardiovasc Dis* 2007: 50 (2): 151–165.
13. McFadden EP, Stabile E, Regar E, Cheneau E, Ong AT, Kinnaird T, et al. Late thrombosis in drug-eluting coronary stents after discontinuation of antiplatelet therapy. *Lancet* 2004; 364: 1519–1521.
14. Waters RE, Kandzari DE, Phillips HR, Crawford LE, Sketch MH Jr. Thrombosis following treatment of in-stent restenosis with drug-eluting stents after discontinuation of antiplatelet therapy. *Catheter Cardiovasc Interv* 2005; 65: 520–524
15. Thomas JJ , Taylor LL, Camp T, Ghaemmaghami CA. Delta measurements, using an ultrasensitive troponin I assay, reliably diagnose acute coronary syndromes and predict adverse cardiac events within 30 days of ED visits. (abrst) *Annals Emerg Med.* 2007; 50(3): S29.
16. Anderson JL. Adams CD. Antman EM. Bridges CR, et al. ACC/AHA 2007 guidelines for the management of patients with unstable angina/non-ST-elevation myocardial infarction. *Circulation* 2007; 116(7): e148–304.
17. Naples R, Ghaemmaghami CA. Emergency Department Patients Scheduled for outpatient stress testing have a very good compliance rate. (abstr) *Acad EmergMed.* 2008; 15 (s1): S77.

Chapter 15
Examples of Patient Discharge Instructions, ACS Rule Out Protocols, and Order Sheets

Kay S. Holmes

Abstract The Society of Chest Pain Centers (Society) is a non-profit international society that bridges cardiology, emergency medicine, emergency medical services and other professions focused upon improving care for patients with acute coronary syndromes (ACS) and acute heart failure. The Society promotes protocol-based medicine, often delivered through a Chest Pain Center model, to address the diagnosis and treatment of ACS and acute heart failure, and to promote the adoption of process improvement science by healthcare providers. (Visit www.scpcp.org for more information.)

The Chest Pain Center is promoted by the Society as an Operational Model for ACS care. Within this model, facilities can plan and organize the delivery of care in a systematic manner conducive to a process improvement and patient safety approach.

Chest Pain Center Accreditation was developed using the principles of improvement science that are widely known and used successfully in many areas of endeavor. To improve patient outcomes, the upstream care processes need to be improved. All patient care is a process and can be enhanced.

The Society's approach to Accreditation is radically different from other certification processes that set specifications and then measure compliance. In contrast to more traditional certification models, our Accreditation Review Specialists are collaborative and provide feedback, education and resources to assist the facility in addressing gaps and improving processes.

K.S. Holmes (✉)
Society of Chest Pain Centers, 770 Jasonway Ave, Ste 1B, Columbus OH 43017, USA
e-mail: kholmes@scpcp.org

W.F. Peacock, C.P. Cannon (eds.), *Short Stay Management of Chest Pain*,
DOI 10.1007/978-1-60327-948-2_15,
© Humana Press, a part of Springer Science+Business Media, LLC 2009

ACS Flowchart

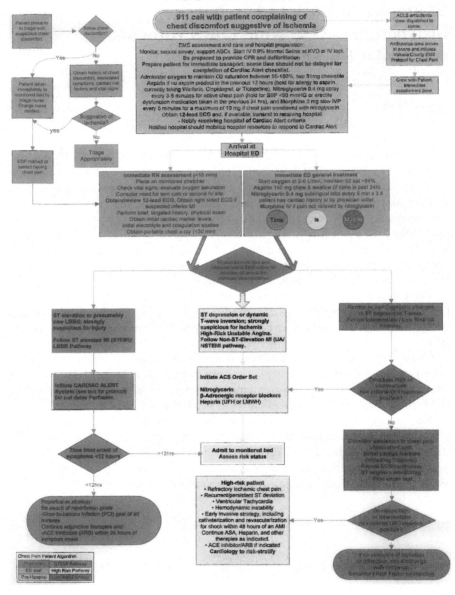

ACS Flowchart

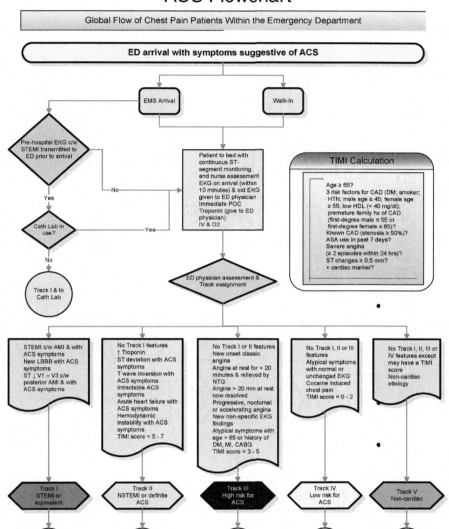

Global Flow of Chest Pain Patients Within the Emergency Department

ED arrival with symptoms suggestive of ACS

EMS Arrival

Walk-In

Pre-hospital EKG c/w STEMI transmitted to ED prior to arrival

Yes

No

Cath Lab in use?

Yes

No

Track I & to Cath Lab

Patient to bed with continuous ST-segment monitoring and nurse assessment EKG on arrival (within 10 minutes) & old EKG given to ED physician Immediate POC Troponin (give to ED physician) IV & O2

TIMI Calculation

Age ≥ 65?
3 risk factors for CAD (DM; smoker; HTN; male age ≥ 45; female age ≥ 55; low HDL (< 40 mg/dl); premature family hx of CAD (first-degree male ≤ 55 or first-degree female ≤ 65)?
Known CAD (stenosis ≥ 50%)?
ASA use in past 7 days?
Severe angina (≥ 2 episodes within 24 hrs)?
ST changes ≥ 0.5 mm?
+ cardiac marker?

ED physician assessment & Track assignment

STEMI c/w AMI & with ACS symptoms
New LBBB with ACS symptoms
ST ↓ V1 – V3 c/w posterior AMI & with ACS symptoms

No Track I features
↑ Troponin
ST deviation with ACS symptoms
T wave inversion with ACS symptoms
Intractable ACS symptoms
Acute heart failure with ACS symptoms
Hemodynamic instability with ACS symptoms
TIMI score = 5 - 7

No Track I or II features
New onset classic angina
Angina at rest for < 20 minutes & relieved by NTG
Angina > 20 min at rest now resolved
Progressive, nocturnal or accelerating angina
New non-specific EKG findings
Atypical symptoms with age > 65 or history of DM, MI, CABG
TIMI score = 3 - 5

No Track I, II or III features
Atypical symptoms with normal or unchanged EKG
Cocaine induced chest pain
TIMI score = 0 - 2

No Track I, II, III or IV features except may have a TIMI score
Non-cardiac etiology

Track I
STEMI or equivalent

Track II
NSTEMI or definite ACS

Track III
High risk for ACS

Track IV
Low risk for ACS

Track V
Non-cardiac

Cath Lab

ICU or Tele

CDU or Tele

CDU or Tele

Home or Admit

Chest Pain Flowchart
Low Risk ACS

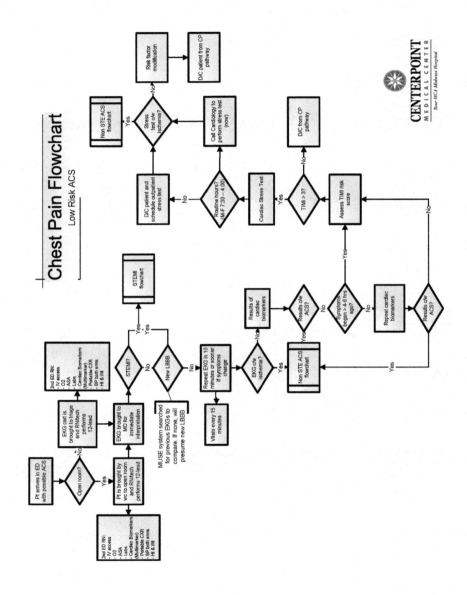

ACS Flowchart

Chest Pain Flowchart
Non ST Elevation ACS

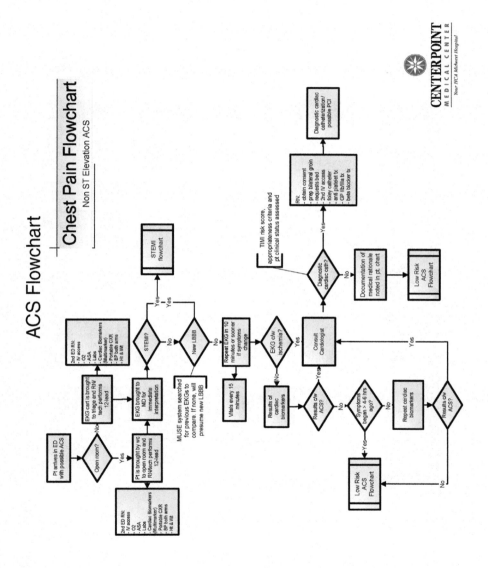

ACS Flowchart

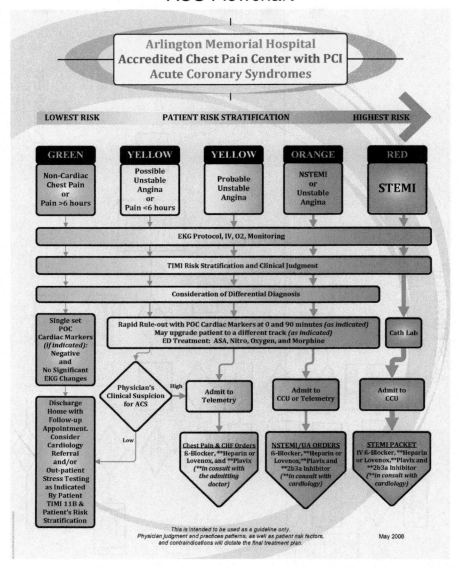

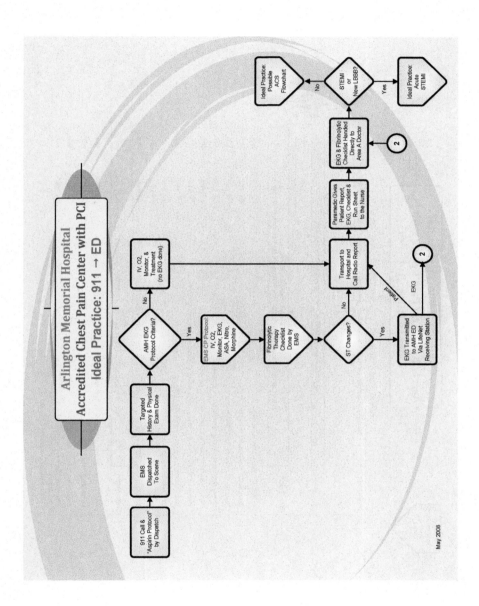

Arlington Memorial Hospital
Accredited Chest Pain Center with PCI
Ideal Practice: 911 → ED

May 2008

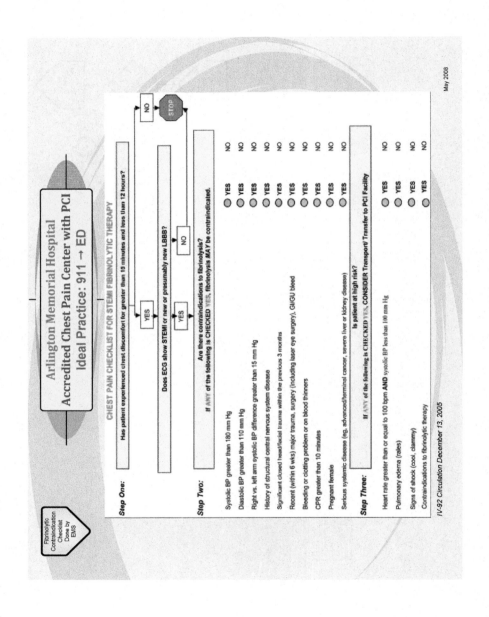

Fibrinolytic Contraindication Checklist Done by EMS

Arlington Memorial Hospital
Accredited Chest Pain Center with PCI
Ideal Practice: 911 → ED

CHEST PAIN CHECKLIST FOR STEMI FIBRINOLYTIC THERAPY

Step One: Has patient experienced chest discomfort for greater than 15 minutes and less than 12 hours?

YES

Does ECG show STEMI or new or presumably new LBBB?

YES   NO

Step Two: Are there contraindications to fibrinolysis?
If ANY of the following is CHECKED YES, fibrinolysis MAY be contraindicated.

	YES	NO
Systolic BP greater than 180 mm Hg	YES	NO
Diastolic BP greater than 110 mm Hg	YES	NO
Right vs. left arm systolic BP difference greater than 15 mm Hg	YES	NO
History of structural central nervous system disease	YES	NO
Significant closed head/facial trauma within the previous 3 months	YES	NO
Recent (within 6 wks) major trauma, surgery (including laser eye surgery), GI/GU bleed	YES	NO
Bleeding or clotting problem or on blood thinners	YES	NO
CPR greater than 10 minutes	YES	NO
Pregnant female	YES	NO
Serious systemic disease (eg, advanced/terminal cancer, severe liver or kidney disease)	YES	NO

Step Three: Is patient at high risk?
If ANY of the following is CHECKED YES, CONSIDER Transport/ Transfer to PCI Facility

	YES	NO
Heart rate greater than or equal to 100 bpm AND systolic BP less than 100 mm Hg	YES	NO
Pulmonary edema (rales)	YES	NO
Signs of shock (cool, clammy)	YES	NO
Contraindications to fibrinolytic therapy	YES	NO

NO

STOP

IV-92 Circulation December 13, 2005

May 2008

ACS Flowchart

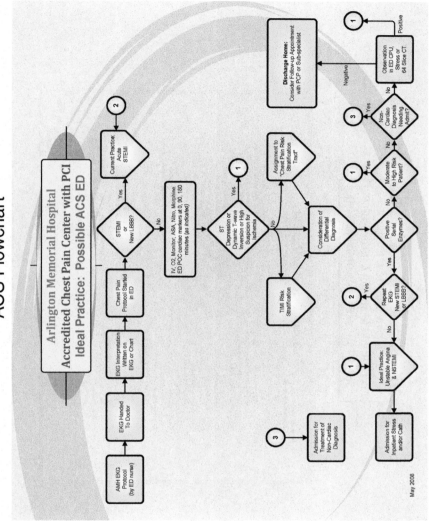

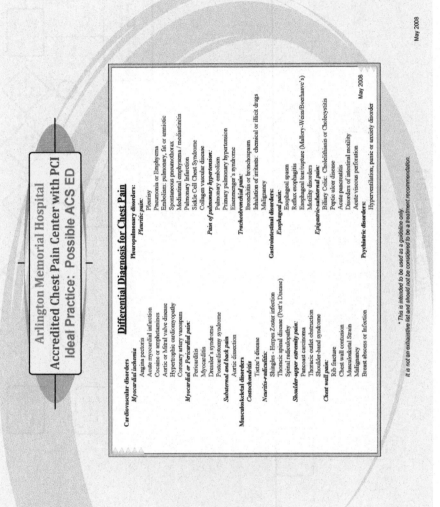

Arlington Memorial Hospital
Accredited Chest Pain Center with PCI
Ideal Practice: Possible ACS ED

Differential Diagnosis for Chest Pain

Cardiovascular disorders

Myocardial ischemia
  Angina pectoris
  Acute myocardial infarction
  Cocaine or amphetamines
  Aortic or Mitral valve disease
  Hypertrophic cardiomyopathy
  Coronary artery vasospasm

Myocardial or Pericardial pain:
  Pericarditis
  Myocarditis
  Dressler's syndrome
  Postcardiotomy syndrome

Substernal and back pain
  Aortic dissection

Musculoskeletal disorders

Costochondritis
  Tietze's disease

Neuritis-radiculitis:
  Shingles - Herpes Zoster infection
  Thoracic spinal disease (Pott's Disease)
  Spinal radiculopathy

Shoulder-upper extremity pain:
  Pancoast carcinoma
  Thoracic outlet obstruction
  Shoulder-hand syndrome

Chest wall pain:
  Rib fracture
  Chest wall contusion
  Musculoskeletal Strain
  Malignancy
  Breast abscess or Infection

Pleuropulmonary disorders:

Pleuritic pain:
  Pleurisy
  Pneumonia or Emphysema
  Embolism: pulmonary, fat or amniotic
  Spontaneous pneumothorax
  Mediastinal emphysema / mediastinitis
  Pulmonary Infarction
  Sickle Cell Chest Syndrome
  Collagen vascular disease

Pain of pulmonary hypertension:
  Pulmonary embolism
  Primary pulmonary hypertension
  Eisenmenger's syndrome

Tracheobronchial pain:
  Bronchitis or bronchospasm
  Inhalation of irritants: chemical or illicit drugs
  Malignancy

Gastrointestinal disorders:

Esophageal pain:
  Esophageal spasm
  Reflux esophagitis
  Esophageal tear/rupture (Mallory-Weiss/Boerhaave's)
  Motility disorders

Epigastric-substernal pain:
  Biliary Colic: Cholelithiasis or Cholecystitis
  Peptic ulcer disease
  Acute pancreatitis
  Disorders of intestinal motility
  Acute viscous perforation

Psychiatric disorders:
  Hyperventilation, panic or anxiety disorder

May 2008

* This is intended to be used as a guideline only
it is not an exhaustive list and should not be considered to be a treatment recommendation.

May 2008

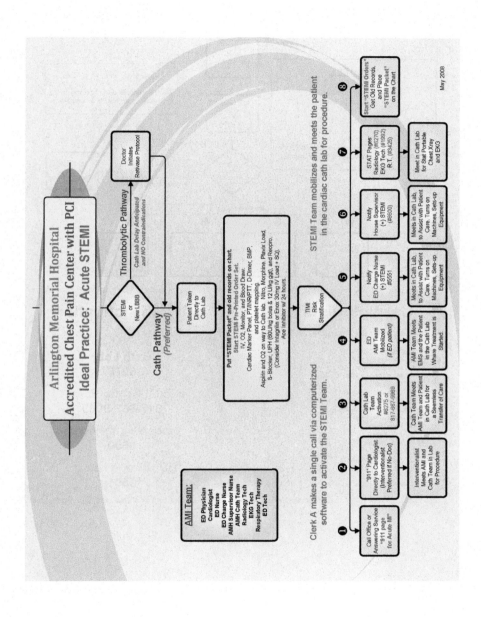

Arlington Memorial Hospital
Accredited Chest Pain Center with PCI
Ideal Practice: Acute STEMI

AMI Team:

ED Physician
Cardiologist
ED Nurse
ED Charge Nurse
AMH Supervisor Nurse
AMH Cath Team
Radiology Tech
EKG Tech
Respiratory Therapy
ED Tech

STEMI or New LBBB

Thrombolytic Pathway

Cath Lab Delay Anticipated and NO Contraindications

Doctor Initiates Retavse Protocol

Cath Pathway *(Preferred)*

Patient Taken Directly to Cath Lab

Put "STEMI Packet" and old records on chart. Start STEMI Pre-Printed Order Set. IV, O2, Monitor, and Blood Draw: Cardiac Marker Panel, PT/INR/PTT, D-Dimer, BMP, and platelet mapping.

Aspirin and O2 on way to Cath lab. Nitro, Morphine, Plavix Load, B-Blocker, UFH (60U/kg bolus & 12 U/kg gtt), and Reopro. (Consider Integrilin or Enox 30mg IV Load + SQ). Ace inhibitor w/ 24 hours.

TIMI Risk Stratification

Clerk A makes a single call via computerized software to activate the STEMI Team.

STEMI Team mobilizes and meets the patient in the cardiac cath lab for procedure.

❶ Call Office or Answering Service "911 page for Acute MI"

❷ "911" Page Directly to Cardiologist (Interventionalist Preferred if No-Doc)

Interventionalist Meets AMI and Cath Team in Lab for Procedure

❸ Cath Lab Team Activation #6275 or 817-867-9869

Cath Team Meets AMI Team and Patient in Cath Lab for a Seamless Transfer of Care

❹ ED AMI Team Mobilized *(if ED patient)*

AMI Team Meets EMS and the Patient in the Cath Lab Where Treatment is Started

❺ Notify ED Charge Nurse (+) STEMI #5551

Meets in Cath Lab, to Assist with Patient Care. Turns on Machines, Sets-up Equipment

❻ Notify House Supervisor (+) STEMI #6600

Meets in Cath Lab, to Assist with Patient Care. Turns on Machines, Sets-up Equipment

❼ STAT Pages Radiology (#5270) EKG Tech (#1982) R.T. (#3425)

Meet in Cath Lab for Stat Portable Chest Xray and EKG

❽ Start "STEMI Orders" Get Old Records, and Place "STEMI Packet" on the Chart

May 2008

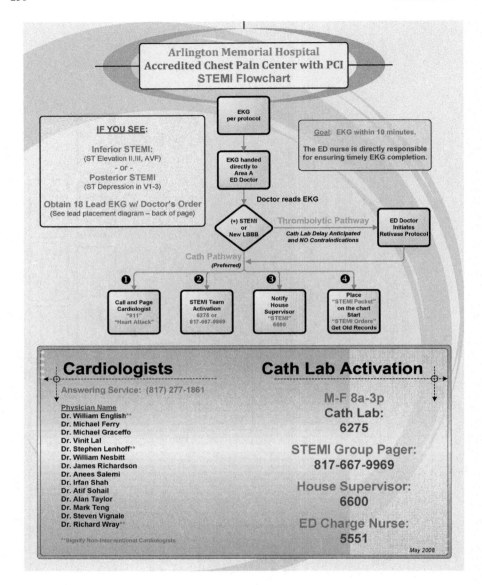

Arlington Memorial Hospital
Accredited Chest Pain Center with PCI
STEMI Flowchart

EKG per protocol

IF YOU SEE:

Inferior STEMI:
(ST Elevation II,III, AVF)
- or -
Posterior STEMI
(ST Depression in V1-3)

Obtain 18 Lead EKG w/ Doctor's Order
(See lead placement diagram – back of page)

EKG handed directly to Area A ED Doctor

Goal: EKG within 10 minutes.

The ED nurse is directly responsible for ensuring timely EKG completion.

Doctor reads EKG

(+) STEMI or New LBBB

Thrombolytic Pathway

Cath Lab Delay Anticipated and NO Contraindications

ED Doctor Initiates Retivase Protocol

Cath Pathway
(Preferred)

❶ Call and Page Cardiologist "911" "Heart Attack"

❷ STEMI Team Activation 6275 or 817-667-9969

❸ Notify House Supervisor "STEMI" 6600

❹ Place "STEMI Packet" on the chart Start "STEMI Orders" Get Old Records

Cardiologists

Answering Service: (817) 277-1861

Physician Name
Dr. William English**
Dr. Michael Ferry
Dr. Michael Graceffo
Dr. Vinit Lal
Dr. Stephen Lenhoff**
Dr. William Nesbitt
Dr. James Richardson
Dr. Anees Salemi
Dr. Irfan Shah
Dr. Atif Sohail
Dr. Alan Taylor
Dr. Mark Teng
Dr. Steven Vignale
Dr. Richard Wray**

**Signify Non-Interventional Cardiologists

Cath Lab Activation

M-F 8a-3p
Cath Lab:
6275

STEMI Group Pager:
817-667-9969

House Supervisor:
6600

ED Charge Nurse:
5551

May 2008

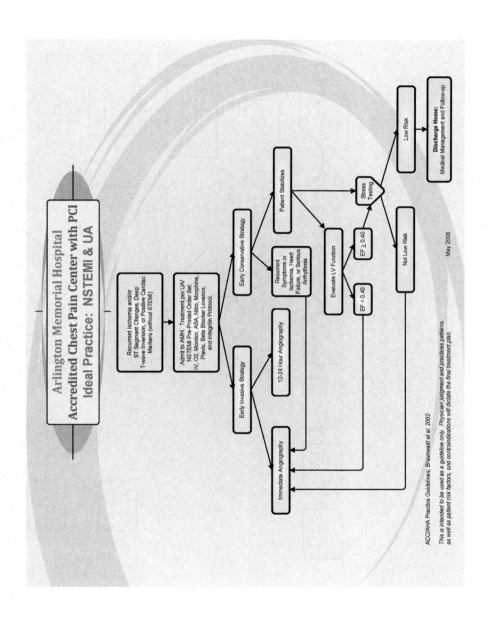

Arlington Memorial Hospital
Accredited Chest Pain Center with PCI
Ideal Practice: NSTEMI & UA

Recurrent Ischemia and/or ST Segment Changes, Deep T-wave Inversion, or Positive Cardiac Markers (without STEMI)

Admit to AMH. Treatment per UA/ NSTEMI Pre-Printed Order Set: IV, O2, Monitor, ASA, Nitro, Morphine, Plavix, Beta Blocker Lovenox, and Integrilin Protocol.

Early Conservative Strategy

Early Invasive Strategy

Recurrent Symptoms or Ischemia, Heart Failure, or Serious Arrhythmia

Patient Stabilizes

12-24 Hour Angiography

Immediate Angiography

Evaluate LV Function

EF < 0.40

EF ≥ 0.40

Stress Testing

Not Low Risk

Low Risk

Discharge Home: Medical Management and Follow-up

ACC/AHA Practice Guidelines; Braunwald et al. 2002

May 2008

This is intended to be used as a guideline only. Physician judgment and practices patterns, as well as patient risk factors, and contraindications will dictate the final treatment plan.

ACS Flowchart

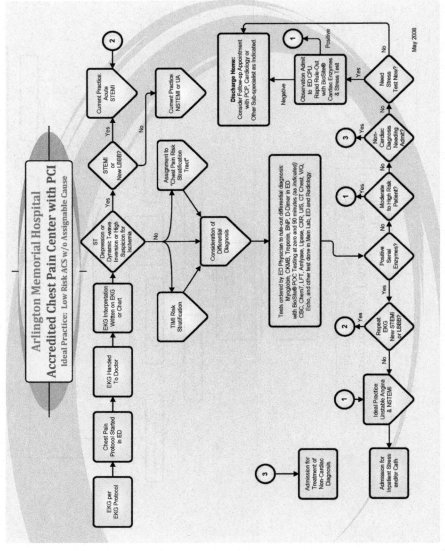

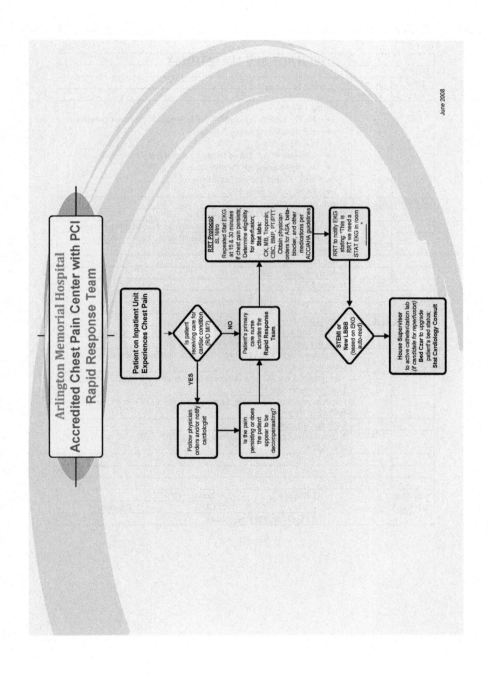

Arlington Memorial Hospital
Accredited Chest Pain Center with PCI
Rapid Response Team

Patient on Inpatient Unit
Experiences Chest Pain

Is patient receiving care for cardiac condition (R/O MI?)

YES

Follow physician orders and/or notify cardiologist

Is the pain persisting or does the patient appear to be decompensating?

NO

Patient's primary care nurse activates the Rapid Response Team

RRT Protocol:
SL Nitro
Repeated Stat EKG at 15 & 30 minutes if chest pain persists;
Determine eligibility for reperfusion;
Stat labs:
CK, MB, Troponin, CBC, BMP, PT/PTT
Obtain physician orders for ASA, beta-blocker, and other medications per ACC/AHA guidelines

RRT to notify EKG stating "This is RRT we need a STAT EKG in room _____"

STEMI or New LBBB (based on EKG auto-read)

House Supervisor to active catheterization lab (if candidate for reperfusion)
Bed Czar to upgrade patient's bed status;
Stat Cardiology Consult

June 2008

ACS Flowchart

Wilson N. Jones Medical Center   **Track III**

\multicolumn{2}{c}{}	HIGH RISK FOR ACS PATHWAY
Date:	
Time All Entries	

Ordered	Done	
		Standing Orders: • EKG, continuous cardiac, ST segment & pulse-ox monitoring • BP monitoring every 5 minutes • Saline lock x 2 • Oxygen @ 2 l/min or to maintain $SaO_2 \geq 92\%$ • Apply radiolucent fast patches • NPO except for medications • Most recent prior EKG
		Diagnostic Testing
		CBC, ERBMP, PT/PTT, portable CXR
		Point of Care Testing: Cardiac Panel (myoglobin, MB, troponin)
		Point of Care Testing: Cardiac Profile (Cardiac Panel + BNP)
		Magnesium
		Urine toxicology screen
		Serum pregnancy test
		Repeat EKG
		Medications
		ASA 81 mg x 4 chewed if not given by EMS or immediately PTA
		NTG 0.4 mg SL q 5 minutes PRN chest pain
		Morphine 3 mg IV q 5 minutes for chest pain not relieved by NTG (max = 3 doses)
		Metoprolol 5 mg IV now & repeat q 5 minutes x 2 (total = 15 mg). Hold for heart rate < 60
		Heparin protocol (Unstable Angina/Late onset DVT & PE version) bolus and drip
		Lovenox 1 mg/kg SC
		Normal saline fluid bolus 250 ml now & PRN SBP < 90 mmHg then 100 ml/hr

Allergies: □ NKDA	Room #	Admit to: Dr.
		□ CDU □ Telemetry
	\multicolumn{2}{l}{Physician/MLP Signature:}	

Track III
Initial Recognition & Management in the Emergency Department
Of Patient At High Risk For ACS

High Risk For ACS

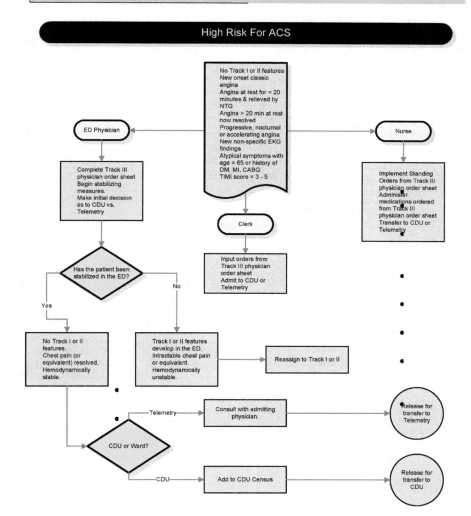

Wilson N. Jones Medical Center   **Track IV**

LOW RISK FOR ACS PATHWAY		
Date:		
Time All Entries		
Ordered	Done	
		Standing Orders: • EKG, continuous cardiac, ST segment & pulse-ox monitoring • BP monitoring every 15 minutes • Saline lock x 2 • Oxygen @ 2 l/min or to maintain $SaO_2 \geq 92\%$ • Apply radiolucent fast patches • NPO except for medications • Most recent prior EKG
▨	▨	Diagnostic Testing
		CBC, ERBMP, PT/PTT, portable CXR
		Point of Care Testing: Cardiac Panel (myoglobin, MB, troponin)
		Point of Care Testing: Cardiac Profile (Cardiac Panel + BNP)
		Magnesium
		Urine toxicology screen
		Serum pregnancy test
		Repeat EKG
▨	▨	Medications
		ASA 81 mg x 4 chewed if not given by EMS or immediately PTA
		NTG 0.4 mg SL q 5 minutes PRN chest pain
		Morphine 3 mg IV q 5 minutes for chest pain not relieved by NTG (max = 3 doses)
		Metoprolol 5 mg IV now & repeat q 5 minutes x 2 (total = 15 mg). Hold for heart rate < 60.
		Normal saline fluid bolus 250 ml now & PRN SBP < 90 mmHg then 100 ml/hr
Allergies: ☐ NKDA	Room #	Admit to: Dr. ☐ CDU ☐ Telemetry
	Physician/MLP Signature:	

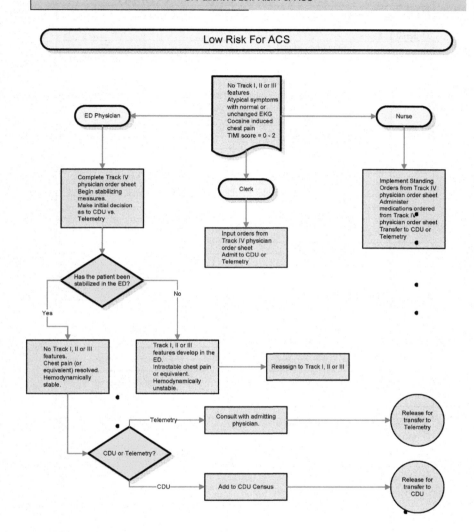

Track IV
Initial Recognition & Management in the Emergency Department
Of Patient At Low Risk For ACS

Low Risk For ACS

No Track I, II or III features
Atypical symptoms with normal or unchanged EKG
Cocaine induced chest pain
TIMI score = 0 - 2

ED Physician

Nurse

Clerk

Complete Track IV physician order sheet
Begin stabilizing measures.
Make initial decision as to CDU vs. Telemetry

Implement Standing Orders from Track IV physician order sheet
Administer medications ordered from Track IV physician order sheet
Transfer to CDU or Telemetry

Input orders from Track IV physician order sheet
Admit to CDU or Telemetry

Has the patient been stabilized in the ED?

No

Yes

No Track I, II or III features.
Chest pain (or equivalent) resolved.
Hemodynamically stable.

Track I, II or III features develop in the ED.
Intractable chest pain or equivalent.
Hemodynamically unstable.

Reassign to Track I, II or III

Telemetry

Consult with admitting physician.

Release for transfer to Telemetry

CDU or Telemetry?

CDU

Add to CDU Census

Release for transfer to CDU

Wilson N. Jones Medical Center   **Track V**

SUSPECTED NON-CARDIAC CHEST PAIN PATHWAY		
Date:		
Time All Entries		
Ordered	Done	
		Standing Orders: • EKG, continuous cardiac, ST segment & pulse-ox monitoring • BP monitoring every 15 minutes • Oxygen @ 2 l/min or to maintain $SaO_2 \geq 92\%$ • Apply radiolucent fast patches • NPO except for medications • Most recent prior EKG
/////	/////	Diagnostic Testing
		CBC, ERBMP
		Liver profile
		CXR *portable* *single view* *two view*
		Point of Care Testing: Cardiac Panel (myoglobin, MB, troponin)
		Point of Care Testing: Cardiac Profile (Cardiac panel + BNP)
		Urine toxicology screen
		Serum pregnancy test
		CT-A chest with IV contrast
		d-dimer
		Repeat EKG
/////	/////	Medications
		ASA 325 mg chewed if not given by EMS or immediately PTA
		NTG 0.4 mg SL q 5 minutes PRN chest pain
		Morphine 3 mg IV q 5 minutes for chest pain not relieved by NTG (max = 3 doses)
		Green slider 60 ml PO x 1
Allergies: ☐ NKDA	Room #	
	Physician/MLP Signature:	

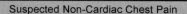

Track V
Initial Recognition & Management in the Emergency Department
With Suspected Non-Cardiac Chest Pain

Suspected Non-Cardiac Chest Pain

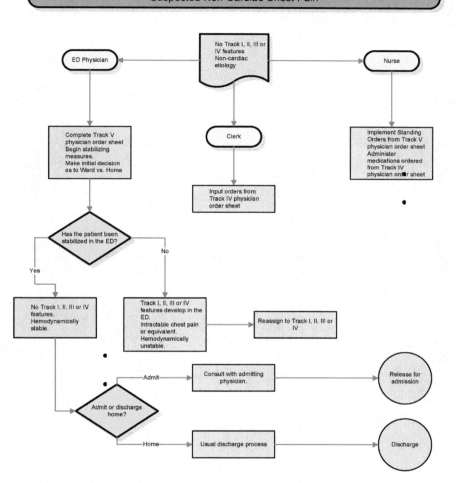

ACS Risk Stratification Tool

Arlington Memorial Hospital
Accredited Chest Pain Center with PCI
Ideal Practice: Possible ACS ED

TIMI 11B RISK SCORE
UNSTABLE ANGINA and NSTEMI

Predictor Variable	Point Value
Age ≥ 65 years	1
≥ 3 risk factors for CAD	1
• Family history of CAD	
• Hypertension	
• Hypercholesterolemia	
• Diabetes	
• Current smoker	
Aspirin use in last 7 days	1
Recent, severe symptoms of angina	1
• ≥ 2 anginal events in last 24 hours	
Elevated cardiac markers	1
ST deviation ≥ 0.5 mm	1
Prior coronary artery stenosis ≥ 50%	1

TIMI Risk Score	Risk of Death, MI, or Urgent Revasc. Within 14 Days	Patient's Risk Status
0 or 1	5%	Low
2	8%	Low
3	13%	Intermediate
4	20%	Intermediate
5	26%	High
6 or 7	41%	High

TABLE 4. TIMI 11B Risk Score for Patients With Unstable Angina and Non–ST-Segment Elevation MI: Predictor Variables. IV-97 Circulation December 13, 2005

May 2008

ACS Order Set

Wilson N. Jones Medical Center
Clinical Decision Unit

TRACK III PATHWAY	
Date:	Transfer to the Clinical Decision Unit
Time:	Primary Dx: Possible Acute Coronary Syndrome
	Secondary Dx:
	Assign To: Dr: and MLP:
	Vital Signs q 4 hrs
	Allergies:
	Activity: Bedrest with bedside commode privileges for BM
	Diet: NPO
	Nursing:

	• Continuous cardiac, ST segment & pulse-ox monitoring
	  • Saline lock x 1 (x 2 if Heparin drip ordered)
	  • Apply radiolucent fast patches
	  • Gather ED physician & nurse templates, ED lab & x-ray results, ED EKGs, most recent prior EKG & old chart
	  • Notify physician or MLP for:
	    ○ T > 101; SBP > 190; SBP < 90; HR > 120; HR < 50; RR > 28; RR < 10; SaO2 < 92%
	    ○ Recurrent chest pain
	    ○ Elevated cardiac enzymes
	  • Guaiac all stools while on heparin or LMWH

	Standing Orders:

	T0: On Arrival to the CDU
	  • EKG #1
	  • Add on lipid profile and magnesium to ED lab
	  • Oxygen @ 2 l/min or to maintain $SaO_2 \geq 92\%$
	  • Aspirin 81 mg x 4 chewed if not given by ED or EMS
	  • Metoprolol Tartrate 5 mg IV x 1 – 3 doses then 25 mg PO if not given in the ED. Follow with 25 mg PO q 6 hours. Hold if HR < 60 or SBP < 100.
	  • NTG paste 2% sliding scale q 4 hrs if not on NTG drip.
	    ○ For SBP < 100: remove nitropaste
	    ○ For SBP 100 – 120: apply 1".
	    ○ For SBP 121 – 140: apply 2".
	    ○ For SBP > 140: apply 3".
	  • ☐ Heparin protocol or ☐ Enoxaparin 1 mg/kg SC
	  • Potassium sliding scale.
	  • Order nutrition & social services consultations

	T4: Four Hours After Arrival to the CDU
	EKG #2
	Point of Care Testing: Cardiac Panel (myoglobin, MB, Troponin)
	Magnesium Sulfate sliding scale. Hold if creatinine > 1.9.
	  o For Mg < 1.2: notify physician or MLP
	  o For Mg < 1.4: give 5 g MgSO4 IV
	  o For Mg < 1.6: give 4 g MgSO4 IV
	  o For Mg < 1.8: give 3 g MgSO4 IV
	  o For Mg < 2.0: give 2 g MgSO4 IV

	T6: Six Hours After Arrival to the CDU Metoprolol Tartrate 25 mg PO. Hold if HR < 60 or SBP < 100.
	T12: Twelve hours After Arrival to the CDU EKG #3 Point of Care Testing: Cardiac Panel (myoglobin, MB, Troponin) Metoprolol Tartrate 25 mg PO. Hold if HR < 60 or SBP < 100. Enoxaparin 1 mg/kg SC if not on Heparin
	T18: Eighteen Hours After Arrival to the CDU Metoprolol Tartrate 25 mg PO. Hold if HR < 60 or SBP < 100. Call physician if he/she has yet to see patient.
	T23: Twenty Three Hours After Arrival to the CDU Discharge or prepare for hospital admission
	PRN Orders
	EKG prn chest pain or ST segment elevation on monitor
	NTG 0.4 mg SL q 5 minutes prn chest pain.
	Morphine 3 mg IV q 5 minutes prn chest pain resistant to NTG. Maximum total dose = 15 mg.
	Serax 10 mg PO q 6 hrs prn for anxiety or restlessness.
	Colace 100 mg PO q 12 hrs prn.
	Tylenol 650 mg PO q 4 hrs prn.
	Physician/MLP Signature:

ACS Order Set

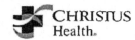 **CHRISTUS**
Health.

Revised 11/05 ,10/07   Patient ID Sticker

Acute Coronary Syndrome

Guideline III Low to Moderate Risk (Non-Diagnostic or Normal EKG)

Order Set

Time of symptom onset _____ Arrival time to the ED _____

Orders and Treatments

- 12 Lead EKG on arrival
- Notify Emergency Department Physician STAT
- Continuous cardiac monitoring and pulse oximetry upon arrival
- O2 at 2-4 Liters per minute nasal cannula or 15 Liters per minute NRB to SaO2 above 96%
- Stat Portable Chest X-ray
- Initiate PIV Saline Lock (20 ga or larger)
- Vital Signs every 15-30 minutes as needed
- Obtain Patients Weight _____ Kg
- Repeat EKG if rhythm changes or in 30 min if pain continues
- Notify physician for increasing Chest pain, arrhythmias, SBP below 90 or greater than 160
- Notify physician if chest pain continues
- Notify physician of positive cardiac enzyme

Physician Orders/ Holding Orders

	Nurse	Initial/Time
• CBC, CMP, CKMP, Troponin		____ / ____
• Repeat CKMB, Troponin every 6 hours x 2		____ / ____
• Fasting lipid profile		____ / ____
____ Myoglobin		____ / ____
____ Aspirin 325mg by mouth stat then Daily (if no aspirin allergy)		____ / ____
____ Nitroglycerin 0.4 mg SL,If currently experiencing chest pain, may repeat every 5min x2		____ / ____

Notify Physician if patient is Currently taking Viagra, Cialis or Levitra Prior to administering NTG

____ Morphine Sulfate 2-4 mg IVP every 5 minutes as needed for chest pain		____ / ____
maximum dose of 10mg per hour (If no morphine allergy)		____ / ____
____ Metoprolol 25 mg by mouth Daily.		____ / ____
(contraindicated for HR below 60 or SBP below 110, history of asthma)		
____ Phenergan Interchange policy IV in 10ml NS slow IV Push every 4 hrs as needed for N/V		____ / ____
____ Heparin Nomogram		____ / ____
____ Lovenox 1 mg per kg (____ mg) subcutaneous now and then every12 hours		____ / ____
____ Echocardiogram ____ STAT _____ Today _____ Routine		____ / ____
____ Repeat CXR in AM		____ / ____
____ Diet _____ Cardiac _____ Cal ADA Diet Other _____		____ / ____
____ See Home Medication Reconciliation Form		____ / ____
____ Stress Test		____ / ____

Cardiology consult – Dr. _____ paged @ _____ , If no response in 15 minutes,
Repaged @ _____

Admit to ___ Telemetry ____ Observation ____ Regular Admit ____ICU

Dr. _____ Transfer to _____ Dr. _____ accepting

Physician Signature: _____

RN Initial/Signature ( ) _____
Care is transferred to the admitting physician at the time the patient leaves the emergency department.
Contact the admitting physician on arrival for additional problems or changes in the patient's condition.

AUTOMATIC STOP ORDERS

ORAL ANTICOAGULANTS	AFTER 24 HOURS
ALBUMIN	AFTER 24 HOURS
LARGE VOLUME INTRAVENOUS	AFTER 24 HOURS
INJECTABLE ANTICOAGULANTS (SC)	AFTER 5 DAYS
CONTROLLED SUBSTANCES	AFTER 5 DAYS
CORTISONE PRODUCTS	AFTER 5 DAYS

Addressograph

MD Date of Order	Hour of Order	Nurse's Signature	

NURSE: PLEASE X IN COLUMN ON LINE, FOR MEDICATIONS REQUIRED FROM PHARMACY
PHYSICIAN MUST ENTER DATE, HOUR, AND SIGN EACH SET OF ORDERS

ALLERGIES:

INITIAL ORDERS FOR **ACUTE CORONARY SYNDROME (Non ST Elevation)**

(Check appropriate boxes and fill in the blanks)

1. Admit Dr. _____ 's Service
   - ☐ Cardiologist _____
   - ☐ Admit to Teaching Service
   - ☐ CCU
   - ☐ Telemetry
2. Diagnosis: ☐ Unstable angina ☐ M.I. (type): _____
   ☐ Other: _____
3. Code Status:
   - ☐ Full Code ☐ DNR ☐ Partial DNR (See DNR Order Sheet)
4. Essential Tests:
   - ☒ 12-lead ECG Reason: _____
   - ☐ Repeat ECG Reason: _____
   - ☐ Right sided ECG if IWMI
   - ☒ Chem screen, Magnesium
   - ☒ PT, PTT, CBC
   - ☒ Troponin Stat then q 8hrs X 2
   - ☒ Cholesterol, HDL, direct LDL and Triglyceride
   - ☐ TSH (if patient is in Atrial Fibrillation)
   - ☐ Portable chest x – ray Reason: _____
   - ☐ UA
5. Activity (check one):
   - ☐ Complete bed rest ☐ Bed rest with bathroom privilege ☐ Up as tolerated
6. Diet:
   - ☐ NPO ☐ 2 Gm Na+ Low Cholesterol ☐ Diabetic
   - ☐ Other _____
7. IV Access:
   - ☐ Saline Lock ☐ Other: _____ @ _____ cc/h
8. Vital Signs every: _____
9. Medications (include name, dose, frequency and route of administration):
   Weight: _____ lbs. or _____ kg.
   - ☐ O₂ (check one): ☐ Nasal cannula @ _____ Liters per minute
   - ☐ _____ FiO₂ by mask
   - ☐ Baby ASA 81 mg X 2 chewable tablets X 1 dose: ☐ Given in the field
     (If not administered, give reason: _____)

ETD Attending Signature: _____

Attending Physician Signature: _____

These orders are good for 8 hours only unless countersigned by the Primary Care Physician

PLEASE DO NOT RETURN CHARTS WITH NEW ORDERS TO RACK-FLAG CHART
HACKENSACK UNIVERSITY MEDICAL CENTER
PHYSICIANS ORDERS AND TREATMENTS

Page 1 of 3

AUTOMATIC STOP ORDERS

ORAL ANTICOAGULANTS	AFTER 24 HOURS
ALBUMIN	AFTER 24 HOURS
LARGE VOLUME INTRAVENOUS	AFTER 24 HOURS
INJECTABLE ANTICOAGULANTS (SC)	AFTER 5 DAYS
CONTROLLED SUBSTANCES	AFTER 5 DAYS
CORTISONE PRODUCTS	AFTER 5 DAYS

Addressograph

MD Date of Order	Hour of Order	Nurse's Signature	NURSE: PLEASE X IN COLUMN ON LINE, FOR MEDICATIONS REQUIRED FROM PHARMACY PHYSICIAN MUST ENTER DATE, HOUR, AND SIGN EACH SET OF ORDERS

ALLERGIES:

INITIAL ORDERS FOR **ACUTE CORONARY SYNDROME (Non ST Elevation)**

(Check appropriate boxes and fill in the blanks)

9. Medications (continued):

☐ Clopidogrel (Plavix) 300 mg PO X 1 dose

☐ Metoprolol (Lopressor) 5 mg IV X 1 dose given by MD

☐ Additional Metoprolol (Lopressor) 5 mg IV X 1 dose 5 minutes after the previous dose given by MD

☐ Additional Metoprolol (Lopressor) 5 mg IV X 1 dose 5 minutes after the previous dose given by MD

Heparins / Low Molecular Weight Heparin (check one):

☐ **Cardiology** Heparin Weight-Based Nomogram (use Nomogram order)

☐ Heparin Bolus _____ units IV, then Heparin Drip of 25,000 units/250cc of D_5W start at _____ units/hr

☐ Enoxaparin (Lovenox) (1 mg /kg sc q 12 hrs.) _____ (not recommended if creatinine > 2.5 mg / dl)

☐ Nitroglycerin ointment _____

☐ Nitroglycerin drip 50 mg/250cc of D_5W start at _____ mcg/min (titrate to Chest pain free, maintain SBP> _____)

☐ Eptifibatide (Integrilin) – see HUMC dosing chart

   ☐ IV push 180 mcg/kg over 5 seconds = _____ mL X 1 dose

   ☐ IV infusion 75 mg/100 mL premix (check one):

      ☐ Creatinine < 2 mg/dL: 2 mcg/kg/min = _____ mL/h X _____ hrs

      ☐ Creatinine 2 – 4 mg/dL: 1 mcg/kg/min= _____ mL/h X _____ hrs

      ☐ Creatinine > 4 mg/dL: Not recommended (consider Abciximab)

☐ Abciximab (Reopro) – see HUMC dosing chart

   ☐ IV push 0.25 mg/kg over 5 seconds = _____ mL X 1 dose

   ☐ IV infusion 3.7mL/250mL D_5W (7.4 mg/250mL D_5W) at 0.125 mcg/kg/min = _____ mL/h (maximum 20mL/h) X _____ hrs

☐ ACE Inhibitor: _____

☐ ASA _____

☐ Beta-Blocker: _____

☐ Clopidogrel (Plavix) 75 mg PO daily

☐ Famotidine (Pepcid) 20 mg PO bid

☐ Statin _____

ETD Attending Signature: _____

Attending Physician Signature: _____

These orders are good for 8 hours only unless countersigned by the Primary Care Physician.

PLEASE DO NOT RETURN CHARTS WITH NEW ORDERS TO RACK-FLAG CHART
HACKENSACK UNIVERSITY MEDICAL CENTER
PHYSICIANS ORDERS AND TREATMENTS

Page 2 of 3

Acute Coronary Syndrome Orders   Medical Record   HUMC INV # 5010225 Rev. 9/30/05

AUTOMATIC STOP ORDERS

ORAL ANTICOAGULANTS	AFTER 24 HOURS
ALBUMIN	AFTER 24 HOURS
LARGE VOLUME INTRAVENOUS	AFTER 24 HOURS
INJECTABLE ANTICOAGULANTS (SC)	AFTER 5 DAYS
CONTROLLED SUBSTANCES	AFTER 5 DAYS
CORTISONE PRODUCTS	AFTER 5 DAYS

Addressograph

MD Date of Order	Hour of Order	Nurse's Signature	
			NURSE: PLEASE X IN COLUMN ON LINE, FOR MEDICATIONS REQUIRED FROM PHARMACY PHYSICIAN MUST ENTER DATE, HOUR, AND SIGN EACH SET OF ORDERS

ALLERGIES:

INITIAL ORDERS FOR **ACUTE CORONARY SYNDROME (Non ST Elevation)**
(Check appropriate boxes and fill in the blanks)

9.   Other Medications (continued)
☐ _____
☐ _____
☐ _____
☐ _____
☐ _____
☐ _____
☐ _____
☐ _____

10.   If patient develops chest pain:
☐ Call Admitting Physician STAT
☐ Nitroglycerin 1/150 SL q 5 minutes X 3 prn if SBP >100 mmHg
☐ Stat ECG

11. ☒ Patient to be seen by Cardiac Rehab Team, EXT # 3792

12. ☒ Assess patient for Smoking Cessation Education prior to discharge

13.   Other Orders:

ETD Attending Signature: _____

Attending Physician Signature: _____

These orders are good for 8 hours only unless countersigned by the Primary Care Physician.

PLEASE DO NOT RETURN CHARTS WITH NEW ORDERS TO RACK-FLAG CHART
HACKENSACK UNIVERSITY MEDICAL CENTER
PHYSICIANS ORDERS AND TREATMENTS

Page 3 of 3

ACS Order Set

STAT
Place X in box if STAT Medication Order.
(If STAT box is marked, a new order
sheet is required for future orders).

Generic substitution and therapeutic interchange are authorized unless prohibited by the prescriber according to hospital policy

PATIENT STATUS: ☒ Place in Observation Bed

CLINICAL DECISION UNIT CHEST PAIN EXCLUSION CRITERIA
(Check all that apply – if any checked patient EXCLUDED from Clinical Decision Unit)

UNSTABLE Vital Signs
- ☐ Temperature greater than 36 C or 100.5 F
- ☐ Heart Rate less than 50 or greater than 130
- ☐ Systolic Blood Pressure less than 90 or greater than 190
- ☐ Respiratory Rate less than 10 or greater than 30
- ☐ O_2 Saturation less than 88%
- ☐ Unstable Airway

☐ **Prolonged, ongoing or recurrent chest pain**
☐ **Pulmonary edema**

Dysrythmias or evidence of Cardiac Ischemia
- ☐ Ventricular Tachycardia
- ☐ 2nd or 3rd Degree Heart Block
- ☐ New ST elevation consistent with acute infarction
- ☐ New BBB
- ☐ New or dynamic ST depression in several leads
- ☐ Rapid Atrial Fibrillation

☐ **NTG drip**
☐ **Active DNR**
☐ **Dementia or altered mental status**
☐ **Previous MI or revascularization procedure (exceptions at the discretion of the Cardiologist)**

CLINICAL DECISION UNIT CHEST PAIN INCLUSION CRITERIA
(Check all that apply)

☐ Chest Pain that is possibly angina in origin, but is relieved with rest, oxygen or SL NTG
☐ Must be an Emergency Department Patient assessed by the Emergency Department Physician

DO NOT WRITE IN THIS SECTION

OR THE MARGINS OF THIS PAGE

☒ **SEE PAGE 2 FOR ADDITIONAL ORDERS**

DATE: _____ TIME: _____ PHYSICIAN: _____ **M.D.**

Forsyth MEDICAL CENTER
Remarkable People. Remarkable Medicine.

FMEMD0005C

CLINICAL DECISION UNIT CHEST PAIN ORDERS
Page 1 of 3

R: 03/04/2008

Name/MR#/Label

☐ **STAT**
Place X in box if STAT Medication Order.
(If STAT box is marked, a new order
sheet is required for future orders).

Generic substitution and therapeutic interchange are authorized unless prohibited by the prescriber according to hospital policy

PATIENT STATUS: ☒ Place in Observation Bed

BED TYPE: ☒ CDU   Time:_____

ED Physician:_____

EMERGENCY DEPARTMENT PHYSICIAN CONSULTED WITH CARDIOLOGIST: ☐ Yes   ☐ No

Time:_____

Physician:_____

☒ **TELEMETRY MONITOR**
DIAGNOSIS:_____

CODE STATUS:_____   CONDITION:_____

LABS: If not done in the Emergency Department
☒ Cardiac Enzymes:
    ☒ CKMB every 3 hours X 3 (presentation to the ED then 3 hours then 6 hours) | If initial enzymes or second set of
    ☒ Troponin every 3 hours x 3 (presentation to the ED then 3 hours then 6 hours) | enzymes normal, Cardiologist
☒ Cardiac Platelets | may elect to order a treadmill and
☒ CBC with differential | discharge patient if normal
☒ CMP
☒ Fasting Lipid Panel
☒ Magnesium

CARDIOPULMONARY SERVICES:
☒ EKG every 3 hours X 3 (presentation to the ED then 3 hours then 6 hours)   **REASON: CHEST PAIN**

CARDIAC NON-INVASIVE:
☐ Dobutamine Stress Echocardiogram after confirmation with cardiology: **REASON: CHEST PAIN**   Cardiologist:_____
☐ Stress Echocardiogram after confirmation with cardiology: **REASON: CHEST PAIN**   Cardiologist:_____
☐ Other:_____   **REASON:**_____   Cardiologist:_____

FOOD AND NUTRITION:
☒ 2 gm Sodium Cardiac Prudent Diet
☒ Keep NPO – 2 hours prior to treadmill

NURSING CARE AND TREATMENTS:
☒ Vital Signs per CDU protocol
☒ Activity: Bed rest – up to bathroom as tolerated with assistance
☒ Provide education regarding Cardiac Risk Factors and Emergency Access for cardiac events

DO NOT WRITE IN THIS SECTION OR IN THE MARGINS OF THIS PAGE

☒ **SEE NEXT PAGE FOR IV AND MEDICATION ORDERS**
DATE:_____   TIME:_____   PHYSICIAN:_____   **M.D.**

Forsyth) MEDICAL CENTER
Remarkable People. Remarkable Medicine   **FMEMD0005C**

CLINICAL DECISION UNIT CHEST PAIN ORDERS
Page 2 of 3
R: 03/04/2008

Name/MR#/Label

STATEMENT STAT
Place X in box if STAT Medication Order.
(If STAT box is marked, a new order
sheet is required for future orders).

Generic substitution and therapeutic interchange are authorized unless prohibited by the prescriber according to hospital policy

IV'S AND MEDICATIONS:

☒ Insert Saline lock for IV Access **(complete Heplock NS Flush Order Set and transmit to Pharmacy)**
☒ Aspirin 325 mg PO x 1 dose STAT (if not given in ED)
☒ Aspirin 300 mg PR **if unable to tolerate PO** x 1 dose STAT (if not given in ED)
   Do not give Aspirin because: ☐ Allergy   ☐ Active Bleed   (deleted   " ☐ given in ED")

WITH THE ONSET OF CHEST PAIN:

☒ Nitroglycerin 0.4 mg sublingual every 5 minutes X 3 doses (After the third dose consider Morphine)
☒ O$_2$ at 3L/min via nasal cannula

☒ **Notify Emergency Department Physician**
☐ Beta Blocker _____

   (Beta blocker is required within 24 hours of arrival time for the AMI patient unless contraindicated)

☐ Beta Blocker contraindicated due to **(REASON)**:
   ☐ Allergy
   ☐ Hypotension
   ☐ Bradycardia with heart rate of _____ prior to administration
   ☐ Heart Failure
   ☐ Shock
   ☐ Bronchospasm/Asthma/COPD

PRN'S:

☒ Morphine 2mg IV every five minutes as needed for chest pain (maximum dose = 20mg in four hours)
☒ Propoxyphene-N 100 mg/ Acetaminophen 650 mg (Darvocet-N 100) one tablet PO every 4 hours as needed for pain,
   may repeat x 1 tablet in 30 minutes (Maximum dose = 6 tablets / 24 hours)
☒ Ondansetron (Zofran) 4 mg IV every 6 hours PRN nausea / vomiting
☒ Metoclopramide (Reglan) 10 mg IV every 6 hours as needed for nausea
☒ Acetaminophen (Tylenol) 650 mg PO every 4 hours as needed for pain / fever
☒ Mag/Al/Simethicone (Double strength Mylanta) 15 mL PO every 2 hours as needed for indigestion
☒ Milk of Magnesia 30 ml PO Daily as needed for constipation
☒ Alprazolam (Xanax) 0.25 mg PO every 6 hours as needed for anxiety
☒ Zolpidem (Ambien) 5 mg PO At bedtime. May repeat dose x 1 tablet

DO NOT WRITE IN THIS SECTION

OR IN THE MARGINS OF THIS PAGE

☐ SEE PHYSICIAN ORDER SHEET FOR ADDITIONAL ORDERS
DATE: _____ TIME: _____ PHYSICIAN: _____   M.D.

Forsyth) MEDICAL CENTER
Remarkable People. Remarkable Medicine.   **FMEMD0005C**

   CLINICAL DECISION UNIT CHEST PAIN ORDERS
              Page 3 of 3
R: 03/04/2008

                                                    Name/MR#/Label

ACS Clinical Pathway

A Pathway ( ) not represent the standard of care. Clinical judgment may supersede these g( )es.

Beaumont®
William Beaumont Hospital

CLINICAL PATHWAY - ACUTE CORONARY SYNDROME /MYCARDIAL INFARCTION

PATIENT PROBLEMS	ADMISSION DAY	HOSPITALIZATION PHASE	DISCHARGE OUTCOMES
Alteration in tissue perfusion R/T decreased coronary artery perfusion	Patient is free of S/Sx of decreased tissue perfusion; no angina, or ECG changes	With increased activity, med adjustments: patient remains free of angina.	With med adjustments, increased activity: patient remains free of angina.
Potential for pain R/T coronary artery ischemia	Patient able to identify angina and evaluate it on a 1-10 scale, or non-verbal indicators.	Patient is pain free as evidenced by verbal and non-verbal indicators.	Patient is pain free as evidenced by verbal and non-verbal indicators.
Potential alteration in rhythm disturbance.	Patient is free of symptomatic arrhythmia.	Patient is free of symptomatic arrhythmia.	Patient is free of symptomatic arrhythmia.
Knowledge deficit R/T disease process	Patient/S.O. verbalizes understanding of hospital regime.	Patient/S.O. verbalizes understanding of CAD, risk factors, tests/procedures and meds.	Patient/S.O. verbalizes understanding of discharge instructions.
Alteration in vascular integrity R/T invasive procedure		No bleeding, bruit, bruit, hematoma. Peripheral pulses at baseline.	Dressing remains dry with no oozing from the cath site on ambulation.
Alteration in mobility R/T procedure		Bedrest maintained per orders and patient progresses per activity orders.	Activity at pre-admission level.

	HOSPITALIZATION PHASE			
TESTS	-CK-MB Q 8hrs x 3	-Stress test (if CK-MB negative)	**Treatment Options**	-Repeat abnormal labs
	-Troponin Q 8 hrs x 3	-DM : IIT / FBS & 4PM		
	-12 Lead EKG x 3 days	-Lipid Panel, fasting within 24 hrs	1. Stress Testing	
	-CBC with platelets Q AM x 3	-Heparin aPTT Q 8 (if on IV Heparin)		
	-Consider Echo	-CXR if not done in EC & PRN	2. Cath Lab testing/procedure	
	-Basic Metabolic Panel			
CONSULTS	-Cardiology	-Continuing Care	3. Medical Treatment	-Evaluate need for home care - Follow up care
	-Cardiac Rehab			-VS per unit routine
	-Endocrinologist		4. CVS consult (if indicated)	-Weight
	-Primary Care Physician			-HTN Control
TREATMENTS	-I & O	-Smoking Cessation		-Diabetes Control
	-O2 per resp	-Teaching documented		-Dietary Counseling
	-VS Q 2-4° & PRN	-Medication teaching		-Smoking Cessation
	-Cardiac Monitor	-Risk factor teaching		
	-Weight	-Diet teaching		-Cardiac Rehab
	-Bleeding Precautions			
	-Diet: Low Fat, Low Chol, 2-4 gm Na			-IVL discontinued prior to discharge
MEDICATIONS	-IV	-IV to IVL (Day 3)		Discharge Medications Include:
	-Heparin IV	-Nitroglycerin: IV / PO / ointment		-ASA / Clopidogrel
	-ASA (soluble) / Clopidogrel	(DC IV / ointment at least		-Beta blocker
	-Enoxaparin (Lovenox)- no cath planned	2 hours before stress test)		-ACE Inhibitor / ARB if EF < 40%
	-Eptifibatide (Integrelin)- for high risk patients only			-Lipid management
	-Beta Blocker (within 24 hrs) if not contraindicated			-NTG SL or Spray
	-Lipid management			
	-ACE Inhibitor / ARB if EF<40%	-Stool softener		
ACTIVITY	-Patient progresses to a new activity as tolerated			

7354 JAN 08 R

White Copy: Physician • Yellow Copy: Patient • Pink Copy: Hospital Records • Blue Copy: Primary Care Physician

Unstable Angina
Non-ST-Segment Elevation MI (NSTEMI)
CARDIAC DISCHARGE CHECKLIST

Patient name: _____

Discharge Date: _____

Designated cardiologist: _____

BRIEF HISTORY: *Check duration of medication for each agent*

Discharge Medications	Y ☑	N ☑	30d	6 mos	9mos	Indef.	Comments	Initials
Aspirin (____mg/d po) *please fill in ASA dose* + Clopidogrel (75 mg/d po)	❏	❏						
Aspirin alone (____mg/d po) *please fill in dose*	❏	❏						
Clopidogrel alone (75 mg/d po)	❏	❏						
Nitrates	❏	❏						
β-blocker	❏	❏						
ACE inhibitor/ARB	❏	❏						
Calcium channel blocker	❏	❏						
Warfarin (Specify INR in comments)	❏	❏						
Lipid-lowering agent(s)	❏	❏						

Interventions and counseling	Y ☑	N ☑	Initials	Date	Comments
Risk stratification at discharge	❏	❏			
Disease and treatment education	❏	❏			
Risk-factor modification counseling (general)	❏	❏			
Blood pressure controlled	❏	❏			
Diabetes controlled	❏	❏			
Smoking cessation recommended	❏	❏			
Dietitian/nutritionist interview	❏	❏			
Cardiac rehabilitation interview and enrollment	❏	❏			
Physical activity counseling	❏	❏			

Scheduled follow-ups	Y ☑	N ☑	Initials	Date	Comments
Cardiologist follow-up	❏	❏			Date:
Primary care follow-up	❏	❏			Date:
Cardiac rehabilitation	❏	❏			Begins:
Stress test follow-up	❏	❏			Date:
Lipid profile follow-up	❏	❏			Date:
Anticoagulation service follow-up	❏	❏			Date:
Clinical summary and patient education record faxed to appropriate physicians	❏	❏			

ACTION Registry™

NSTEMI and STEMI DISCHARGE FORM
PATIENTS SHOULD GIVE A COPY OF THIS FORM TO THEIR DOCTOR AT THEIR NEXT VISIT

Aspirin	❑ Yes – _____ mg per day ❑ No – Why? _____	*Aspirin* helps prevent blood components (platelets) from sticking together to help prevent future heart attacks and strokes.
Clopidogrel	❑ Yes – 75 mg per day If Yes, duration of therapy _____ months ❑ No – Why? _____	*Clopidogrel* helps prevent platelets from sticking together. Used together with aspirin inpatients with and without stents to prevent future heart attacks. Also, should be used in patients who cannot tolerate aspirin.
Angiotensin-converting enzyme inhibitor (ACE-I) or Angiotensin receptor blocker (ARB)	❑ Yes – Drug prescribed _____ mg per day ❑ No – Why? _____ Your left ventricular ejection fraction (LVEF) is _____ %. *This is a measure of how well your heart is pumping. The normal LVEF > 55%. If your LVEF < 40%, an ACE-I/ARB is indicated.*	*ACE-I/ARBs* lower blood pressure, prevent complications of diabetes, and treat congestive heart failure.
Beta blocker	❑ Yes – Drug prescribed _____ mg _____ times per day ❑ No – Why? _____	*Beta blockers* slow heart rate, lower blood pressure, and prevent abnormal heartbeats (arrhythmias).
Aldosterone receptor blocker	❑ Yes – Drug prescribed _____ mg per day ❑ No – Why? _____ *Indicated if your LVEF<40%, your creatinine is less than 2.5 mg/dL, your potassium level is less than 5.0meq/L, and you are having symptoms of heart failure or have diabetes.*	*Aldosterone receptor blockers* help to lower blood pressure and treat congestive heart failure when used in conjunction with ACE-I/ARB in patients with heart failure symptoms or diabetes.
Nitroglycerin	1. For chest pain lasting 2 to 3 minutes, place one nitroglycerin tablet under your tongue. 2. If the 1st dose does not provide relief within 5 minutes, repeat the dose at 5 minute intervals, up to a total of 3 doses. 3. If pain is still not relieved after 1st dose, call 911 or go to the nearest emergency room, preferably by ambulance.	*Nitroglycerin* is used as needed for chest pain. Carry it with you at all times.

Lipid management	I have been prescribed the following drug: Drug: _____ mg daily My lipid profile this hospitalization: Total cholesterol: _____ mg/dL Low-density cholesterol (LDL) _____ mg/dL High-density cholesterol (HDL) _____ mg/dL Triglycerides: _____ mg/dL	Regardless of your LDL level, you should be started on a statin to prevent future heart attacks.
Smoking Cessation	❏ Not applicable ❏ I currently smoke and have been counseled to stop. I will stop smoking by _____/_____/_____. ❏ I have been prescribed the following medications to help me stop: Drug: _____. ❏ I have been referred to a smoking cessation program: Program name: _____ Program number: _____	
Diabetes management	❏ Not applicable My hemoglobin A1c is: _____ % My fasting blood sugar during this hospitalization was: _____ mg/dL	The *hemoglobin A1c* is a measure of blood sugar control over the past 3 months. If your hemoglobin A1c is greater than 7.0% or your *fasting glucose* was greater than 110mg/dL, you should be started on diabetic medications.
Nutrition, weight, and blood pressure management	❏ I have been counseled about modifying my diet. My current weight is _____ lb. My target weight is _____ lb. My Body Mass Index (BMI) is _____ My current blood pressure is _____/_____ mmHg. I may contact _____ in Nutrition Services at phone number _____.	Your goal Body Mass Index should be < 25. Your goal blood pressure should be 140/90 mmHg or less (or less than 130/80 mmHg for patients with diabetes mellitus or chronic kidney disease).
Exercise program	❏ I have received exercise instructions for the next 4 to 6 weeks, before I start cardiac rehabilitation. ❏ I have received a referral to an outpatient cardiac rehabilitation program: Name of program: _____ Phone: _____	Exercise improves stamina and quality of life, strengthens the heart and other muscles, and improves blood circulation. It can also be beneficial for weight loss.

```
┌─────────────────────────────┐
│                             │
│    Your hospital            │
│    logo/address             │
│                             │
└─────────────────────────────┘
```

Dear Dr. _____:

Your patient, _____, has been discharged on (date) _____
following treatment for _____ days with a diagnosis of acute coronary syndrome
(unstable angina ___ or non–ST-segment elevation myocardial infarction ___).
Risk stratification at discharge was _____.
                                   (Hospital discharge report attached)

The patient underwent the following procedures: PCI _____ CABG _____
The following medications have been prescribed postdischarge:
Aspirin + clopidogrel:
Aspirin at a dose of _____ mg/d
Clopidogrel at a dose of 75 mg/d   Planned duration _____
Nitrates (_____) at a dose of _____ mg/d
Beta-blocker (_____) at a dose of _____ mg/d
ACE inhibitor/ARB (_____) at a dose of _____ mg/d
Calcium channel blocker (_____) at a dose of _____ mg/d
Lipid-lowering agent(s)(_____) at a dose of _____ mg/d
Other: _____

The following counseling concerning risk modification was provided:_____
_____
_____

Follow-up is strongly recommended in these areas: _____
_____
_____

If you have questions, please contact me at: telephone_____ fax_____
voice mail _____ e-mail _____

Sincerely,

Heart Education	❑ I have received cardiac education during my hospital admission.
	❑ I know the warning signs and symptoms of a heart attack and the action to take if they occur.
	❑ I have received instructions on my discharge medications.

Follow-up Appointments

I have a follow-up appointment with my primary care physician _____ phone _____
on: _____/_____/_____

I have a follow-up with my cardiologist _____ phone _____
on: _____/_____/_____

I may contact _____ MD/RN at phone _____ with any questions or concerns.

Patient signature: _____ Date: _____/_____/_____

Physician/nurse signature: _____ Date: _____/_____/_____

ACS Mock Drill

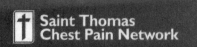

Accreditation Mock Drill   Saint Thomas
                                                Chest Pain Network

Review Team:

Saint Thomas
Health Services Staff
ED Director
EMS Director

Length:

Approximately 2 Hours

Location:

Local EMS
ED
Cardiac Cath Lab if Applicable

Participants:

ED Staff
Medical Staff
EMS
Lab Technologist
Cath Lab Staff
Unit Clerks
Volunteer Patients
CPC Committee

I. Local EMS
   a. Process – from 911 call to patient care and patient transport
   b. Protocols – chest pain protocol
   c. Report – content
   d. Initial EKG – ability to transmit
   e. Relationship with hospital – education opportunities,
      CPC committee, case reviews

II. Patient Arrival
   a. EMS Arrival
      i. Bed Availability
   b. Walk in:
      i.   True time of arrival (clock synchronization)
      ii. Triage process: Initial EKG
      iii. Transport from triage to bed
      iv. Bed availability

III. Chest Pain Pathways
   a. STEMI Pathway
      i.   Cardiologist on-call (call returned within 10 minutes)
      ii. Fibrinolytics or PCI (>37 per year)
      iii. If fibrinolytics:
           1. Type, dosing, reperfusion
           2. Ordered by Cardiologist or ED Physician
      iv. If PCI
           1. Will follow cath lab process
           2. Who alerts cath lab team? (ED physician or cardiologist)
           3. Cath Lab/ED relationship (CPC committee)
           4. Cath Lab/ED cross training
   b. NSTEMI or US pathway
      i.   Serial EKG's/Cardiac Markers
      ii. Fibrinolytics or PCI
   c. Low Risk for ASC or not assignable cause pathway
      i.   Rule out process
      ii. Stress testing availability
      iii. Discharge Instructions/Patient follow-up

IV. Review
   a. Metrics
   b. Process for improvement – flow charts
   c. Personnel, competencies and training
   d. Functional facility design and commitment
      (signage, traffic patterns, access to ED and triage)
   e. Community outreach/wellness education

V. Recommendations

ACS Activation Tool

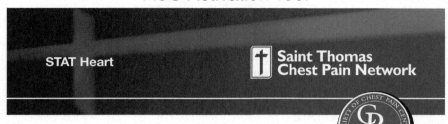

STAT Heart

✝ **Saint Thomas Chest Pain Network**

Saint Thomas Hospital: 877.374.1914 · Baptist Hospital: 877.456.4585

Initial Treatment

- Cardiac Monitor, Oxygen, IV X 2, Vital Signs
- Aspirin 324 mg PO ONCE, if not given PTA

- Nitroglycerin: 0.4 mg SL for CP every 5 mins. X 3 if SBP > 90
  Consider Ntg paste 1-2 inches PRN CP
  Consider Ntg drip IV 10 mcg/min up to 200 mcg / min

- Clopidogrel (Plavix) 300-600 mg PO ONCE
- Metoprolol (Lopressor) 5 mg IV every 5 min X 3
  Unless Contraindicated: Oral dose already given or HR < 50 or SBP < 90

- Morphine Sulfate 2-4 mg IV titrated for CP every 5 - 10 mins. Keep SBP > 90.

- CBC, INR, Cardiac Enzymes, BMP, Portable CXR

Decision Point

- STEMI or New LBBB
- ≤ 12 hours of Symptoms Onset

Any of the variables below present:

- 1st Door to Balloon < 90 minutes
- Symptoms Onset > 3 hours
- Contraindications to Thrombolytics
- Cardiogenic Shock
- High Risk of Bleeding

 Yes

 No

Primary PCI Regimen

Eligible Associates
- Within 12 hours of symptom onset
- ST-Segment elevation in 2 or more contiguous leads > 1mm or new onset LBBB

Additional Medications
- Heparin: 60 units/kg IV Bolus
  — or —
- Lovenox: 30 mg single IV Bolus plus 1 mg/kg SQ for patients < 75 years of age with normal renal function.

No maintenance infusion during transfer.

FAX Lab Results, ECG & Face Sheet

Saint Thomas Hospital:	615.222.3189
Baptist Hospital:	615.284.3854

For Air Transport, call

AirEvac Lifeteam: 800.247.3822 (800.Air.Evac)

FIBRINOLYSIS Regimen

Eligible Associates
- Within 12 hours of symptom onset
- ST-Segment elevation in 2 or more contiguous leads > 1mm or new onset LBBB
- Absence of contraindications

Fibrinolytic (tenecteplase (TNK) or retaplase (rPA)
- Note exact time of lytic administration and repeat ECG 30 mins. after administration
- TNK: Single IV Bolus over 5 seconds per TNK dose chart
  — or —
- rPA: 10 units over 2 mins. given twice at 30 min. intervals

Additional Medications
- Heparin: 60 units / kg IV Bolus, max 4,000 units Bolus, with lytic administration followed by maintenance drip at 12 units/kg/hr maximum 1,000 units/hr.
  — or —
- Lovenox: 30 mg single IV Bolus plus 1 mg/kg SQ for patients < 75 years of age with normal renal function.

sths.com/chestpainnetwork

ACS Staff Education

IMPORTANT: label both EKG copies as "RIGHT SIDED EKG"

STEP #1 – Obtain a Standard 12 lead EKG *(pink leads)*

STEP #2 – Obtain a Right Sided (R4-6) and Posterior (P7-9) EKG *(yellow leads)*

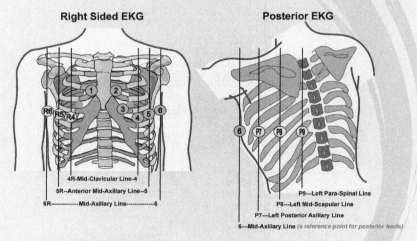

Right Sided EKG   **Posterior EKG**

4R-Mid-Clavicular Line-4
5R--Anterior Mid-Axillary Line--5
6R--------------Mid-Axillary Line-------------6

P9---Left Para-Spinal Line
P8---Left Mid-Scapular Line
P7---Left Posterior Axillary Line
6---Mid-Axillary Line *(a reference point for posterior leads)*

Right Sided Leads (R4-6):
1. Move lead 1 to R4 position (right mid-clavicular line at 5th inter-costal space)
2. Move lead 2 to R5 position (right anterior mid-axillary line)
3. Move lead 3 to R6 position (right mid-axillary line)

Posterior EKG Leads (P7-9) *Note: use lead 6 as a reference point for posterior lead placement*
4. Move lead 4 to P7 position (left posterior axillary line, next to the old V6 lead)
5. Move lead 5 to P8 position (left mid-scapular line)
6. Move lead 6 to P9 position (left para-spinal line)

IMPORTANT: label both EKG copies as "RIGHT SIDED EKG"

CT Decision Algorithm

64 Slice CT with Cardiac Angiography

Arlington Memorial Hospital - Accredited Chest Pain Center with Angioplasty
Appropriate use criteria for CTA

APPROPRIATENESS CRITERIA FOR CARDIAC CT*
AMERICAN COLLEGE OF CARDIOLOGY AND RADIOLOGY

APPROPRIATE
- Acute Chest pain- Intermediate pre-test probability
  - No ST-elevation/cardiac enzymes
  - Chest Pain syndrome
  - Stress test uninterpretable or equivocal
  - EKG uninterpretable OR unable to exercise
- Coronary anomaly or congenital heart disease
  - New CHF for possible CAD
- R/O Aortic dissection or thoracic aneurysm
  - Electrophysiology
  - Pulmonary vein anatomy
  - Coronary vein anatomy
- Cardiac mass or pericardial disease
  - Technically poor echo, MRI or TEE

POSSIBLY APPROPRIATE
- Acute pain syndrome
  - Low or High pre-test probability
  - "Triple R/O"
- Chest pain syndrome
  - Intermediate prob - EKG interpretable
  AND able toexercise
  - Prior CABG
  - Prior stents
- Asymptomatic
  - CTA - High Framingham risk
  - Calcium score - High or Inter Framingham risk
- Preop - High or inter risk surgery
  - Intermediate peri-op risk
- LV function or Heart valve evaluation
  - Technically poor echo, MRI or TEE

INAPPROPRIATE
- Acute chest pain - High pre-test probability
  - EKG ST - elevation or positive cardiac enzymes
- Chest pain syndrome
  - High pre-test probability
  - Positive stress test - moderate to severe
- Pre-op CTA - Low risk surgery
- Asymptomatic - for CTA
  - Mod or Low Framingham risk
  - Prior CABG
  - Prior stents
- Asymptomatic - for calcium score
  - Low Framingham risk
  - Prior within 5 years
  - Normal cath within 2 years
  - Prior calcium score >400

64 Slice CT with Cardiac Angiography

Arlington Memorial Hospital – Accredited Chest Pain Center with Angioplasty
Flow Diagram for Appropriate Use

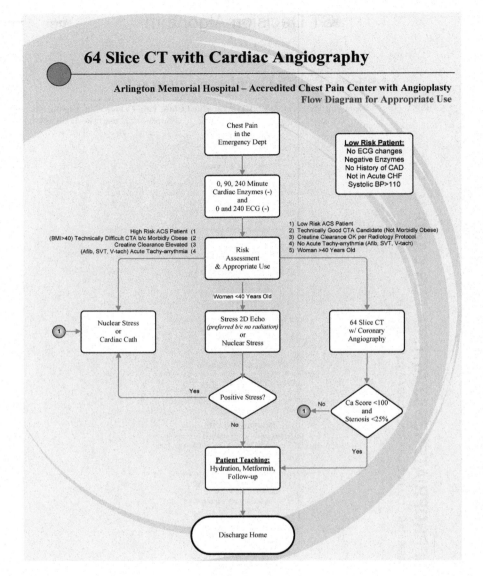

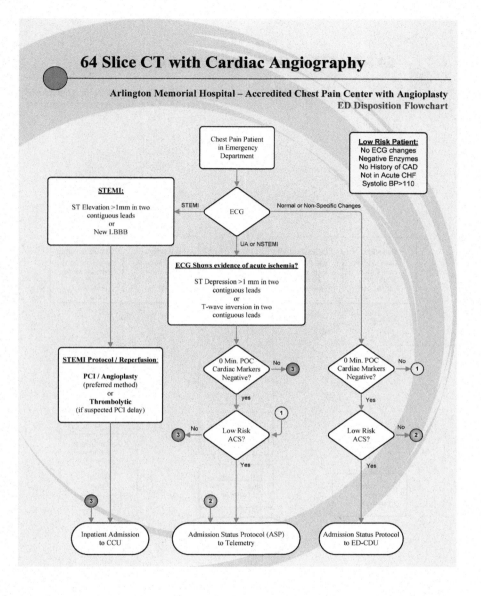

64 Slice CT with Cardiac Angiography

Arlington Memorial Hospital – Accredited Chest Pain Center with Angioplasty
ED Disposition Flowchart

64 Slice CT with Cardiac Angiography

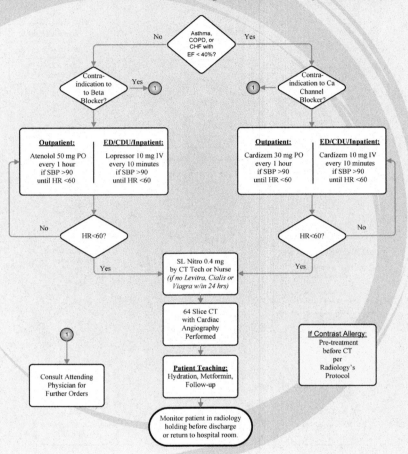

Arlington Memorial Hospital – Accredited Chest Pain Center with Angioplasty
Flow Diagram for: ED, CDU, Inpatient and Outpatient

Asthma, COPD, or CHF with EF < 40%?

No — Yes

Contra-indication to to Beta Blocker?   Yes — ①

① — Contra-indication to Ca Channel Blocker?

Outpatient:
Atenolol 50 mg PO every 1 hour if SBP >90 until HR <60

ED/CDU/Inpatient:
Lopressor 10 mg IV every 10 minutes if SBP >90 until HR <60

Outpatient:
Cardizem 30 mg PO every 1 hour if SBP >90 until HR <60

ED/CDU/Inpatient:
Cardizem 10 mg IV every 10 minutes if SBP >90 until HR <60

HR<60?   No

HR<60?   No

Yes

SL Nitro 0.4 mg by CT Tech or Nurse
(if no Levitra, Cialis or Viagra w/in 24 hrs)

Yes

64 Slice CT with Cardiac Angiography Performed

①

If Contrast Allergy:
Pre-treatment before CT per Radiology's Protocol

Consult Attending Physician for Further Orders

Patient Teaching:
Hydration, Metformin, Follow-up

Monitor patient in radiology holding before discharge or return to hospital room.

Index

CPSIA information can be obtained
at www.ICGtesting.com
Printed in the USA
LVOW01s1425281116

514773LV00002B/38/P